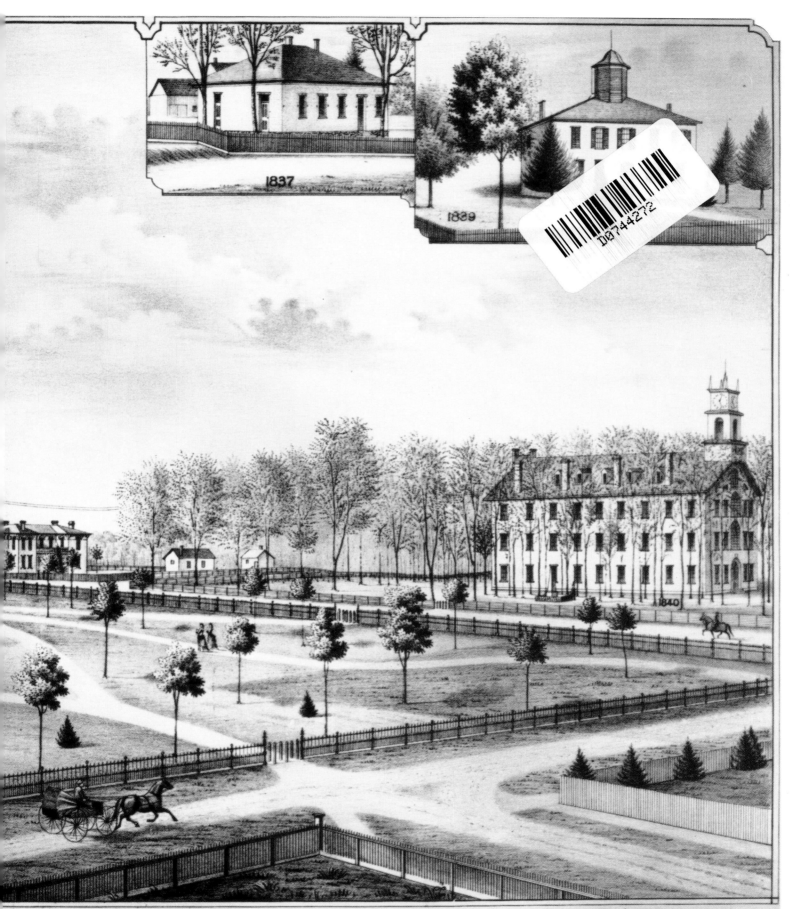

1837

1839

1840

RY UNIVERSITY,

ASTLE, IND.

REV. PATTERSON McNUTT, A.M.,
Professor of Mathematics.

JOHN BREWER DeMOTTE A.M.,
Principal, Preparatory Dept. and Inst'r in Mathematics.

S. S. HAMILL, A.M., *Teacher of Elocution.*

C. H. HAINES, A.B., *Tutor.*

THOMAS JEFFERSON BASSET, A.M.,
Instructor in Ancient Languages.

PHILLIP S. BAKER, A.M.,
Instructor in Natural Science and English.

CAPT. D. D. WHEELER, U. S. A.,
Professor of Military Science and Tactics.

DEPAUW
A PICTORIAL HISTORY

Clifton J. Phillips and John J. Baughman,
with the assistance of
Harold O. Spicer, John T. Schlotterbeck, and Wesley Wilson

Introduction by John Jakes

DePauw University

1987

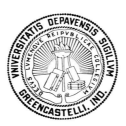

ISBN 0-936631-12-0

CONTENTS

SESQUICENTENNIAL
1837 — 1987

DEPAUW

PREFACE

This book was conceived in discussions of the sesquicentennial planning committee called together by President Richard F. Rosser in the spring of 1985 to begin preparations for the celebration of the 150th anniversary of the founding of Indiana Asbury-DePauw University. An editorial committee was appointed to supervise the writing and publication of a series of departmental and school histories as well as a larger pictorial history of the university as a whole. Both President — later Chancellor — Rosser and his successor, President Robert G. Bottoms, encouraged and supported this project from its inception.

DePauw: A Pictorial History owes much to its predecessors: Belle A. Mansfield's *DePauw University – a Historical Sketch* (1901); Irving F. Brown's *Indiana Asbury-DePauw University: A History* (1914); William W. Sweet's *Indiana Asbury-DePauw University, 1837-1937* (1937); and George B. Manhart's *DePauw Through the Years* (1962). Besides bringing the story down to the present, this volume attempts to present the history of the institution in a new light by combining an analytical narrative with carefully selected illustrations. Each chapter contains, in addition to the main text, several word-and-picture vignettes and pictorial layouts highlighting significant episodes, personalities, and other features.

Most of the text is the work of the two chief authors, who have been colleagues in the history department at DePauw for more than 30 years. John Baughman prepared the initial draft of the first chapter as well as an administrative history of the institution since 1884. He also wrote nearly all the picture captions and some of the vignettes, and played an active editorial role throughout. Clifton Phillips, who serves as the editor of DePauw's sesquicentennial historical publications, was largely responsible for drafting the remaining text and making the final revisions.

Former Professor of English Harold Spicer contributed many of the items on student life in both the main text and the vignettes. Associate Professor of History John Schlotterbeck was a member of the editorial committee from the outset and provided the valuable quantitative analysis found in the appendices. Another member of the editorial committee, University Archivist Wesley Wilson, helped to select the illustrations and prepare them for publication. Finally, DePauw alumnus and novelist John Jakes wrote the lively introduction.

The authors wish to thank the many persons whose efforts helped to make this volume possible. Several of them are attached to the university's office of public relations: Gregory Rice, university editor; Dian D. Phillips, director of publications; and Mary Rector, photographer. Janae Berry, a freelance layout artist, also contributed to the book.

Members of the staff of the university archives, past and present, who furnished research assistance during the project include Eleanor Cammack, David Horn, Julia D. Young, Sharon Cheslik, Susan Moore, Laura Clymer, Joan Cunningham and the late Virginia Brann. We are also grateful to the spouses and families who patiently endured the strains and stresses of a protracted enterprise.

We have tried to avoid most of the usual pitfalls of college histories. This has meant resisting the temptation to recount nostalgically the funny stories told around the fraternity house fireplace, faculty eccentricities, presidents' and deans' follies, and the last-minute football victory over Old Siwash, or to flatter wealthy donors and influential alumni and overpraise recent administrations. We have attempted to be fair and evenhanded, noting both trials and triumphs, praising the strengths of the university where appropriate and admitting occasional weaknesses and misadventures.

What finally emerges from these pages, we believe, is a late 20th century interpretation of the history of Indiana Asbury-DePauw University that strives for objectivity while necessarily reflecting to some degree the special perspectives of the authors.

It is our hope that this volume will make a useful contribution to DePauw's sesquicentennial celebration by providing its readers with a valid record in words and pictures of the institution's first 150 years. It is dedicated to all those who have had a part as students, members of the faculty and administration, trustees, or benefactors, living and dead, in molding the university during the past century and a half.

Clifton J. Phillips
John J. Baughman
Greencastle, Indiana
June 30, 1987

INTRODUCTION

DePauw, they say, is rich with traditions.

You hear it so often from alumni, faculty, administration, trustees, and students, you almost expect Tevye the dairyman to come dancing from behind one of the trees near East College, leading a line of villagers from Anatevka in the singing of the famous opening lyric from "Fiddler on the Roof."

Perhaps all the enthusiasm's justified. Reflecting, you do find a great many traditions that combine to make DePauw a singular and well-loved school. In the pages of this lively history of her first 150 years you'll see the wellsprings of many of those traditions, in an evocative array of photographs and a splendid text prepared for the anniversary celebration by Clifton Phillips, John Baughman and their colleagues.

So by way of introduction, let me avoid any mention whatsoever of all of those traditions except two, which you might not discover through pictures. They happen to be the two I believe are most responsible for DePauw's special and lasting place in the world of American universities, and the hearts of her graduates.

The first tradition is the university's commitment to the liberal arts.

Now "liberal arts" is a term tossed around so freely and so frequently at DePauw, it might be well to pin it down. In the universities of medieval Europe, the liberal arts were seven in number, divided in two groups. The lower, or elementary grouping, was the trivium ("place where three roads meet"). It consisted of grammar, rhetoric, and logic, all of which had to be mastered for a bachelor's degree. The higher grouping was the quadrivium ("four roads"): arithmetic, astronomy, geometry and music. These were required for the master's degree.

What is most significant is this. The liberal arts were generalized bodies of knowledge thought to be essential for the living of any good and useful life—and never mind the occupation of the person doing the living. Further, the disciplines required to master the liberal arts—hard work, reasoning, judgment—were considered just as important as any "facts" that were presented. This was education to improve—actually *create*— the adult human being. It was not career education; not physician training, for example. If that was to be undertaken, it could only come later. The basics were more important.

Centuries passed, and the Indiana Methodists chartered "a seminary of learning ... in the town or vicinity of Greencastle, in Putnam County, and State of Indiana." When they did so, they wisely upheld the tradition of the liberal arts—general, as opposed to technical or vocational, education. Professor Manhart's fine two-volume history of DePauw reports that the first 22 students enrolled in 1839-40 were offered a four-year curriculum of Latin, Greek, Mathematics (algebra, geometry, trigonometry), History, Rhetoric, Science (including astronomy), some sort of government course, and another course dealing with "Moral Science" and "Evidences of Christianity." Not bad for a religious denomination in the early 19th century; of the original seven, only music was sacrificed, probably thought slightly pagan.

You can clearly see that this DePauw tradition kept faith with the sort of education long upheld as the ideal. Education to create the whole person. To this day, the tradition continues.

Of course the statement is not pure truth. There are presently courses very much skewed toward specific, even technical knowledge. The Methodist founders accomplished a lot, but you can't expect them to have predicted TV studios, or what a "manager" might be and do. The stunning changes in modern society dictate a certain flexibility. But the underlying tradition has never caved in. It is the same now as it was in 1837, and it was the same in 1837 as in the Middle Ages.

Still, I doubt DePauw could claim distinction if that tradition was the only basis for the claim. It takes a second tradition, working in tandem with the first, to account for the university's extraordinary success.

To get at this second tradition, let's glance at the people instrumental in founding the school. I find vivid and significant parallels between the lives of some of those early Methodists and the nature of DePauw life today.

The Methodist church, largely the creation of the English revivalist clergyman John Wesley, was a somewhat simpler, warmer, less doctrinaire faith than Wesley's own Church of England. It arose in parallel with British colonialism, and its tenets seemed particularly adaptable to, and appreciated by, those men and women living in isolation on the North American frontier. Methodism said an intimate relationship with God was possible even though the believer was miles and miles from any great cathedral or priestly interpreter.

The men who spread and taught this doctrine were recognized on the 18th and 19th century frontier by what one scholar describes as "the hair, the hat and the horse." The clergyman's hair was usually shoulder length, his hat a familiar black broad-rim, and his horse very strong. Strong because the preacher was almost always on it—"itinerating" as they called it.

The men were the circuit riders. It isn't pejorative to call them macho. They had to be macho, or something very close, to spend the greater part of a lifetime wending along trails where no roads existed, subject to attack by Indians and desperadoes, crossing mountains, fording rivers, enduring sleet, heat, downpours, blizzards, poverty and saddle sores without complaint; without letup; and with joy ("Live or die, I must ride!" exclaimed John Wesley's American right hand, Bishop Asbury, who calculated that he itinerated at least 275,000 miles in his career, crossing the Allegheny Mountains 62 times.)

These ardent and hardy men visited the faithful at stops along a regular route—the circuit. They customarily visited and preached to small groups. If there was as established church, it was called a station; the riders bypassed it. Usually stations were found only in larger towns. The faithful awaited the circuit riders in settings more remote, and less grand—"friendly farmhouses, commodious barns, carpenter shops, courthouses, taverns, warehouses."

Consider these circuit riders, then. They were, one, highly dedicated. It isn't hard to say the same thing about those called to the secular faculty at DePauw. If they don't have a dedication to teaching—as opposed to a wish to sequester themselves with scholarly research, leaving the teaching to graduate degree candidates—they are well advised to look elsewhere for employment. This is a *teaching* institution.

Two, the circuit riders dealt with very small groups. DePauw necessarily began on a small scale—22 enrolled that first year. All males, I regret to say. In 1837 the conventional wisdom not only denied an education to women, it proclaimed that they couldn't absorb it if they got it. They said it, I didn't.

In any case, I see a resemblance between the circuit rider's tiny wilderness congregation and the traditionally small teacher-student groups at DePauw. Over the years, while the school has certainly gotten bigger, it hasn't gotten that much bigger. Neither have classes. (In my freshman year, spent at Northwestern, one of the the main English survey courses played to a hall that held over 1,200 bodies; I say played because class size made it more like a performance than an educational experience.)

Third, and lastly, because they dealt with small groups of people whom they saw regularly, the circuit riders were naturally involved and familiar with almost every aspect of the lives of their charges. The preacher not only taught, he broke bread with his listeners. He advised, he sympathized, he came to share a good part of the life of each person to whom he ministered. A similar sort of relationship exists today between many a teacher and pupil at DePauw, because DePauw is small enough for it to happen.

I can testify that it does happen; it happened to me. I had just that sort of fine, close, interactive experience with any number of professors ... Virginia Harlow, Fred Bergmann, Ermina Mills, Oliver Robinson, Edna Taylor, and the beloved bulldog, Raymond Pence. (I regret I was never fortunate enough to have a course with the other giant of that era, Jerome Hixson).

That faculty knew me well enough to help me survive a bumpy first year on the campus, discover and exploit my few strengths and minimize my many weaknesses (which included a wretched inability to memorize German vocabulary; I did it, but just barely).

So there are the two traditions: the liberal arts ... and an almost perfect environment for teaching them. I sometimes mentally shorthand the whole process as "large ideas, served small." For me, the traditions are the heart of DePauw, and the reason for her excellence.

Having said that, let me commend to you the pages that follow ... a remarkable visual journey through DePauw's first century and a half.

As with any institution which lasts that long, there were good times and not so good times. Washington C. DePauw had to be brought in with a bunch of bail-out money he earned in the Civil War and was willing to use to save the struggling little Indiana Asbury. The deal cannily worked out was the exchange of Washington's cash for the attachment of his name to the college.

More recently, the school seemed to draw in upon itself for a while. Good students still came here, but from a steadily shrinking geographic area. I count as one of the outstanding accomplishments of Dick Rosser's administration the recognition of this threat to DePauw's status as a national university, and the steps taken to nullify that threat.

Such ups and downs are to be expected. What's lucky, and remarkable, is that our two most important traditions have not been eroded or blown away by the winds of time. I trust they will remain strong, the underpinning of the university, for the next 150 years, too.

But now, instead of forward, look backward with Professors Phillips and Baughman and your other highly expert guides.

I promise that you're going to love the trip.

John Jakes
Hilton Head Island
April 6, 1987

Copyright © John Jakes 1987

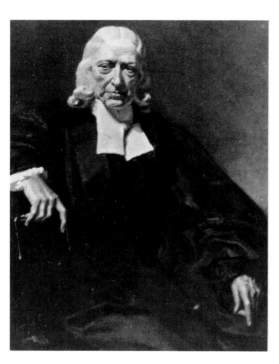
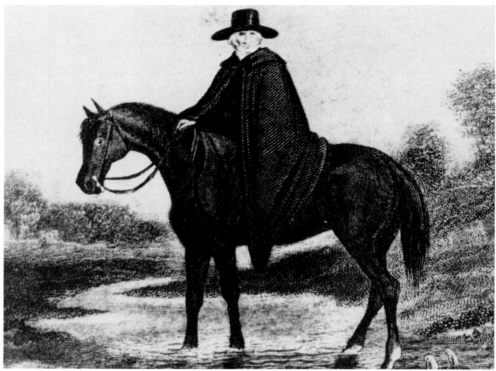
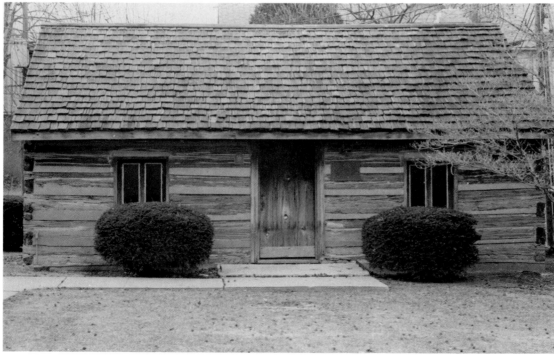
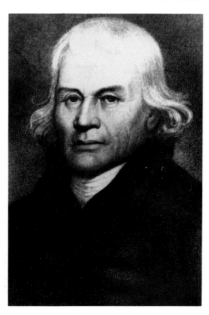

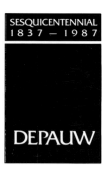
Chapter I

THE INDIANA ASBURY YEARS

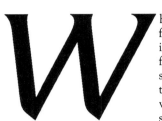

When DePauw University opened its doors in 1837, it had not only a different name and setting but also a quite different ethos from today. Located in a frontier community of the Old Northwest, Indiana Asbury, as its founders named it, stressed Christian character and piety over scholarship or social adaptation. Yet a unique spirit was created that has pervaded the institution for 150 years, surviving the change in name in 1884 as well as the various shifts in emphasis taking place before and after that date. It is this spirit, or mystique, that the authors of this new history of the university seek to identify and interpret in word and picture.

To attempt to record the mind of the founders and recapture the essence of the university's beginnings in the spring and summer of 1837 requires a vivid imagination as well as historical sensitivity. Preceding the advent of modern photography and the typewriter, the era is poorly documented by either written or pictorial materials and is also subject to the peculiar biases of that romantic and optimistic age. Moreover the story of the founding and first years of Indiana Asbury is part of the larger history of American higher education as well as of Methodism and its struggle to establish an educational system appropriate to its needs.

Methodism, which had begun in the 18th century as a movement within the Church of England stressing personal piety and evangelistic fervor, was led by an Oxford-educated Anglican minister, John Wesley, and quickly spread to the British colonies in North America. By the close of the American Revolution its adherents were numerous enough and its leaders ready to organize as an independent religious body. On Christmas 1784, delegates meeting in Baltimore created the Methodist Episcopal Church of the United States and named Francis Asbury as its first bishop. Methodist circuit riders reached Indiana Territory by 1801, and within 30 years Methodists comprised the largest single religious denomination in the State of Indiana with an estimated membership of 20,000.

Methodism spoke to the spiritual needs of a frontier state where the prospects for both material success and personal longevity were precarious. For many, the teachings of Methodist Christianity provided a favorable spiritual and moral climate to undergird the difficult task of hewing out a new civilization in the wilderness. With its emphasis on charismatic leadership the Methodist Church had initially frowned upon formal education, and a number of early attempts to establish its own colleges had only mixed success. But by 1820 a shift was taking place in the thinking of Methodist leaders. A resolution of their General Conference of that year recommended that local conferences establish "literary institutions, under their own control, in such way and manner as they may think proper," a measure reaffirmed four years later. Besides a number of academies and seminaries successfully launched in the 1820s, a few Methodist colleges began to appear in the next decade, beginning with Wesleyan University in Connecticut in 1831.

The very first session of the newly created Indiana Conference in 1832 appointed a committee "to take into consideration the propriety of building a Conference Seminary." The committee's report, noting that most of the literary institutions were in the hands of other denominations, argued for the desirability of "an institution under our own control from which we can exclude all doctrines which we deem dangerous; though at the same time we do not wish to make it so sectarian as to exclude or in the smallest degree repel the sons of our fellow citizens from the same."

What the Hoosier Methodist leaders were chiefly concerned about in the 1830s was the prevailing Presbyterian preponderance in the state's formal educational institutions. Not only had the rival denomination founded its own sectarian schools—the forerunners of Hanover and Wabash Colleges—but also constituted the dominant influence among the faculty and trustees of the publicly funded Indiana College founded in 1825, later named Indiana University in 1838. After a futile attempt to persuade the Indiana General Assembly to force the Presbyterians to share with the Methodists in the management and faculty of the state college at Bloomington, the Indiana

Conference fell back on the notion of creating its own institution. Taking into account the continuing prejudice against formal education among many Methodists, there is justifiable confusion about what was really meant by such terms as literary institutions, seminaries, or colleges and universities—all still poorly defined in the American educational lexicon of that era. But clearly Indiana Methodist leaders were now ready to launch some kind of venture in higher education.

The Conference took final action on the proposal at its Indianapolis meeting in October 1836, when it decided to establish "an institution of the first order...upon an extensive plan of operation and equal to any College or University in the valley of the Mississippi." A committee was appointed to draw up a charter and see to its approval by the state legislature. Another committee would evaluate the offers of the various towns competing for the location of the institution, considering such matters as the amount of money subscribed by each community as well as the general state of health and morals! Somehow the small Putnam County town of Greencastle managed to raise $25,000 to induce the committee to select it over Indianapolis, Lafayette, Madison, Rockville, and Putnamville as the site for the new college. Another factor was its alleged healthfulness. One local booster, Dr. Tarvin Cowgill, is supposed to have said that "people never die in Greencastle, although for convenience they have a cemetery there."

The charter for Indiana Asbury University, as the new institution was officially named in honor of Bishop Francis Asbury, was prepared and on January 10, 1837, duly approved by the Indiana General Assembly. Despite its sectarian sponsorship, the "Seminary of learning" was to be founded "for the benefit of the youth of every class of citizens, and of every denomination, who shall be freely admitted to equal advantages and privileges of education." Again the charter refers to "an extensive University or College Institution...to be conducted on most liberal principles, accessible to all religious denominations and designed for the benefits of the citizens in general." While some historians point to this statement as reflecting the liberality of the founders' intentions, others suggest that it merely represents the lip service to nonsectarianism required to win legislative approval.

The charter named 25 trustees to be invested with the direction of the university, particularly to appoint the president and his assisting faculty, and to begin the enterprise. Vacancies were to be filled by the Indiana Conference of the Methodist Church or such other annual conferences as might be established in the state. In addition, the conference or conferences were authorized to appoint nine visitors, who would report annually on the condition of the university and, together with the trustees, make up the Joint Board or governing body of the institution. Clearly Indiana Asbury University was conceived at its origin as a creature of the Methodist Episcopal Church.

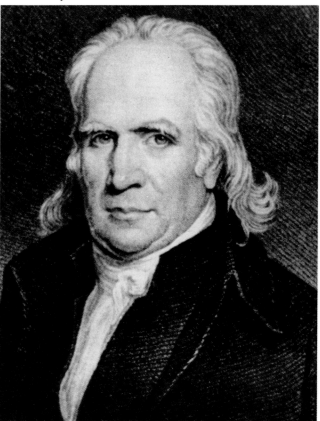

Robert R. Roberts, presiding bishop of the Indiana conference of the Methodist Episcopal Church in 1834-35-36, during whose tenure Indiana Asbury was founded. Of his annual salary of $200 he gave $100 to the new college and named it a residuary legatee of his will. He and Mrs. Roberts are buried on the campus. In 1961 Bishop Roberts Hall was completed and named for him.

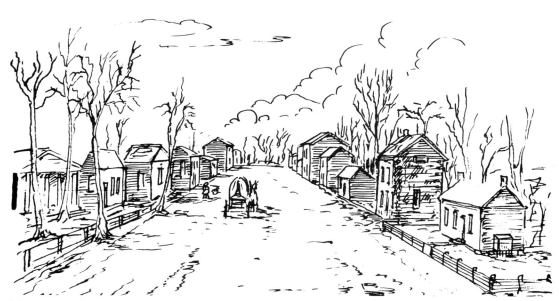

Main street of a typical small Hoosier town during the first decade of Indiana Asbury history. This sketch comes from the diary of E. E. Edwards, a student from 1849-52. (Courtesy Colorado State University)

An Indiana frontier cabin, typical of the Putnam County log cabins most Indiana Asbury students came from. The 1839 painting is by George Winter (Tippecanoe County Historical Association).

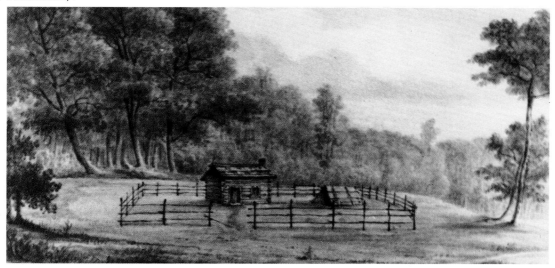

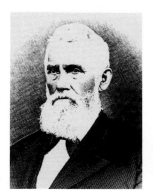
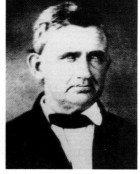
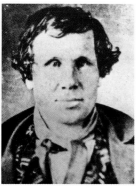
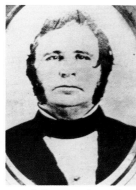

Early trustees, clockwise from top left: Dr. Alexander C. Stevenson, first president of the board; John Cowgill, Greencastle lawyer, judge and mayor; William H. Thornburgh, Greencastle merchant and former steamboat captain; and Martin M. Ray, a lawyer from Shelbyville..

In 1837 Greencastle, the site for the new university, was still a raw frontier village. It was formed from land given to the newly created Putnam County for its seat of government by pioneer settler Ephraim Dukes in 1823. Surrounded by small log or frame houses scattered along unpaved streets and about 20 or so stores located in a square, the one-story, brick, hip-roofed courthouse was the focus of business activity.

In his diary, first teacher Cyrus Nutt records his impression on arrival in 1837:

Greencastle was only about ten years old, small and rough. The site was by no means the most pleasant, it being a succession of hills and hollows, the streets were without grading, or side walks except about the public square. Six months in the year mud was an abundant article. The population was about five hundred. Yet this place and its vicinity subscribed twenty five thousand dollars to obtain the location of the University and it was exceedingly fortunate for that place that it succeeded in its application. Had it failed the county seat would probably have been moved to Putnamville, and Greencastle would to day have been numbered with the things that were....

Likewise President Matthew Simpson shares this revealing impression of the community when he arrived in 1839.

The houses were primitive, and the people largely from Kentucky, Tennessee, and North Carolina. There were three church edifices, a Baptist, a Presbyterian, and a Methodist, all of them very plain....While the people were both respectable and pious, society was in almost every sense in a very primitive condition.

The first meeting of the trustees was held in the still-unfinished Methodist church building the first week of March 1837. Of the 16 men present, 15 were from Greencastle or Putnam County. Bishop Robert R. Roberts, who had presided over the 1834, 1835, and 1836 sessions of the Indiana Conference which had taken the decisive steps to establish the university, was absent, as were other trustees from parts of the state too remote for easy access to Greencastle. The board chose three Greencastle men as its first officers: Dr. Alexander Stevenson, a physician and farmer, was named president and served twice from 1837-1839 and again 1840-1841; Dr. Tarvin Cowgill, who had headed the group that successfully presented Greencastle's case before the Indiana Conference, secretary; and Rees Hardesty, a local businessman, treasurer. Hardesty later served twice as president (1839-1840, 1841-1843), as did prominent Greencastle businessman William H. Thornburg (1843-1848) and lawyer John Cowgill (1848-1853). Largely because of travel conditions, a group of relatively young Methodist farmers, merchants, and professional men of Greencastle were dominant in the early planning and direction of Indiana Asbury University.

Among the first business transacted by the trustees, who met 17 times during 1837, was the selection of a building site in the southern part of the town plat of Greencastle. Two Methodist clergymen, John C. Smith and Aaron Wood, were chosen as agents to raise money for

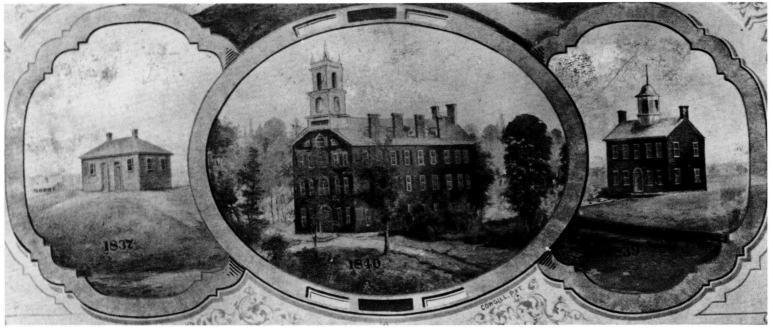

Drawings of the early Indiana Asbury campus buildings, probably by local Greencastle artist Elisha Cowgill. At left is the town seminary, located on west Washington St., used for primary and preparatory classes in the spring and summer of 1837. In the center is a drawing of the Edifice, located on the present site of the Roy O. West Library and facing north. At right is the county seminary building on the southeast corner of Seminary and College streets. It was used for all classses until 1840 and for the preparatory department until 1875, when it was removed to make way for the College Avenue Methodist Church (later Speech Hall).

the university by stumping the state and selling scholarships enabling the purchaser to enroll students in its classes. They frequently received more goodwill and prayer than cash. Leasing the county seminary building for the anticipated preparatory department, the board complied also with a requirement of a loan of $200 by opening an "ABC Spelling reading writing and Arithmetic School" in a small two-room "town seminary" on Washington Street on March 20. The pastor of the local Methodist Church, John Newell, taught a handful of children here until mid-June, when he was succeeded by James McCachran, who turned the teaching duties back to Newell again sometime during the following year. This initial educational venture at Old Asbury is not mentioned in the records after September 1838, when it apparently came to an end.

More enduring was the preparatory department, essential to any institution of that day hoping to obtain students qualified to undergo the rigor of the classical college curriculum. The preparatory department opened on June 5, 1837, under the direction of Cyrus Nutt, a Methodist minister and recent graduate of Allegheny College in Pennsylvania. He used a room in the town seminary until August, when he moved to the more commodious county seminary on the southeast corner of the present Seminary Street and College Avenue, which remained the site of the new university's activities for the next three years.

By November 1837, the infant institution boasted 40 students, ranging in age from 13 to 28. As early as December the trustees began making appointments to the college faculty. They elected the Rev. Joseph S. Tomlinson professor of mathematics, but the Transylvania University graduate declined to leave the presidency of Augustana College in Kentucky for what seemed an uncertain future in Greencastle. A few months later he also rejected the board's offer of the presidency. The first regular member of the faculty, then, was Cyrus Nutt, who accepted an appointment as professor of languages in addition to his post as principal of the preparatory department. For the moment he also served as acting president and was assisted in the preparatory classes by the Rev. John Weakley. Finally in

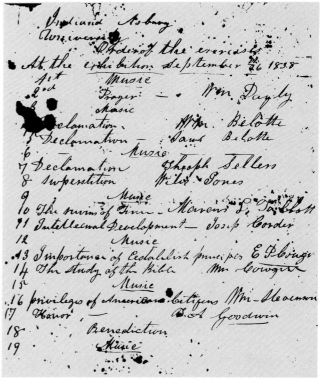

A handwritten program from September 1838 "exhibition" of student oratory at Indiana Asbury.

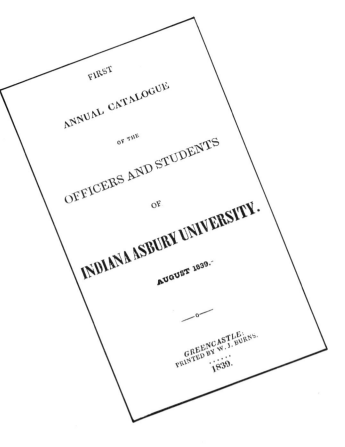

COURSE OF STUDY.

In the preparatory department will be taught English Grammar, Geography, Book-keeping, Arithmetic, Introduction to Algebra, and the rudiments of the Latin and Greek languages.

The requisites for admission into the Freshman Class are, a knowledge of Geography, English Grammar, Arithmetic, First Lessons in Algebra, Latin Grammar, Historia Sacra, Cæsar's Commentaries, Virgil, Greek Grammar, and Greek Testament.

FRESHMAN YEAR.
FIRST SESSION.
1. Sallust.   Roman Antiquities.
2. Græca Minora.
3. Algebra—Davies' Bourdon.
SECOND SESSION.
1. Cicero—Horace begun.—Exercises in writing Latin.
2. Græca Majora—Excerpta Historica.   Grecian Antiquities.
3. Legendre's Geometry.

SOPHOMORE YEAR.
FIRST SESSION.
1. Horace finished—Latin Prosody.
2. Græca Majora—Excerpta Rhetorica—Greek Exercises.
3. Trigonometry—Mensuration—Surveying.
SECOND SESSION.
1. Tacitus—Juvenal.
2. Græca Majora, 1st vol. finished.
3. Analytical Geometry.

JUNIOR YEAR.
FIRST SESSION.
1. Ancient and Modern History with Chronology.
2. Græca Majora (2d vol.)
3. Differential and Integral Calculus.
SECOND SESSION.
1. Natural and Experimental Philosophy, (Olmstead.)
2. Chemistry—Turner's.
3. Rhetoric—Logic—Criticism.

SENIOR YEAR.
FIRST SESSION.
1. Natural Philosophy finished—Astronomy.
2. Mineralogy—Geology.
3. Mental Philosophy—Upham.
SECOND SESSION.
1. Political Economy—Political Grammar.
2. Law of Nations—Paley's Theology.
3. Moral Science—Evidences of Christianity.

Through the entire course particular attention will be paid to Composition and Declamation, and the Seniors will be regularly exercised in Forensics.

Instructions will also be given in the Hebrew, French, and German Languages, when either the inclination of

CYRUS NUTT

The Rev. Cyrus Nutt, Indiana Asbury's first professor, was born in a log cabin near Southington, Ohio in 1814. Before coming to Greencastle to open the little preparatory school at Old Asbury he had graduated from Allegheny College in Pennsylvania and taught for a year in its preparatory department. In his diary in 1853 he described the journey to his new post and his first experiences there:

From Indianapolis was a stage route forty miles to Putnamville which was the nearest point which could be reached by public conveyance to Greencastle. I left Indianapolis at day break in the morning and arrived at Putnamville at about four, P.M. From Putnamville I rode in a wagon that was going out for hay some two miles; the remainder of the distance was three miles which I walked, reaching my journey's end at 12, A.M. on the 16th of May 1837.

I found boarding at Brother W.K. Cooper's who was a member of the Board of Trustees, a very worthy member of the Church. Here I found a very kind home for six months. The Preparatory Department was to open on the fifth of June and as yet the county seminary building was not ready and would not be, for two months. As the time for the commencement neared, a room in the old town school house, a one story Brick about thirty by twenty was obtained. The West end of this building, long since demolished, was the birth place of the literary department of Indiana Asbury University. On the Day appointed, and announced through the public journals for the opening, I repaired to the room appointed in the delapidated building. Five pupils appeared, barefooted, and without coats; they were boys from town.

Some six weeks had passed from the commencement of the Literary Department, when we moved our quarters to the County Seminary building, a two-story Brick about thirty-six feet by twenty. This held us nearly three years. The number of students increased to fifteen before the close of the first term, which ended with an exhibition about the middle of September.

By 1839 he was appointed professor of Greek and Latin in the college department and had helped organize the first literary society, the Platonean. After his marriage in 1843 he left the university briefly to enter the pastoral ministry but returned as professor of Greek language and literature from 1846 to 1849. In the latter year he again resigned in order to become president first of Fort Wayne Female College and then of Whitewater College, as well as presiding elder of the Richmond district of the Methodist Church. In 1857 he came back to Indiana Asbury as professor of mathematics and vice president, even serving as acting president for the following year during the interval between the Curry and Bowman administrations. For this latter service he was granted a bonus of $500, which went unpaid for 10 years! In 1860 Nutt resigned from Indiana Asbury for the last time to accept the presidency of neighboring Indiana University, which he guided successfully through the Civil War years and the following decade. Upon his death in 1875 a special train brought friends and associates from Bloomington to Greencastle for the funeral of the first Indiana Asbury professor and his burial in Forest Hill Cemetery. Descendants continue to enroll at DePauw to this day.

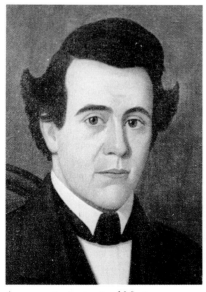

A romantic portrait of Nutt as a young man.

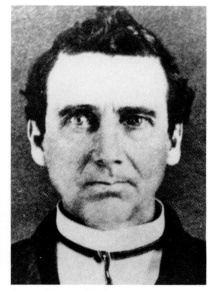

Cyrus Nutt in his later years.

Charles C. Downey attended Indiana Asbury but graduated from Wesleyan in Connecticut. He returned to become tutor in the preparatory department, professor of natural science, professor of chemistry and pharmacy, and professor of mathematics. Below him is John Wheeler, who joined the faculty in 1842 after being a member of the first graduating class in 1840. After leaving Asbury, Wheeler became president of Baldwin University and then Iowa Wesleyan. Bottom: Benjamin Franklin Tefft served as professor of Greek and Hebrew at Indiana Asbury fom 1843-46. His inaugural address at the college so impressed the board that it ordered 1000 copies printed.

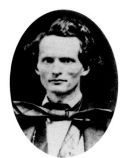

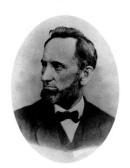

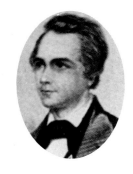

February 1839, Matthew Simpson of Allegheny College, after earlier turning down the professorship of mathematics, accepted the presidency of Indiana Asbury University. The first official listing of Indiana Asbury faculty in 1839 included Simpson, Nutt, and Weakley, plus John Wheeler, a member of the senior class, as tutor in mathematics.

The 1839-40 catalogue, the first to be issued, outlined a prescribed course for the college of recitations leading after four years to the degree of bachelor of arts. The course outline closely followed the established pattern of the older liberal arts colleges to the east. Arranged in two semesters of 21 weeks each, it comprised a heavy dose of Latin, Greek, and mathematics in the first two years, alleviated by a variety of subjects such as rhetoric, logic, ancient history, political economy, and the law of nations in the final two years. The capstone of the entire educational program was the study of mental and moral philosophy and "Christian evidences" in the senior year. This part of the curriculum was directed by the president himself, who was indeed often called upon to teach other courses as well. This major course was in no way a formal philosophy course, but rather, a practical course in "right living." In 1839-40 only 22 students were registered for the full classical course, while 43 were listed as irregular, or non-degree, students; and the largest number, 58, were pupils in the preparatory department. Two literary societies, the Platonean and Philological—usually called Plato and Philo for short—had been organized, affording students both social fellowship and an opportunity to supplement the rather thin prescribed curriculum with oratorical exercises on issues of current interest.

By September 1840 the new classroom building, under construction since 1837 and generally known simply as the Edifice, was far enough along to provide a suitable place for the university's first commencement and the belated inauguration of President Simpson. On the 16th of that month, chosen because it was the eve of the meeting of the

Indiana Methodist Conference, the chapel was crowded with visitors from around the state as Asbury's first three graduates were recognized—Thomas A. Goodwin, Finley L. Maddox, and John Wheeler. Joseph E. McDonald, who left college before graduation, was later awarded a degree as a member of the class of 1840. Indiana's governor, David Wallace, delivered the charge and presented the keys of the university to President Simpson, who made a lengthy inaugural address outlining the aims and objectives of higher education in terms not altogether unlike those often heard in the university's later history. In addition to furnishing general knowledge, colleges should promote "a capacity for close and thorough investigation, ability to communicate information in an interesting and successful manner, and a disposition

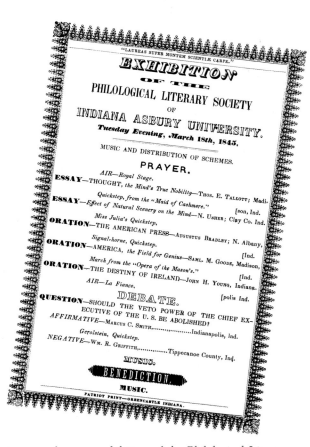

A program from an exhibition of the Philological Literary Society (Philo for short).

to use the utmost exertions for the amelioration of the conditions of mankind." The ceremony concluded with an evening lecture to the literary societies by the 26-year-old Henry Ward Beecher of the Second Presbyterian Church in Indianapolis. The university was launched.

Soon additional instructors were appointed and replacements named for those departing, as the student body gradually expanded. Most, like their predecessors, were ordained ministers in the Methodist Episcopal Church with little more than a classical college background. In 1840 William C. Larrabee became professor of mathematics and natural sciences, Simpson shifting from that field to the professorship of mental and moral philosophy. In 1842 Charles G. Downey, a graduate of Wesleyan University who had served

THE EDIFICE

On June 20, 1837, the cornerstone was laid for the college "Edifice," as it was generally known for the first 35 years of its existence, before a crowd estimated at 10,000 people—and at an incredible 20,000 by some—on a cold day marked by rain and snow flurries. Trustee Calvin Fletcher of Indianapolis spoke briefly, but the Rev. Henry B. Bascom, reputedly the greatest orator in the West, gave the main address lasting nearly two hours. Three years later the three-story brick building located on the present site of the Roy O. West Library, but facing north, was in use. Completed in 1842, it cost about $20,000 and was, according to college tradition, designed by a Greencastle architect from Connecticut named Elisha Braman. The first floor of the original Edifice contained three recitation halls and a large chapel. On the second floor were additional classrooms and on the third floor the library and two large halls for the student literary societies. Several chimneys from the numerous stoves used for heating protruded from the roof, which was also graced by a short tower housing the reportedly very melodious college bell. In 1852 a large clock was installed in the tower's cupola with dials on all four sides. For the times it was truly a magnificent structure and provided more than adequate quarters for all college activities until the erection of East College in the 1870s.

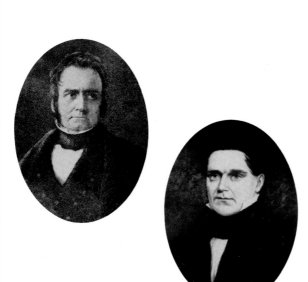

The Reverend Dr. Henry Bascom (left), chaplain of the Congress and president of Transylvania University, delivered a two-hour oration at the laying of the cornerstone. He was elected bishop of the Methodist Episcopal Church in 1846 but died in 1850 (Indiana Historical Society).

Calvin Fletcher (right), president of the Indiana State Bank, also spoke. An Indianapolis lawyer, farmer and "man of affairs," Fletcher served on the first board of trustees from 1837-39 and later became its treasurer (1848-55). His son, Miles Fletcher, would later teach at Asbury.

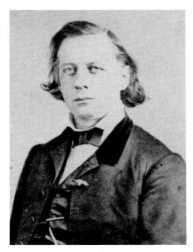

Henry Ward Beecher, a young minister of the Second Presbyterian Church in Indianapolis, addressed the literary societies on the occasion of the first commencement and the inauguration of President Simpson in 1840.

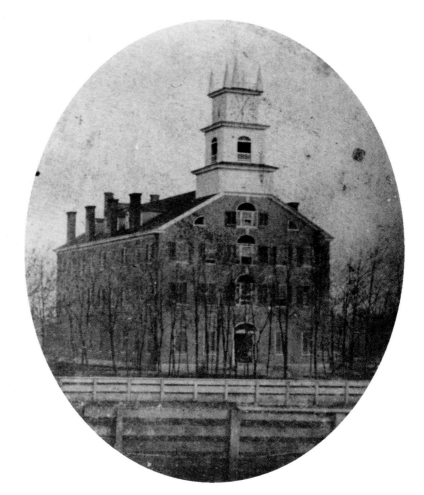

This photograph of the Edifice prior to the Civil War is the earliest extant photograph of the campus in the DePauw collection.

11

FACULTY

Left hand column:
Left column, from top: John W. Locke, professor of mathematics from 1860-65 and 1866-72. He then became president of McKendree College. Middle: Lewis L. Rogers, principal of the preparatory department from 1861-69 and professor of Latin 1863-79. A graduate of Asbury, he served as treasurer, recorder and faculty secretary. Bottom: John Clark Ridpath, popular professor and later vice president at Indiana Asbury and DePauw from 1869-85. He enjoyed a national reputation for his popular volumes of history.

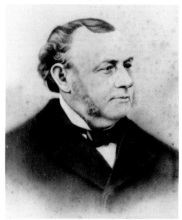

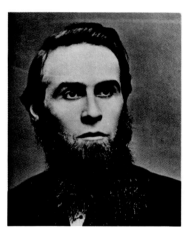

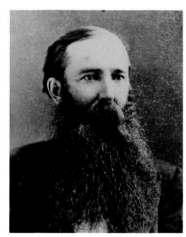

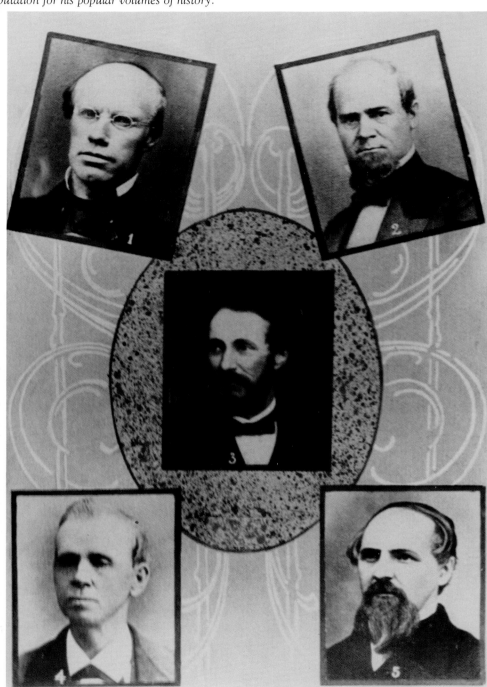

This composite shows pre-Civil War Indiana Asbury faculty. In the center is Miles J. Fletcher, professor of English literature and normal instruction, belles lettres, and history from 1852-54 and 1857-61. Top left: E. E. Bragdon, professor of Latin from 1854-58. Top right: Bernard H. Nadal, professor of belles lettres and history from 1854-57. Lower left: Henry C. Benson, professor of Greek language and literature from 1850-52. Lower right: Benjamin T. Hoyt, professor of Latin, belles lettres, and history from 1858-67.

Below: This faculty composite is from 1869. In the center is President Thomas Bowman. Clockwise from top left around him are John W. Locke, professor of mathematics from 1860-72; Philander Wiley, professor of Greek from 1860-80; Benjamin T. Hoyt, professor of Latin, belles lettres, and history from 1858-67; Lewis L. Rogers, professor of Latin and principal of the preparatory department from 1861-79; John A. Reubelt, professor of modern languages and Latin from 1863-69; and Joseph Tingley, professor of natural science from 1847-79.

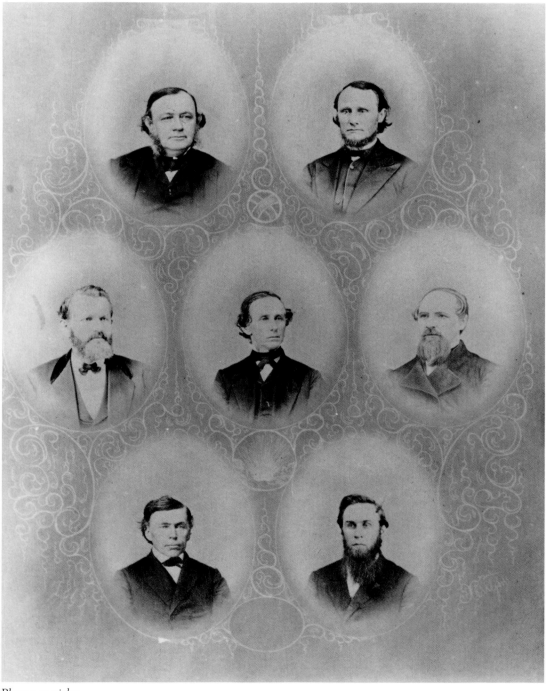

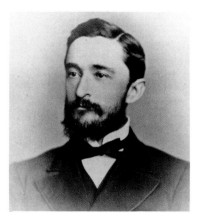

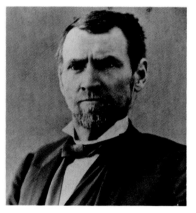

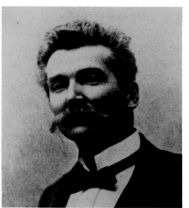

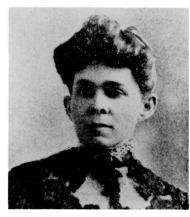

Photos at right:
Top: Professor John E. Earp was professor of modern languages, Hebrew, history, rhetoric and English literature from 1869-86. He helped organize the Music School, and left in 1886 to become president of Southwestern College. Second: The Rev. Patterson McNutt, Asbury class of 1855, became professor of mathematics from 1872-83. A Civil War captain, McNutt became president of both Baker University in Kansas and Marshall College in Illinois. Third: John B. Demotte, an Asbury graduate, was principal of the preparatory department from 1874-83, professor of mathematics from 1880-82, and professor of physics from 1882-91. He also conducted the early orchestra. DeMotte received the second Ph.D. awarded by DePauw in 1887. Bottom: Alma Holman (Burton), another Asbury graduate, became its first woman professor in the college. She taught modern languages from 1882-85.

as tutor in mathematics at Asbury in 1840-41, was appointed professor of natural science, relieving Larrabee of that portion of his responsibilities. He remained for 15 years, including a stint in the short-lived medical college. Another who began his career as tutor in mathematics was Joseph Tingley, an Asbury graduate in the class of 1846 who held the professorship of natural sciences from 1849 to 1879.

As a professed Christian university, Indiana Asbury may be considered a pioneer in the teaching of the natural sciences within and alongside the traditional classical curriculum. In 1849, for example, the university established a two-year scientific department which permitted students aiming for careers in teaching or business to substitute for Latin and Greek more "practical" subjects such as science and modern languages. Extended to three years in 1854, this new course became a four-year program leading to the degree of bachelor of science in 1858.

The heart of the curriculum, however, remained the classical languages. When Cyrus Nutt resigned in 1843, Benjamin Tefft, a second Wesleyan graduate to join the Asbury faculty, served as professor of Greek and Hebrew for three years. From 1846 to 1849 Nutt was back teaching Greek and after another off-campus interlude ended his Asbury career as professor of mathematics from 1857 to 1860, as well as vice president and acting president. His successors as professors of Greek were Henry C. Benson (1850-1852) and Samuel A. Lattimore (1852-60), both recent graduates. Another pioneer teacher at Indiana Asbury, John Wheeler, was professor of Latin language and literature from 1842 to 1854.

In his "Reminiscences of Thirty Years in Asbury" published in the *Asbury Review* in 1873, Professor Joseph Tingley gave a vivid word-picture of the campus and town

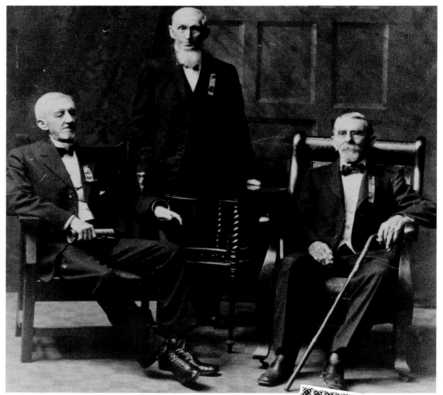

A 1912 reunion of the survivors of the Indiana Asbury class of 1845 brought together (from left) Thomas Talbott, Dr. William H. Larrabee (son of Professor Larabee) and Dr. W. R. Genung.

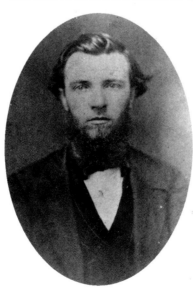

Dr. William R. Genung, a physician and member of the Indiana General Assembly, graduated in 1845. He also delivered the Greek oration.

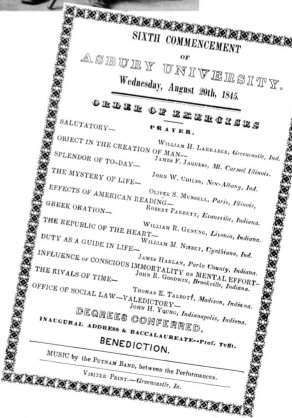

SIXTH COMMENCEMENT
OF
ASBURY UNIVERSITY.
Wednesday, August 20th, 1845.
ORDER OF EXERCISES

SALUTATORY--
PRAYER.

OBJECT IN THE CREATION OF MAN—
WILLIAM H. LARRABEE, Greencastle, Ind.

SPLENDOR OF TO-DAY—
JAMES F. JAQUESS, Mt. Carmel Illinois.

THE MYSTERY OF LIFE—
JOHN W. CHILDS, New-Albany, Ind.

EFFECTS OF AMERICAN READING—
OLIVER S. MUNSELL, Paris, Illinois.

GREEK ORATION—
ROBERT PARRETT, Evansville, Indiana.

THE REPUBLIC OF THE HEART—
WILLIAM R. GENUNG, Livonia, Indiana.

DUTY AS A GUIDE IN LIFE—
WILLIAM M. NISBET, Cynthiana, Ind.

INFLUENCE OF CONSCIOUS IMMORTALITY ON MENTAL EFFORT—
JAMES HARLAN, Parke County, Indiana.

THE RIVALS OF TIME—
JOHN R. GOODWIN, Brookville, Indiana.

OFFICE OF SOCIAL LAW—VALEDICTORY—
THOMAS E. TALBOTT, Madison, Indiana.
JOHN H. YOUNG, Indianapolis, Indiana.

DEGREES CONFERRED.
INAUGURAL ADDRESS & BACCALAUREATE--Prof. Tefft.
BENEDICTION.

MUSIC by the PUTNAM BAND, between the Performances.

VISITER PRINT.—Greencastle, Ia.

14

TOMMY GOODWIN COMES TO GREENCASTLE

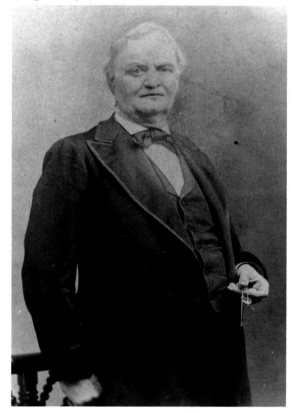

Thomas Goodwin in his later years. A native of Brookville, IN, Goodwin was one of three graduates in the first graduating class of 1840. His reminiscences offer a delightful account of the college in its first moments.

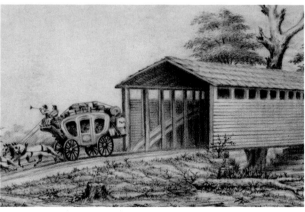

A stagecoach crosses Pogue's Run on the National Road (now U.S. Highway 40) from Indianapolis to Greencastle (The Christian Schrader Collection, Indiana State Library).

The Rev. Thomas Goodwin, a member of the first graduating class and first out-of-town student, recalled 50 years later his arrival in Greencastle from Brookville, Ind. in 1837:

At last November came. The fall term was to open on the first Monday. There was but one way to get to Greencastle, and that was by stage to Putnamville, and from that place to Greencastle as best I could....

It was nearly night when we reached Putnamville, about twenty hours from Indianapolis. My first inquiry of Mr. Townsend, the tavern keeper, was for a conveyance to Greencastle. He informed me that there was none, but if I would wait till Sunday morning he would take me in his two-horse wood wagon for two dollars. I could have walked, and would, but I was no elephant,—I could not carry my trunk. From supper to bedtime I was entertained by Mr. Townsend with dolorous lamentations because the proposed university had been located at Greencastle instead of Putnamville. Greencastle was an out-of-the-way town anyhow, away off the National road; no stage ran through it or to it; how could it ever amount to anything, not being on the National road? Here, he said, we have a stage each way every day, and he continued in this strain, with short intervals for sleeping, until about ten o'clock Sunday, when he landed me at Lynch's tavern, on the east side of the square, and I was at Greencastle, lacking about two hours of four days from Brookville, one hundred and ten miles away....

Gladly dismissing Mr. Townsend, with his two dollars, I turned for comfort to Mr. Lynch, my new landlord.... In answer to my question where the University was, he said, "I don't know for certain. It was last summer, at the deestrict school house, but I have hearn that they have moved it to the county siminary. Be you come to go to it? You will not find it much of a university, I reckon"...

But I went to my room and dressed for church. My prudent mother had told me not to travel in my best, but to save them for Sunday. It was now Sunday and I donned my new suit of blue mixed jeans, as handsome a piece of homemade as ever came from a weaver's loom; doubly precious to me because my mother had spun the yarn from choice fleeces from our own sheep. The coat was of the box pattern with a long tail, coming to below the knees, with immense outside pockets, and made roomy, for the boy would grow much before that Sunday suit would be worn out; and the pants were even more roomy, for the days of tights had not yet cursed society. The new pastor, Rev. James L. Thompson, preached his first sermon that morning in the little hipped-roofed church about thirty-five by forty-five feet in size. After sermon...I went to the preacher and introduced myself. I told him who I was, where I came from, and what I had come for. "Hold, stop, brothers! Here, Brother Dangerfield, Brother Thornburg, Brother Cooper, Brother Hardesty, Brother Nutt, here is Brother Tommy Goodwin; he has come all the way from Brookville to attend the institution," said the ardent preacher at the top of his voice, and then followed handshakings such as I never had been the victim of before, and no student has ever had since. It was the first realization of their hopes. They had never seen a sure enough student before, except their own children and neighbors....

After finding his way to his first class on Monday morning, Goodwin returned to his room in the tavern on the square somewhat homesick and desperately hoping for a letter from home. The next evening his "case" came before the official meeting:

The preacher had undertaken to find a boarding house for me, and he inquired of the brethern. No one had thought of keeping boarders. There had been no demand, hence there was no supply. ...'Here, brethern, what about boarding this student? Something must be done. Here they come flocking in and no place to board; we are expected to look after this.' At last William K. Cooper said that if the young man would sleep with Professor Nutt he would take him until a better place could be found. Some one suggested that the professor might have something to say about sleeping with the young man. The result of the negotiations was that the young man and professor slept together for several months, and several families began to adjust their domestic affairs so as to board students, but less than a dozen "flocked" that winter.

about the time of his arrival as a student 30 years before:

Conspicuous amid the low, white houses, which dotted here and there the fields around, towered the college building. Its newly painted white belfry, with bright green blinds, its ground is bare of trees and exposing patches of the yellow clay which had been loosened by recent grading, testified that the institution was yet in its young life....The remaining portion of the village presented a rude and uninviting appearance. Its nine hundred inhabitants seemed to have expended their whole stock of enterprises and public spirit upon the one object of founding

the University, and to have nothing left for further improvement....

The business centre of Greencastle, then as now, was the public square. It consisted of a group of unsightly houses, mostly built of wood, surrounding a rickety court house in the form of a cube attached to a very tall sharp pointed spire bearing two guilt balls and a weather vane. The maufacturing interests were represented by various establishments devoted to chair-making, shoe-making and carpentering, each employing one hand including the proprietor. There was also a wool-carding mill turned by horse power, which you passed between the college and the

square, and across the ravine over which it was built, stretched a solitary log, flattened upon its upper side for the convenience of footmen. This rustic bridge formed a part of the principal path, (there were no pavements) connecting those two great centres of commerce and literature....

Almost adjoining the college out-lot on the east, was a partially cleared space, [East College yard] overgrown with briars, and south of this a grove containing a dense undergrowth of paw paw bushes....

Hitherward the hilarious students, wearied quite too soon with study, resorted for fun and frolic; and having

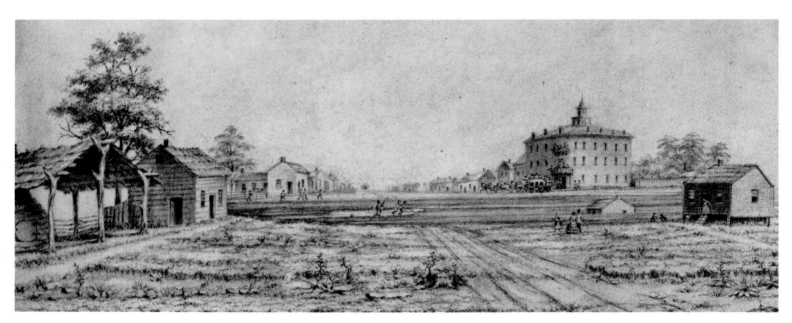

Above: Washington St. in Indianapolis, looking east from the Courthouse in the 1830s or 1840s. The university's Indiana Central Medical College was located in 1849 on the third floor of the Johnson Building between Meridian and Pennsylvania streets on Washington. In 1850 it moved to a two-story brick building on the southeast corner of Washington and East streets, approximately in the upper right of the drawing (The Christian Schrader Collection, Indiana State Library).

At right, a typical Indiana hotel, as drawn by the hand of E. E. Edwards in his diary from 1846-47. (Colorado State University)

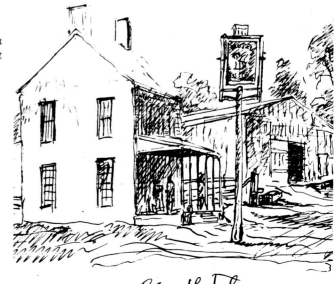

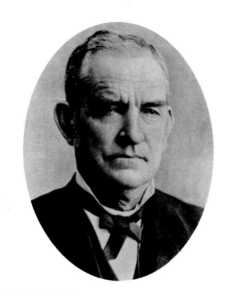

At right, Judge A. C. Downey, who served as professor of law in the short-lived law school.

Below: "Tumbledown", as pictured in the 1846 diary of Asbury student E. E. Edwards. The college provided no dormitories until 1885, so students were frequently found in such lodgings. He rented a room here from Judge Cowgill at $1.50 a month.

"Tumbledown" is the na[me] of the princely palace in which I live

"met and battled with the foe," returned with subdued spirit, scarred and battered clothes, and other evidences of the fact that (if not a veteran) he was, at least, (black) eye witness to the memorable scenes of the Paw Paw war....

Yet a little further westward [Blackstock Field] were the hunting grounds of the snipe hunter, where in midnight darkness, the uninitiated applicant, having been instructed to "put out the light," was left alone to "hold the bag" while the initiated, under cover of a promise to surround and drive the snipes therein, first slyly and then precipitately retreated to their boarding houses.

In the meantime the trustees had decided, with the concurrence of the Indiana Conference of the Methodist Church, to establish a medical department in Indianapolis and appointed eight persons to its faculty in 1848. All were physicians except Charles G. Downey, who was transferred from the professorship of natural science in Greencastle. Known as the Indiana Central Medical College, the school opened in December 1849 but closed after only three years, having graduated 40 of the more than 100 students who attended its classes, including Joshua T. Belles, the grandfather of British Prime Minister Harold MacMillan. Reasons for its demise are hazy, but probably most important was a feeling that the university was over-extending itself in view of its modest financial resources.

More enduring was the law school program which operated in Greencastle from 1853 to 1863. Its faculty consisted of a single professor of law who lectured for a few weeks each term to a handful of would-be lawyers. John A. Matson, Judge A.C. Downey, and John Cowgill each served as law professor at one time or another. The university awarded 54 degrees of bachelor of laws during the decade.

The diary of E.E. Edwards, who enrolled in the preparatory department of Indiana Asbury in 1846 as a boy of 15, presents a vivid picture of student life. He first lived in a rented room in the home of Judge John Cowgill—a member of the board of trustees—located on the northwest corner of the town square and called "Tumbledown." Here were housed four boys on the ground floor and six on the second. All out-of-county students, many in their early teens, had to find both room and board from local landlords, the university providing no dormitory accommodations until 1885. The college bell rang at 4:00 a.m., but Edwards did not rise until about six. At eight he joined with the rest of the student body in a brief religious service in the college chapel, where scripture selections were read, prayers offered, and announcements made; sometimes the choir sang under the direction of Professor Tingley. The rest of the morning was spent in class recitations. Edwards and his fellow students were supposed to study in their rooms after the noon meal until four or five o'clock, when they were free for recreation. After supper they returned to their rooms to study until the college bell rang at 9 p.m., signalling lights out. On Sunday morning students were required to attend one of the Greencastle churches and in the afternoon a lecture at the college by the president or one of the professors.

This rather Spartan routine was occasionally broken by pranks and parties, though students in general came under much more rigorous faculty supervision than imaginable today. Parents were encouraged even to entrust students' spending money with a member of faculty. The young men managed to find time for occasional oyster suppers with ginger beer, but dating local girls was closely monitored. As for pranks, Edwards reports how he and others distributed the university woodpile around town to such effect that classes had to be dismissed the next day because there was no firewood for the classroom stoves.

Some idea of college costs may be obtained from a letter written by student Aden G. Cavins in 1847 to his father:

At present I enjoy remarkable good health, and can cheerfully say that I have so far spent my time since I left old Green [County] in a flow of high spirits. Sickness prevailed here more during the fall than it has for a number of years, the cause of which, I believe, is unknown.

The number of students in attendance during this term is about 175 which exceeds that of any previous term, and of course renders the lower departments of study too much crowded for convenience, or thorough drilling, or rapid improvement. There is some probability that this will be remedied by the creation of another teacher....

I am boarding at Mr. Dicks at 1.75 a week. I commenced boarding at Mr. Talbotts (at 1.50 per week) a very large

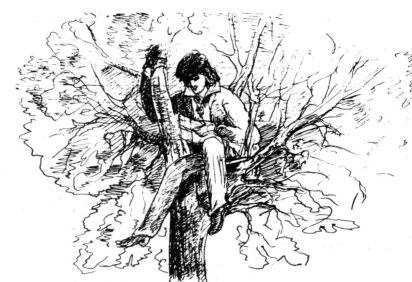

An Asbury student reads in a tree, from a sketch by E. E. Edwards in his 1847 diary. Below: Sketch of a "snipe hunt", the prank of initiation for so many early Asbury students.

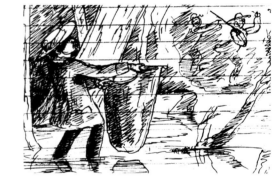

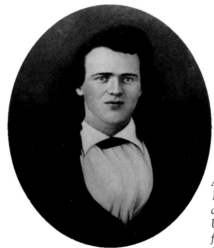

Aden G. Cavins, student from 1845 to 1848. From Bloomfield, Indiana, he completed his law degree at Indiana University. This painting was taken from an original daguerreotype of Cavins near his student days.

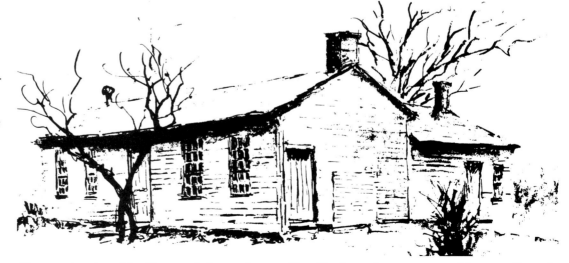

Above, a drawing of the Greencastle home of trustee Rees Hardesty, first treasurer and later president of the board. In this house, Professor Larrabee performed the wedding of Hardesty's daughter in 1850 to recent Asbury graduate and later Indiana congressman and senator Daniel W. Voorhees.

MATTHEW SIMPSON

Matthew Simpson was first president of Indiana Asbury from 1839 to 1848. After leaving the college he was elected a bishop in the Methodist Episcopal Church and became influential in American Protestantism. His wife, pictured below, was Ellen Vernor Simpson.

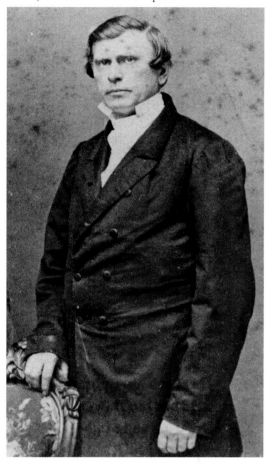

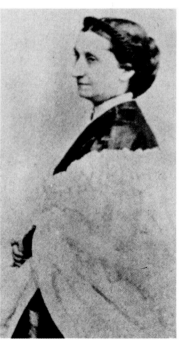

The first president of Indiana Asbury University, the Rev. Matthew Simpson, was born in 1811 in Cadiz, Ohio, where Bishop Francis Asbury himself baptized him while on one of his western journeys. Largely self-educated, young Simpson had taught briefly in a local academy, been admitted to the practice of medicine in his native state, and been ordained into the Methodist ministry, preaching in a small church in Pittsburgh. Deciding to enroll in Allegheny College in 1837, he found himself the recipient of an honorary A.M. degree from the institution and was invited to join the faculty rather than the student body! After two years teaching mathematics and natural science there, he accepted the Asbury presidency in early 1839. At first he taught everything except Greek and Latin while holding the chair of mathematics. Transferring later to the professorship of mental and moral philosophy, he assumed responsibility for that important subject, along with natural theology and "Christian evidences," considered the capstone of the college course and taught by all succeeding presidents for most of the rest of the century.

Like many American college presidents of his time, Simpson combined piety with an innate scholarship despite his lack of formal training. A good speaker with an ingratiating manner, he pleased the entire university constituency during his nine-year tenure. Cyrus Nutt, Asbury's first professor, wrote this in his diary about President Simpson:

The first president, M. Simpson was a man of singular ability in many respects. He was exceedingly popular with both the students and people. He was affable and exceedingly kind in address and conversation, and seldom failed to make a favorable impression upon everyone with whom he conversed. Possessed of some wit, and a smattering of all kinds of learning, and even deeply versed in intellectual science and moral Philosophy, he appeared to advantage in conversation. The elements of popularity were abundant in him. He was emphatically one of the people.... The greatest artlessness and simplicity, with the appearance of great humility were manifest in his deportment.

His pulpit ministration was another source of his great popularity with the masses. A ready utterance in a musical and attractive voice, vividness of fancy, aptness of illustration, and great fervency and glow of feeling, captivated his audience which were always tremendous, when it was known that he was going to preach. His sermons were mostly descriptive. It was seldom that he attempted an argumentative discourse.

By 1848 the infant university was well established, and President Simpson, in somewhat declining health and looking for a less strenuous post, went to Cincinnati to become editor of the *Western Christian Advocate.* Four years later he was elected a bishop of the Methodist Episcopal Church. In that office he soon became an influential national Protestant leader and confidant of Abraham Lincoln, giving one of the funeral addresses for the fallen President.

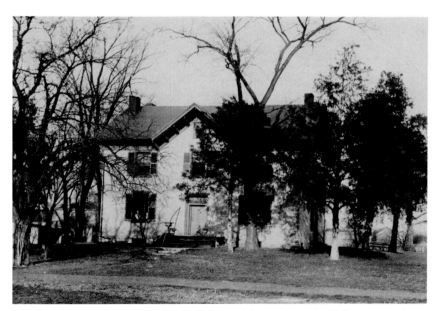

The Simpson home was used for the School of Art in the early DePauw period and later torn down to make way for Rector Hall.

E. E. EDWARDS

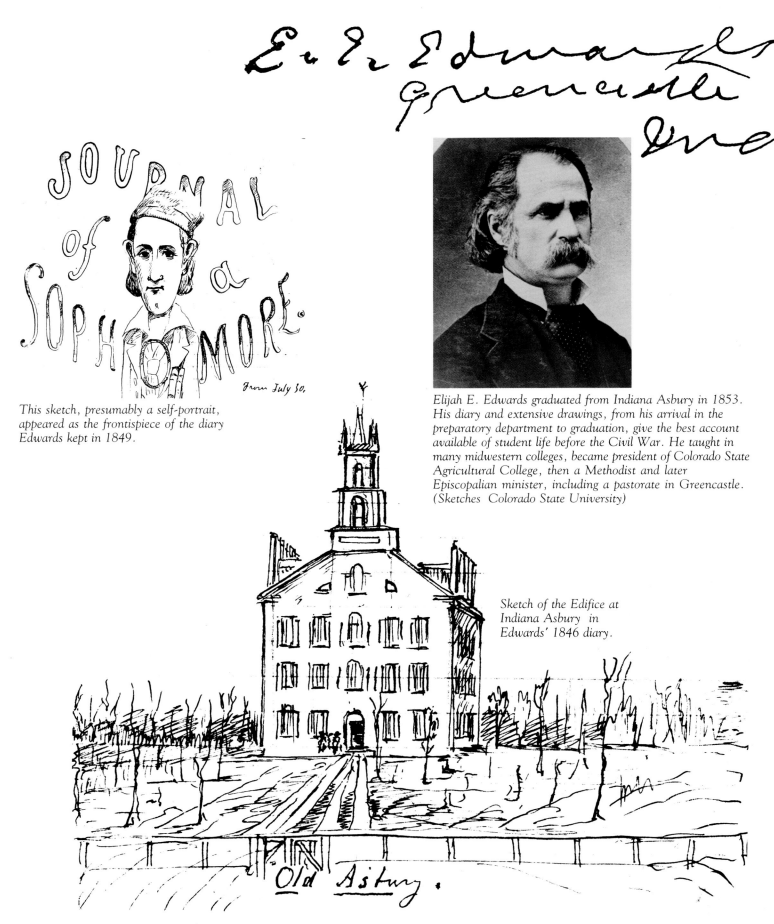

This sketch, presumably a self-portrait, appeared as the frontispiece of the diary Edwards kept in 1849.

Elijah E. Edwards graduated from Indiana Asbury in 1853. His diary and extensive drawings, from his arrival in the preparatory department to graduation, give the best account available of student life before the Civil War. He taught in many midwestern colleges, became president of Colorado State Agricultural College, then a Methodist and later Episcopalian minister, including a pastorate in Greencastle. (Sketches Colorado State University)

Sketch of the Edifice at Indiana Asbury in Edwards' 1846 diary.

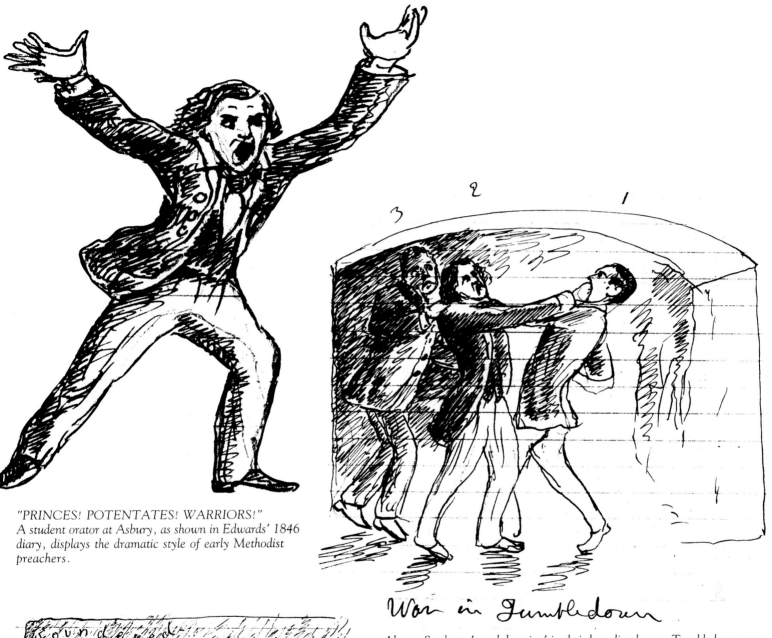

"PRINCES! POTENTATES! WARRIORS!"
A student orator at Asbury, as shown in Edwards' 1846 diary, displays the dramatic style of early Methodist preachers.

War in Tumbledown

Above: Students 'rough housing' in their boarding house, Tumbledown, as pictured in Edwards' 1846 diary.

At left: For out-of-town students, the trip to Greencastle was sometimes an arduous journey. Here, E. E. Edwards' shows himself in the rain waiting for his ride by wagon to the college.

boarding house which accomodates about 22 students but the noise, confusion, and disturbance, was so intense and continuous that it required more concentration of mind than I could command to learn anything save that which if learned ought to be unlearned....

I think it will take about $20 or $21 more to pay my expenses for this term since my books cost me $7.00.

Very early in Indiana Asbury University history the literary societies arrived. These were clubs, semi-independent of the college, which lasted throughout the entire Asbury period and which in their heyday served as a distinctive social and intellectual outlet for the students. Their history was parallel to those of other colleges of this era.

Also early in Asbury history came the new institution of the social fraternity, which challenged the literary society for student interest. The initial excitement of the literary society seemed to wear off after a few years. Older boys in particular began to sense a need for social, as well as intellectual, camaraderie. In 1845 Beta Theta Pi, founded at Miami University in 1839, made its appearance on campus when a few members of Philo held secret organizational meetings in their hall at midnight. Two more fraternity chapters were organized at Indiana Asbury before the Civil War—Phi Gamma Delta and Sigma Chi. In this period, membership in social fraternities was relatively small, limited mainly to upperclassmen. Meetings in the woods, secret ceremony often borrowed from the Masonic movement, boy talk and "horsing around" had appeal over and above the literary society.

The high level of religious interest and personal piety of students and faculty in this period may seem extraordinary to the present-day reader. But it was a national phenomenon in the years following the Second Great Awakening that took place in the United States at the turn of the 18th century. It was what one might expect of boys coming from families that nurtured them for the most part in pietistic Methodism, who grew up in a relatively unsophisticated intellectual

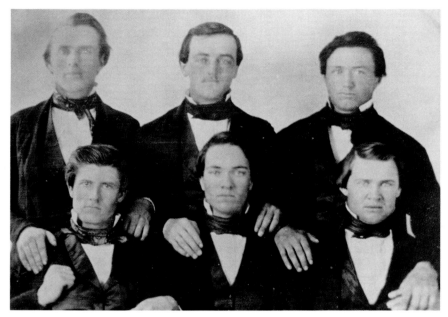

The Philosonian Society, a debating society of the 1850s, was originally anti-fraternity. It later grew into the Secret Ten, a forerunner of Phi Gamma Delta.

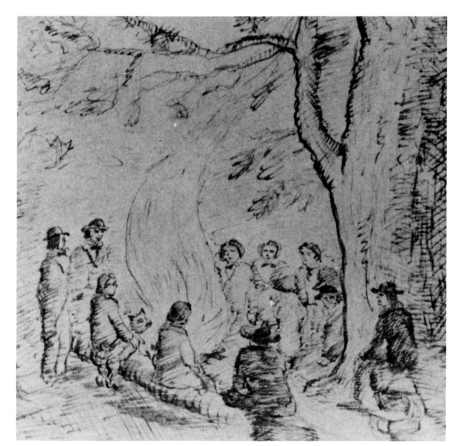

An early chapter meeting of Beta Theta Pi fraternity, held in the woods near Greencastle. Such meetings featured secret ceremonies, boy talk and "horsing around."

milieu. In Greencastle, living away from home for the first time, they found themselves in a sectarian university setting where the adult role models were clergymen-professors who themselves had undergone emotional religious conversion. Student diaries reveal something of the religious turmoil and frequent spiritual rebirth which many students experienced in the frequent church services and camp meetings under faculty influence.

What about faculty life and culture in Greencastle? Many instructors, especially the tutors, were not much beyond the age of the older students and probably socialized with them. Unmarried faculty members lived in boarding houses and had social contacts with each other and young professional men in town. Most of the married professors and their wives were busy raising families, some of them quite large. Pious persons by nature and calling—most of the men were ordained Methodist clergymen—they must have looked to the local Methodist church for much of their social life. Relatively young and receiving miniscule salaries, professors and even presidents often carried on farming activities to augment their income, hauling water, feeding chickens, hewing wood, cultivating gardens, and slopping the hogs before driving the carriage to evening prayer meeting.

Heavier rates of child mortality than today brought frequent tragedy to their homes. The Simpsons were strongly affected by the loss of a son during their Greencastle years, and the Larrabees buried a much-beloved daughter in a beautiful orchard-garden. Rarely a year passed without one or more student deaths also. At the university itself professors had more duties than simply hearing recitations or giving occasional lectures. They were often responsible for such menial tasks as the upkeep and furnishing of their classrooms, repairing the cistern and the lighting system, and calling at saloons and gambling places at 9 p.m. to see if the students were visiting them. Larrabee was an active Mason, as may have been others, and many

THE CONVERSION OF JOHN W. RAY

John W. Ray from Madison, Ind., was a graduate of Indiana Asbury in 1848. An attorney and prominent churchman, he became a colonel in the 49th Regiment, Indiana Volunteers, in the Civil War. A treasurer and cashier in several Indianapolis banks until his death in 1906, he served 27 years as the treasurer of both Indiana Asbury and DePauw University from 1867 to 1894. In his memoirs he left a poignant account of his conversion as a student.

Rev. John C. Smith, who my father had taken into the church at Madison, was the preacher in charge at Greencastle and he announced the beginning of a protracted meeting on the Sabbath to begin Monday night, and for want of something to do I went to church to stay from seven to eight, and then go back to my studies. I understood now why I was drawn there. The Devil had me from 10 that morning.

Now into the House of God, sitting in the pew my whole life rushed before me. Father's life, his gift of his Bible to Mother to be given to me as his only legacy. Mother's prayers, her sweet anxiety for me. My own sinfulness, a rebel against my Father's God. And as I sat there hell seemed to open ready to take me in. No greater torture can the damned endure than came to me in that old church.

As a kind of quietus to my conscience I resolved "if Dr. Simpson preaches tonight I'll join the Church." I had not thought that he would be there. To my surprise he came in, in less than 5 minutes. I was caught in my own resolution. After he preached, Bro. Smith called for mourners. I was the first and at the altar before he spoke a minute.... It seemed it was hell if I stayed in my seat and possibly the mourner's bench would lift me out.

Dr. Simpson at once came down from the pulpit....

The next morning when I went to the Greek lesson at nine o'clock, Prof. Nutt said, "Ray, I want you to tarry after the class is dismissed." ....The class was dismissed and he came from his platform to where I was sitting, took me by the hand, saying, "Ray, were you in earnest in the step you took last night?" Wonderful words to a heart broken sinner.... This second day equal in misery the day before.... Again that night at the mourner's bench.... All the members of the Faculty attended that second night and instead of three at the altar there were more than a dozen.... Miserable night and no pardon. Another day, more sympathy, more earnest words. Another night at the altar.... Dr. Simpson, Larrabee, Nutt, and others took my hand to lead me out of distress, and about 10 o'clock the burden went off.... I know I was then converted. I have not needed that work done since, although I have often fallen short of my duties and often desired more grace and a higher and fuller devotion to God....

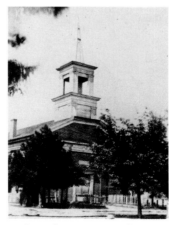 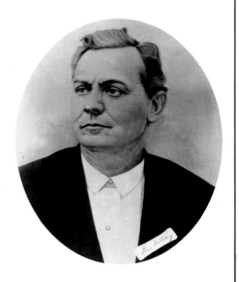

Right: John W. Ray, who became a leading Indianapolis banker, a member of the board of trustees, and treasurer of the university from 1867 to 1894. Above: Roberts Chapel, the third Methodist Episcopal Church in Greencastle, which was built in 1847 on the northwest corner of College and Poplar streets.

participated in literary society activities.

University finances were almost always precarious. Indiana Asbury began with little more of an endowment than the $25,000 raised by Greencastle citizens to bring the university to their community. The original plan of the Indiana Conference was to raise capital by sending out agents to sell shares to loyal Methodist supporters. For $100 a shareholder could send a student to Asbury for six years; for $250, for 20 years; and $10,000 would endow a professorship. The larger sums being hard to come by, subscriptions for $5 and $1 were available. The first student fees were $8.50 per session in the preparatory department and $12 in the college, plus a janitor's fee of $1.25. Over the years these modest fees were slightly increased, until 1874, when tuition charges were abolished and only a contingency fee of $15 per year was assessed each student. Despite low faculty salaries—Professor Nutt began at $400 and President Simpson at $1,000 a year—the university often ended the academic year with substantial deficits and salaries in arrears. Despite faculty salary cuts, by 1844-45 the university owed Simpson $1,164, Larrabee $984, the rest of the staff $3,490. It is a truism that in 19th century higher education professors everywhere subsidized the colleges, often overlooked by the nostalgia the alumni began to have for these "giants" of the classroom.

The first reported audit of university finances in 1855 calculated its total resources at $94,785, including buildings and grounds at $27,000 and railroad bonds at $58,700. In addition unpaid notes due the university came to another $43,516. Clearly Indiana Asbury, and presumably 19th century American higher education as a whole, were low-budget affairs.

In 1848 President Simpson resigned to become editor of the *Western Christian Advocate* in Cincinnati. His nine years of service, much of it spent away from campus speaking to church and other groups and making

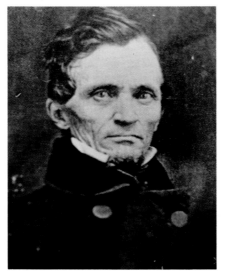

friends for the university like most modern college presidents, were of crucial importance in getting Indiana Asbury established. He was popular with the students and townspeople, perhaps more so than any of his immediate successors. But his star was rising, and he eventually went on to the Methodist espiscopacy and a major role in American Protestantism. Preaching Lincoln's funeral elegy, Simpson later had another Methodist college named after him, but he apparently never lost his interest in Old Asbury.

A year passed in locating a new president. A prominent Methodist minister and later bishop as well as rival of Simpson, E.R. Ames, turned down the proffered appointment; so

Professor Larrabee, who surprisingly was not offered the job, was made acting president for the academic year 1848-49. Finally, in July 1849 Lucien Berry was elected second president of the university. A native of Vermont who had grown up in Ohio and attended Miami University, Berry had held influential pastorates in Knightstown and Indianapolis, where his congregations contained members of the political and economic elite of the state. Berry was a Whig at a time when most Indiana Methodists, including Simpson and Ames, were Democrats. He had been on the Asbury board of trustees since 1842 and was a close friend of Simpson. Seemingly a good choice for the position, Berry was to encounter town-gown conflicts and probably both political and religious rivalry which shortened his presidency.

Though Berry's presidency began well, in a few years problems arose which contributed to his early resignation. Two incidents in 1853 stand out. After a riotous episode in which a black resident was driven from town, Berry expelled a student who admitted his involvement in the affair. In response some Greencastle citizens, including local Democrat leaders, referred to the president and his faculty as a "little coterie of tyrants."

At about the same time a local grocer was suspected of selling liquor to students. Berry tried to retaliate by refusing permission to students to live in the same rooming houses with the grocer's clerks, who supposedly sold the contraband products. The landladies rebelled, supported by most of the town. Both the students and the trustees gave Berry a vote of confidence. But the president, feeling unnecessarily harassed, resigned in July 1854. After a year in a New Albany pastorate, Berry became president of Iowa Wesleyan College but died prematurely in that office in 1858 at the age of 43.

WILLIAM C. LARRABEE

The third professor appointed to Indiana Asbury University was William C. Larrabee, who took over the chair in mathematics in 1841 and also became responsible for teaching the natural sciences. Born in Maine in 1802, he was nine years older than President Simpson and had attended Bowdoin College with Franklin Pierce, who later became president of the United States. His professional experience included teaching posts at Connecticut Wesleyan University and Oneida College Seminary in the state of New York, as well as taking part in the first geological survey of Maine. Historian George Manhart called Larrabee the "most versatile man ever associated with Asbury or DePauw." With his wife, who founded the Greencastle Female Collegiate Seminary, he built a Gothic Revival home near the present site of Bishop Roberts Hall. They named it Rosabower after their beloved daughter Rosa, who died young and was buried in the Dells. In a collection of essays entitled *Rosabower* published in 1852, Larrabee described the scene in mid-19th century romantic prose:

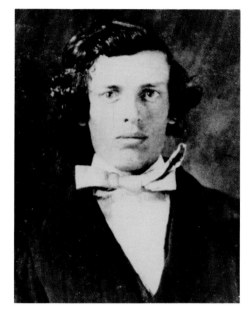

There are voices here, gentle reader: the voices of Nature in her gladness and love. Lots of merry crickets are chirping in the tall grass. The incessant hum of the bee is heard in the air and on the trees overhead. On a little bush by my side sits the sparrow singing to its mate on her nest in the neighboring thicket. From the fence corner comes the plaintive monotone of the robin. From the crevice in the old stump flits the wren twittering emulous. On the topmost branch of the maple sits the mocking-bird, most tuneful of nature's warblers, leaving, in her ecstacies of melody, nothing unimitated. From the adjacent grove comes the cooing of the turtle-dove, mournful and sad. Even the pines, in their waving tassels, furnish a harp for the winds, giving out music soft, soothing, and inimitable....

One evening, in the merry month of May, she was rambling with me about this shady glen, and about the garden walks of home, till the fading twilight sent us to repose. To the night succeeded a morning of intense anxiety. There was hurrying to and fro about the house, and flitting forms of physicians and friends passed and repassed by me, as I was watching intent over my sick and dying child. Another night—a night of bitter agony, a night of intense anguish, a night of dying hope, a night of despair—passed slow and sad away. Another morning came—the morning of the holy Sabbath came bright and beautiful; but I can only remember the voice of wailing and of woe in my once happy home, the melancholy tones of the bell of death pealing on the air, the long funeral procession, the open grave, and by the side of it a coffin with its lid upraised, and in that coffin my own little Emma Rosabelle, with the sunlight of heaven beaming bright on her cold, pale, yet beautiful face. We buried her—buried her here in this rural spot. 'When I am dead' said she, a few days before she fell sick, 'they will not bury me in the cold graveyard, but they will bury me in the bower among the flowers, and my father and my mother will come and sit by me.' So we buried her here, in this lovely bower, and for her sake we call it Rosabower.

After 10 years on the faculty Larrabee left Asbury to become Indiana's first superintendent of public instruction. The university eventually purchased Rosabower, which survived until the 1930s, serving variously as a dormitory, an infirmary, and for other uses.

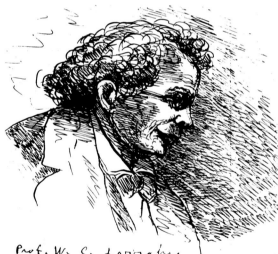

Prof. W. C. Larrabee.

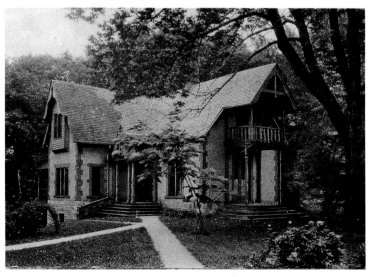

Above: William C. Larrabee, as a young man and as he appeared in E. E. Edwards' diary. He was Asbury's third professor, teaching mathematics and natural science from 1840 to 1850, when he left to become first state superintendent of instruction. His home, Rosabower, was later used as a dormitory and infirmary.

Other changes were affecting the control of Indiana Asbury University at this time as well. In 1844 the Indiana Methodist Conference, which was responsible for naming persons to the board of trustees and visitors, was split in two, creating the new North Indiana Conference; in 1852 and 1853 two more were formed, the Southeast and Northwest Conferences. One result was the weakening of representation on the board from Greencastle and Putnam County. As late as 1847, 15 out of the 25 trustees were residents of Putnam County; by the '50s the county's representation had dropped to three or four. No longer dominated by a group of Greencastle professional men exercising close personal supervision over the university's business, the board was made up of men from all over the state who came together once a year to review and give support to the president's program. In 1854 during the Berry crisis, it was headed for the first time by a non-Greencastle man, Congressman Samuel W. Parker of Connorsville. He was a Whig, originally from New York and president of the Whitewater Canal Company. Town-gown unrest might also be accredited to this loss of Greencastle influence.

In August 1854, the board chose Davis W. Clark, editor of the *Ladies Repository* in Cincinnati, for the presidency, but he refused the position. The board then elected Daniel Curry in a "stormy session" by 11 votes to two for ex-president Berry. A New Yorker and graduate of Wesleyan University in Connecticut, Curry was pastor of a large Methodist church in New York City with academic and pastoral experience in both New York and Georgia. With his experience and maturity—he was 45 years old—he seemed to possess just the right qualifications for the job of putting things back together at Indiana Asbury after the Berry incidents. But Curry came to the university as an outsider with no ties to the community, the state, or Indiana Methodism, and with some reluctance. He lasted just three years.

Curry proved to be an aggressive administrator. 'Old Hippodrome,' as he was soon known on campus, gained strong support from the students in confrontation with town authorities over the stabbing of an undergraduate by a local ruffian. But when he attempted to strengthen college discipline a serious student rebellion erupted. It began in the fall of 1856 with a faculty ruling that the literary societies hold their weekly meetings on Friday afternoon rather than evening. When students resisted the ruling, claiming the right to regulate their own literary society affairs, the president demanded they sign a pledge to obey the regulations of the university or be dismissed. As a result 77 students were suspended including the entire senior class. No one graduated at Commencement in 1857, though defiant seniors were eventually awarded their degrees and recognized as alumni.

In July 1857 the board of trustees voted a lukewarm endorsement of the administration, but Curry resigned anyway, followed by two members of the faculty. Too heavy-handed and tactless for a college president, he went on to successful pastorates in New York and Connecticut and a 12-year stint as editor of the *Christian Advocate* in New York City.

To replace Curry the trustees chose one of their own number, Judge David McDonald, former head of the Indiana University Law School and a layman, who waited a year before declining the post. Cyrus Nutt, who had returned to the Asbury faculty for the third time as vice president, acted as president until the arrival of the Rev. Thomas Bowman, a Pennsylvanian and graduate of Dickinson College whom the board elevated as president in 1858.

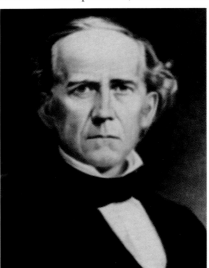

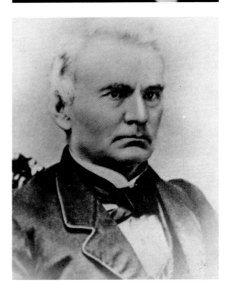

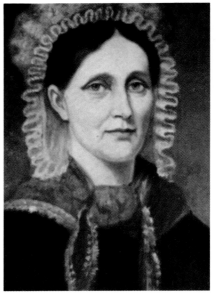

Mrs. Calvin Fletcher (Sarah Hill) was a board member's wife in Indiana Asbury's pre-Civil War era.

REBELLION OF 1856-57

In his booklet *Indiana Asbury University-DePauw University: A History,* Irving Frederick Brown of the class of 1914 wrote the following account of the Curry riots.

The weekly holiday of the school at this time came on Saturday, and for this reason the [literary] society meetings were held on Friday night. After the meetings, the members would sometimes get out and engage in somewhat boisterous fun around the streets, before dispersing for the night. On October 17, 1855, the faculty passed a resolution requiring the societies to hold their meetings on Friday afternoon, and prohibiting such disturbances as they had been causing. President Curry and the faculty claimed that the sessions were protracted to very late hours—usually until after ten o'clock, and not infrequently until nearly midnight—thus endangering the morals and health of the young men, breaking in upon their regular habits, and bringing the college property into increased danger of fire. They also said that the meetings were the occasions of serious disorder, both within and without their halls. The students objected to the above resolutions on the ground, first, that many of their number, who were self-supporting, used Friday afternoons for their work, and, second, that such a plan had been tried and found impracticable. They petitioned the faculty to reconsider their action, but in vain. They then said that they would not meet at all, rather than in the daytime, and both societies accordingly adjourned sine die. A few days later a meeting of students and faculty was called, at which time the students were allowed to present their view of the matter and give their reasons for dissenting. At this meeting they denied all the charges that the faculty had made. The students told the faculty that the meetings rarely varied more than ten minutes either way from ten o'clock, and that only two or three times during the last five years had they been extended beyond eleven o'clock. Moreover, there had never been an accident from fire; and as to the immorality of such a thing, it was better to spend their evenings in literary pursuits, than to spend them in such public resorts as the town afforded. This meeting, however, only made matters worse. On October 25, about one hundred of the students gathered together in what was known as Seller's woods, or in the student term of the time, "Sylva Selleris," which was on the site of McKeen field. Here they talked matters over, and decided that, whatever should happen, they would all stick together. President Curry had, in the meantime, declared the college to be in a state of rebellion, and on Tuesday, October 28, he presented to the students a pledge, on which they were given twenty-four hours to deliberate. At the end of that time, if they decided to accept it, they could remain in school, but if they did not, they were to be suspended.

When the roll was called the next morning at chapel, nineteen answered "yes," eighty-one "no," nineteen asked for further time, and nine were absent. The final result was the suspension of the entire senior class—twenty-two in number—six out of eight juniors, eight sophomores, twelve freshmen, and twenty-nine scientifics. Some went home, some were later allowed to reenter, and some went to other schools, but in later years nearly all of the senior class were enrolled as alumni of the University. This rebellion led directly to President Curry's resignation in July of the following summer.

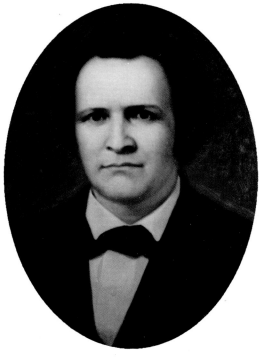

Lucien Berry became second president of Indiana Asbury from 1849-54.

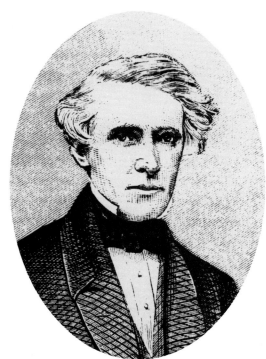

Daniel Curry, third president of Indiana Asbury, from 1854-57.

The '50s were a turbulent period in the university's history, marked by high faculty and administrative turnover as well as a certain amount of alienation. The Berry faculty from 1849 to 1854 consisted of Wheeler, Larrabee, Charles Downey, Tingley, Lattimore, and Benson, plus Miles J. Fletcher, professor of English literature and normal instruction after 1852, and John A. Matson in law, and the president himself. Larrabee left in 1852 and Wheeler, Fletcher, and Matson in 1854 with Berry. Curry replaced Matson with Alexander C. Downey, and brought Edmund E. Bragdon to teach Latin, Bernard Nadal in belles lettres, and Henry B. Hibben to direct the preparatory department and teach foreign languages. Nadal, Hibben, and Charles Downey left in 1857 with Curry, and Bragdon a year later. Tingley and Lattimore were the only leftovers from the Simpson-Berry era; shortly rehired were Matson to replace Downey in law in 1858, Fletcher in Belles Lettres and history in 1857, and Nutt in mathematics with administrative responsibilities in 1857. The Simpson-Berry appointees were back in the saddle on the faculty.

Likewise in the '50s the students were becoming restless under a narrow and rather arbitrary course of

The Imperial Quartet, a group of Indiana Asbury students of 1869.

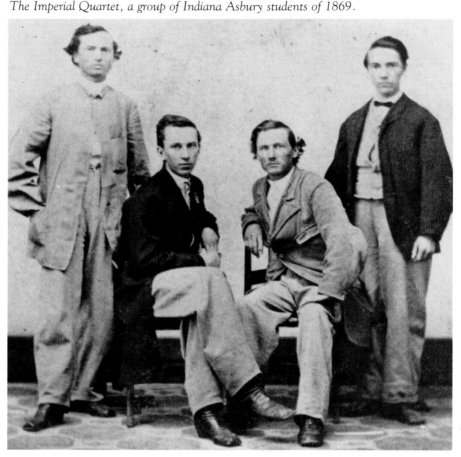

Bottom: Asbury Notes was a semi-monthly journal published from 1852-54 under the auspices of Professors John Wheeler and Joseph Tingley of the Indiana Asbury faculty.

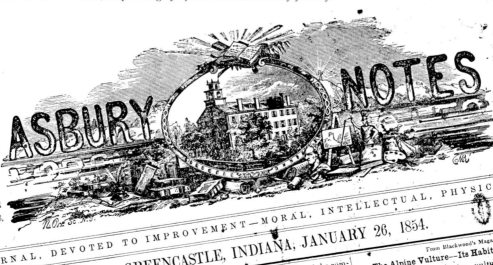

study, which included compulsory chapel attendance plus three or four hours of class recitations each weekday morning, Saturday morning exercises in composition and declamation, and Sunday afternoon faculty lectures. It is surprising that there were not more frequent student uprisings!

The pioneer period had ended in Indiana. In Putnam County and elsewhere self-sustaining pioneer homesteads were giving way to commercial farms and rising industries.

Prosperous members of the new middle class of farmers and professionals were constructing red-brick mansions and sending their children to college to "get ahead." Greencastle was connected to the wider world by the Terre Haute Railroad (later part of the Pennsylvania system) running east and west; and to the north and south by the Louisville, New Albany, and Chicago (The Monon) railroad. While Indiana Asbury experienced some enrollment declines in the '50s, it remained the largest institution of

higher education in the state, with a student body ranging between 200 and 300. Its alumni were successful lawyers, ministers, physicians, editors, teachers, politicians, farmers, and businessmen in Indiana and beyond.

The university, having become firmly established, was now ready for new challenges in the changing conditions of the second half of the 19th century. Perhaps symbolic of the end of pioneer Indiana Asbury was the erection of the Bishop Roberts gravesite monument on the

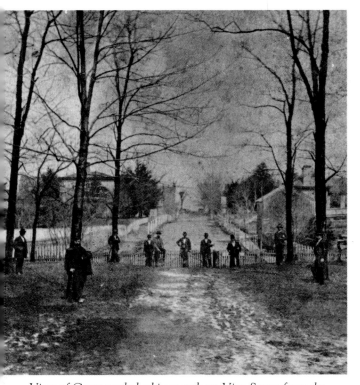

View of Greencastle looking north on Vine Street from the entrance of the Edifice, just right of today's Publications building. A ravine back of the fence was filled in the course of the 19th century. In modern times on the left was the Interurban bus station, later the Fluttering Duck, and now the Walden Inn.

LITERARY SOCIETIES

As in other colleges of the time, the literary societies provided a chief extracurricular outlet for student energies. The first was the Platonean Literary Society, formed in June 1838 under the direction of Professor Cyrus Nutt. Two years later, on President Simpson's advice, it split into two groups, the second taking the name first of the Ciceronian, and finally, the Philological Literary Society. Plato and Philo, as they were generally known, persisted throughout the Asbury period, each with a membership of from 50 to 100 students. After women entered the university in 1867, they formed their own literary society called the Philomathean, and the preparatory department at times had its own, less well developed, society. Most students were to join one or the other of the societies, which were highly competitive but not as exclusive as social fraternities became in later years. Faculty members and selected Greencastle professional men were also connected with the societies, which vied with each other in inviting prominent Americans such as Longfellow, Bryant, Holmes, Agassiz, and Beecher to accept honorary membership.

The literary societies met on Friday evenings in college rooms set aside for them by the university, where their members elected their own officers, conducted business according to parliamentary rules, and debated the issues of the day. Plato and Philo Halls were especially elaborately furnished, with thick carpets, window drapes, and comfortable sofas and chairs. Each had a collection of books which served as a circulating library for its members, who were unable at that time to borrow volumes from the university library. The literary societies obviously served as student retreats where members could relax from the rigid and often sterile atmosphere of the recitation hall, where they were forced to engage in rote, lockstep learning under the stern control of a professor. Here students found an opportunity to organize themselves democratically and thrash out ideas and topics of their own choosing. Perhaps one could say about them what has been said about the playing fields of Eton: that the battles of Shiloh and Antietam were won on the Victorian settees of American college literary societies!

east side of the Edifice. The body of Roberts, who presided over the Indiana Methodist Conference at the time of the granting of the university charter, was returned to campus along with that of his wife to reside under a stone obelisk-type marker. This monument stands today between Harrison and Asbury halls, the only remaining symbol of Indiana Asbury before the Civil War.

The inauguration of Thomas Bowman as president in June 1859 was thought by many to usher in a Golden Age for Old Asbury. The new president, who began a relationship with the institution that was to last for 53 years, had graduated from Dickinson College, studied law and had both business and teaching experience. Before this able leader could preside over major changes in the university, however, he was faced with four crisis years of the Civil War. Despite the near-mass exodus from campus of older boys, the university did not close, though the law school was discontinued in 1862. In 1862-63 enrollment slipped below 200 for the first time since 1846, with 61 in the college and 128 in the preparatory department. Enrollment picked up toward the end of the war, and in 1865-66 reached the highest to date, 407, of whom 159 were in the college. It was obviously the preparatory department, with its large number of boys below the age of military service, which rescued the institution. The number of faculty remained stable, although Professor Fletcher was not replaced when he resigned.

Despite the interruption of the Civil War, the long Bowman administration—it lasted 14 years—produced significant educational progress. Alongside the traditional classical course leading to the bachelor of arts degree and the new scientific department which was extended to a full four-year program culminating in a bachelor of science degree in 1858, were added a Biblical and a normal department, making electives available for students preparing for the ministry or for teaching.

Financial conditions improved somewhat after the war, permitting increases in faculty salaries, which in 1867 were $1,500 per year for professors and $2,000 for the president. While a campaign to raise an endowment in celebration of the centenary of American Methodism in 1866 proved disappointing, several individuals made generous gifts to the university. The John Harmon Chair of Biblical Literature was established in 1865 and four years later the Robert Stockwell Professorship of Greek. Stockwell, from Lafayette, contributed an estimated $77,000 to the university in these years. Lastly, citizens of Greencastle contributed sufficient funds to begin to construct a badly needed new building to supplement the facilities of the Edifice. The cornerstone for this structure, to be located in a large field east of the old campus, was laid on October 20, 1871.

In these years the faculty had expanded to seven positions, including the president, who was also professor of mental and moral philosophy as well as Harmon Professor of Biblical Literature. The veteran Joseph Tingley remained professor of natural science throughout the period, becoming vice-president as well in 1860. The chair of Greek language and literature, after the resignation of Lattimore in 1860, went to Philander Wiley. The Latin chair was held first by Benjamin T. Hoyt and then by Lewis L. Rogers, who also served as principal of the preparatory department for a time. In 1860 John W. Locke succeeded Cyrus Nutt in mathematics and in 1863 German-born John A. Reubelt was appointed to teach modern languages, followed by John E. Earp in 1869. Earp was the first teacher with graduate training, two years at the universities of Tubingen and Berlin. John Clark Ridpath joined the faculty in 1869 as professor of English literature and normal instruction, transferring to the chair of Belles Lettres and history two years later.

The most important innovation of the Bowman years was the admission of women students in 1867, 30 years after the founding of Indiana

This monument to Methodist Episcopal Bishop and Mrs. Robert R. Roberts, which marks their gravesite, was erected in 1859. The stone marker was a gift of the Methodist preachers of Indiana. It is the only remaining object on the DePauw campus from before the civil war.

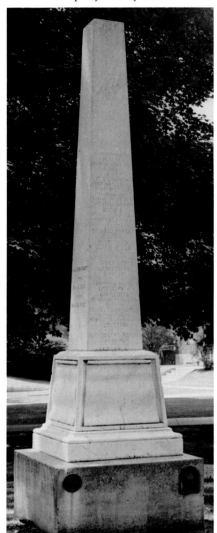

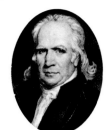

Bishop Robert R. Roberts

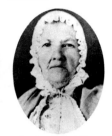

Elizabeth Oldham Roberts

Asbury. During those three decades the higher education of women had been much discussed in the United States and a number of all-female and a few coeducational colleges had been established. Greencastle itself was the site of several "female seminaries," including a very successful one operated by Harriet Dunn Larrabee, wife of Professor William C. Larrabee. As early as 1855 the Asbury trustees went so far as to appoint a committee to consider the establishment of a "Female Department of the University."

THOMAS BOWMAN

The fourth president of Indiana Asbury University was Thomas Bowman. Born in Berwick, Pa. in 1817, he was a member of the first graduating class of Methodist Dickinson College in 1837. He remained at Dickinson for a year studying law, then did some preaching and teaching in an elementary school related to the college. For a while he managed the family farm and flour mill and then for 10 years was principal of Dickinson Seminary (now Lycoming College). He became president of Indiana Asbury in 1858 just as he was about to begin a pastorate in Lewisburg, Pa. At the time of his appointment, Bowman was characterized this way:

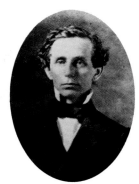

President Thomas Bowman in 1859, the year following his election as president of Indiana Asbury University.

He is graceful enough to be a courtier, simple enough for a Puritan, frank enough for a child, grave as a judge, and pleasant as a woman. His common sense and conciliatory spirit will probably keep him by still waters and in pretty good pastures.

His simplicity, unpretentiousness, and sincerity would help to sustain Bowman through his long tenure in the presidency from 1858 to 1872, including the difficult Civil War years. From May 1864 to March 1865 he also served as chaplain of the United States Senate. After the war Bowman presided with dignity over such important university events as the admission of women students and the initial planning and the laying of the cornerstone of East College. In his *DePauw Through the Years*, George Manhart wrote:

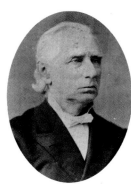

President Thomas Bowman in his later years, when he served as both president of the Board of Trustees (1887-1895), as well as chancellor and chancellor emeritus.

In the classroom, Bowman was said to be 'hailed with delight,' as he made 'everything as clear as a sunbeam.' He seemed to speak equally well before university students, children, or the United States Senate. He was especially popular as speaker at the dedication of churches, on which occasions he was highly 'successful in raising money, having opened the hearts of his hearers until he has free access to their pockets.' ...Of President Bowman as a disciplinarian, one of his students wrote that he had a 'firm but sweet, kind way of controlling.'

Bowman had made a reputation for himself in Methodist circles, and in 1872 at the General Conference he was elected bishop on the first ballot, with the largest vote cast to that time. Bowman continued his interest in Indiana Asbury by serving on its board of trustees, including a term as president from 1887 to 1895. He was also a special lecturer in the School of Theology. He received the largely honorific title of chancellor in 1884 and after 1899 became chancellor emeritus, without duties or salary. As bishop, Bowman traveled to England, Europe, and the Far East and presided over conferences in every state and territory of the United States, as well as in some foreign countries. After 24 years in the episcopacy he retired from active duties in 1896 and lived in retirement until his death in 1914, aged 96. He had eight sons and three daughters, one of whom, Sallie Bowman Caldwell, provided the organ in Meharry Hall and a large part of the funds for the construction of the gymnasium named after her father. Today President Bowman's memory is preserved in the pleasant and dignified park newly created on the south campus.

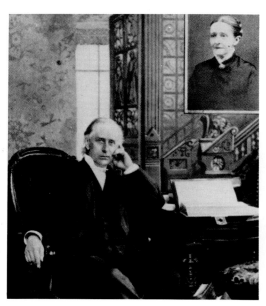

Bishop Thomas Bowman, president of Indiana Asbury University, 1858-72. Matilda Hartman Bowman, 1821-79, wife of the president and mother of his 11 children.

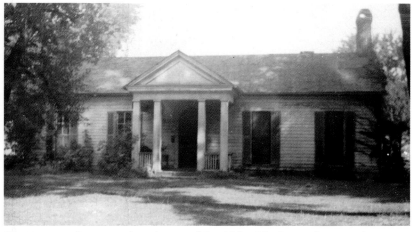

The Bowman home stood on the site of the Alpha Chi Omega house and was torn down in 1952.

31

Nothing, however, came of this or subsequent proposals, though a similar recommendation by President Bowman in 1860 received approval from the board of trustees before being laid aside when war broke out. In July 1864, a meeting of interested persons held in Roberts Chapel in Greencastle proposed to raise funds for a building to house a woman's college in conjunction with Indiana Asbury, but no more was done. At long last, in June 1867 the board of trustees after protracted discussion pro and con opted for a fully coeducational institution by simply voting to "receive Female students into the regular College classes of the University."

That fall five young women, all but one residents of Putnam County, enrolled as freshmen. Four of them—Alice Allen, Laura Beswick, Bettie McReynolds Locke, and Mary E. Simmons—became Asbury's first women graduates in 1871. The fifth, Amanda Beck, dropped out after the freshman year. The coeds had to face the open hostility of a minority of male students resentful of their presence at first. But with the wholehearted support of the faculty, the board, and most Methodist clergy, and the strength of their own resolve they soon won a position of respect and full acceptance in the university. Their numbers grew slowly but surely and in 1871 girls were admitted to the preparatory department as well. Barred from the all-male literary societies, they founded their own Philomathean Literary Society in 1869, and the next year their fellow students were startled to discover that a female social fraternity, or sorority, had been organized on campus—Alpha Chapter of Kappa Alpha Theta, the first of its kind in the United States. Inevitably, perhaps, the first campus wedding took place on Commencement Day 1871, when Laura Beswick married the Rev. Robert N. McKaig of the class of 1870. Officiating was a classmate of the groom, the Rev. Hillary A. Gobin, later to become a professor and then president of the university.

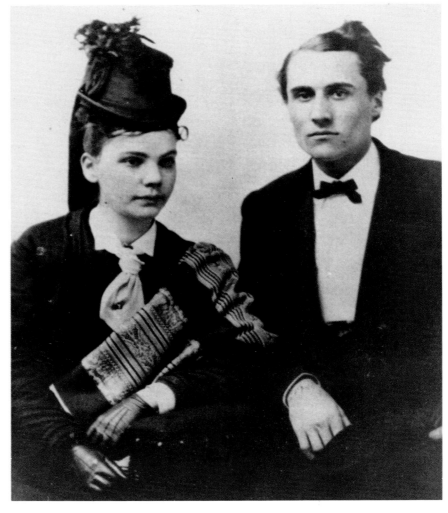

Mary Nelson Stevenson was in the second class to admit women (1869) and graduated in 1873. Henry Augustus Buchtel graduated in 1872, and later became a Methodist pastor, Chancellor of the University of Denver and governor of Colorado. This was one of the earliest student marriages at Old Asbury.

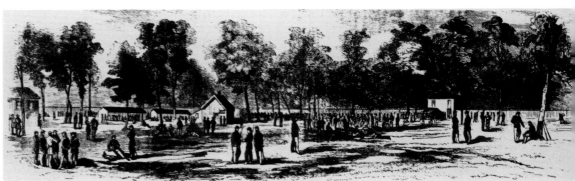

The Asbury Cadets and the Putnam Union Guards of Greencastle first saw service in 1861 at Camp Morton, north of what was then Indianapolis (Indiana Historical Society).

INDIANA ASBURY AND THE CIVIL WAR

Major General Nathan Kimball, a student at Indiana Asbury in 1839, was the highest ranking Asbury man in the Union Army during the Civil War.

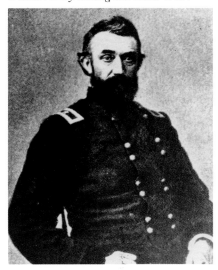

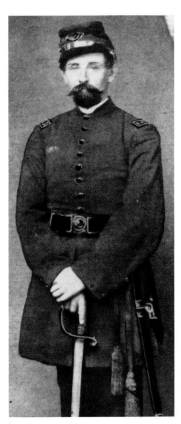

It was difficult to maintain a men's college during the Civil War. Southerners dropped out of school early; in 1860-61 there were two from Louisiana, two from Mississippi, and six from Kentucky. With the fall of Fort Sumpter on April 16, 1861, Lincoln's call for volunteers, supported by Governor Oliver Morton of Indiana, brought confusion to the campus. Classes were immediately dismissed, and students began to sign up. Within five days a company known as the Asbury Guards was drilling on campus. On Sunday, April 21, young men who had joined spoke at morning services in the new Methodist Church, Roberts Chapel. In the regular Sunday afternoon lecture President Bowman gave advice to the youthful volunteers. This was followed by a religious service in Philo Hall in which the volunteers spoke of their home in heaven and their willingness to sacrifice all for country. Fifty guards joined the church that evening and 16 the next morning. On April 24 the Guards left for Indianapolis.

Likewise the Putnam County Union Guards was formed among townspeople in Greencastle; like the Asbury Guards, this group included both college and townsmen. Each had 60 or more privates and a dozen commissioned and non-commissioned officers. Eli Lilly, a local druggist who had attended the preparatory department, was an orderly sergeant. President Bowman and other Greencastle residents visited the volunteers at Camp Morton in Indianapolis. By early May most of the Asbury Guards were back in Greencastle, reluctant to enlist for three years. Those who remained joined the 10th Indiana Volunteer Regiment and fought in Virginia, Kentucky, and Tennessee. Some of the returnees had second thoughts, went to Camp Vigo in Terre Haute and became Company D of the 14th Indiana Volunteer Infantry Regiment. One of President Bowman's own sons was hospitalized while serving in this regiment. Eventually many transferred to other regiments and became officers. Likewise former students and graduates served in units from other states.

The next exodus from campus came during Morgan's Raid on July 1, 1863, when local militia in the "Putnam Blues" were called up. It held a major review in October of that year on the present East College lot. More students left when in 1864 Lincoln called for volunteers for 100 days' service in a relief capacity.

Some 450 Asbury men served. An incomplete list includes 18 colonels, 14 lieutenant colonels, 16 majors, 19 chaplains, 26 surgeons and assistant surgeons, seven adjutants, 64 captains, 42 lieutenants, and 200 non-commissioned officers and privates. One Confederate brigadier general and three colonels, including Reuben Millsaps, who founded Millsaps College, had attended Indiana Asbury. Of the faculty, two short-time teachers served. Former professors Tefft and Hibben were chaplains, two former members of the medical college served as surgeons, and A.C. Downey of the law department became a brigadier general in the militia. Miles Fletcher served as a special aide to Governor Morton and was killed in an accident while on a battlefield trip to take hospital supplies and bring back wounded and sick. Five later members of the faculty served in the war, including President Hillary Gobin. President Bowman was Chaplain of the United States Senate from May 1864 to March 1865.

Right: Captain Alfred J. Hawn was a member of the Asbury Guards in early 1861. Mustered into service later in the year, and commissioned captain in June, he served in both the 16th and 78th Indiana Regiments (Putnam County Historical Society).

Below: A corps of Civil War cadets, probably from Putnam County.

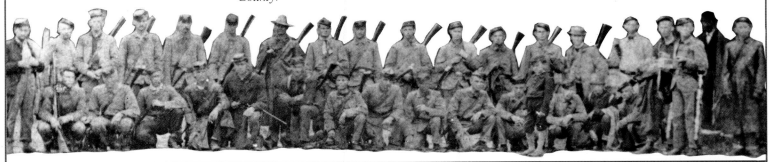

STUDENTS

At right, three students at the close of the Indiana Asbury years. Samuel L. Brengle (at right in photo) graduated in 1883, and later became a Commissioner in the Salvation Army.

Below: Students of the Secret Ten, 1850-51, which was the forerunner of Phi Gamma Delta social fraternity.

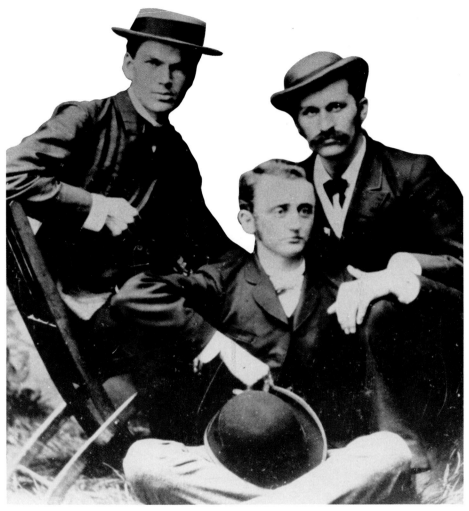

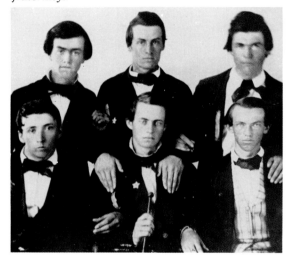

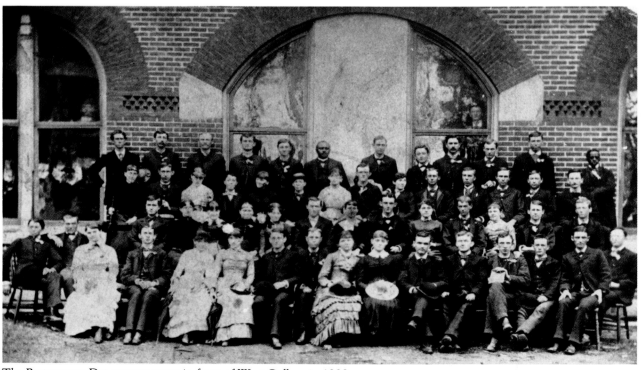

The Preparatory Department poses in front of West College in 1883.

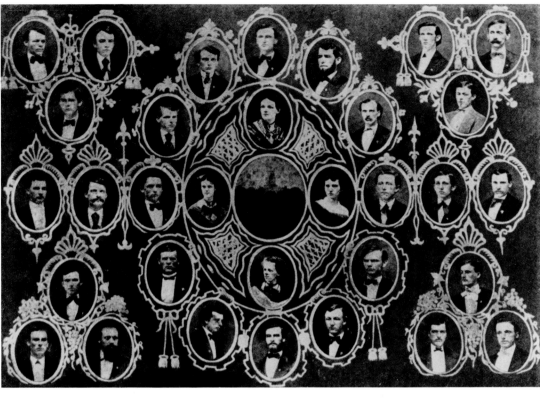

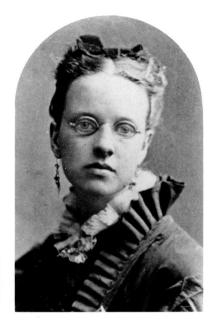

The Indiana Asbury graduating class of 1871 included the first four women graduates — Alice Allen, Laura Beswick, Bettie McReynolds Locke, and Mary Euphemia Simmons — in the center of the class composite.

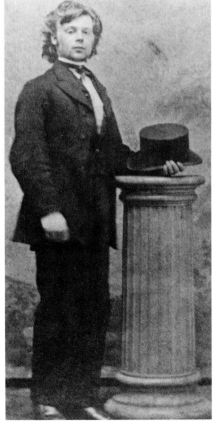

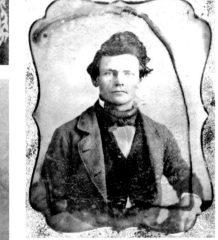

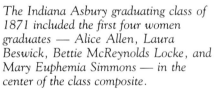

At right: An Indiana Asbury graduate from the class of 1871 poses for the 19th century version of the senior portrait.

Far right column:
Top: Fannie Towne (Stephenson) was a graduate of Indiana Asbury in 1875. She married Clarence W. Stephenson of the class of 1874, a lawyer and judge in Oklahoma. Her son, Rufus T. Stephenson, was professor of Greek at DePauw from 1914-46.
Middle: John Tarkington, class of 1852.
Bottom: Milford B. Rudsill, class of 1852.

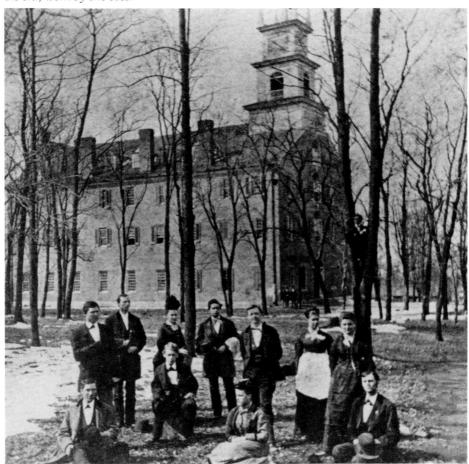

A group poses in front of the Edifice during the 1870s. Note the apron, a student symbol of the era, worn by one coed.

Thomas Bowman's presidency came to an end when the General Conference of the Methodist Episcopal Church elected him bishop on the first ballot in 1872. This able and popular administrator continued to serve Indiana Asbury and DePauw University as a member and president of the board of trustees and later as chancellor and chancellor emeritus before his death in 1914 at the ripe age of 96. A perhaps trivial sidelight is that the Bowmans had the largest presidential family, eight sons and three daughters.

A special meeting of the trustees chose as Bowman's successor Reuben Andrus, a graduate of McKendrie College and pastor of the Meridian Street Methodist Church in Indianapolis. After three years marked by financial problems resulting from the Panic of 1873 and some lack of harmony with both faculty and student body, Andrus returned to the pastoral ministry until his voice failed and he took over the management of a large farm in Howard County, Indiana.

President during the last nine years of Old Asbury's existence was Scottish-born Alexander Martin. A Methodist clergyman who had spent most of his previous career in teaching or administrative posts— most recently as first president of the new West Virginia University—he proved to be a vigorous and competent academic leader at a crucial time in the life of the university.

The faculty experienced some expansion and a good deal of turnover in these years. Asbury graduate Patterson McNutt, who had been a Civil War captain and a college president in Kansas, replaced Locke in mathematics in 1872. Another alumnus, John B. De Motte, headed the preparatory department from 1874 to 1882 before being named professor of mathematics and later professor of physics. Philip S. Baker began in 1875 as tutor in natural science and English and later became the university's first professor of chemistry.

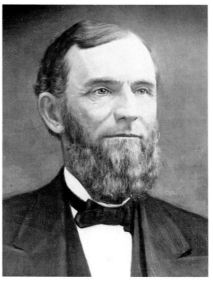

Reuben Andrus, fifth president of Indiana Asbury from 1872-75.

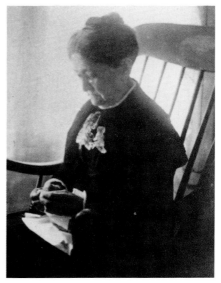

Matilda Stamper Andrus

In 1877 the board of trustees took the extraordinary step, perhaps motivated by indications of faculty-administration dissension going back to the Andrus period, of declaring all chairs but that of the president vacant, with annual elections to the faculty thereafter. Though this draconian measure was quickly rescinded, the board adopted a recommendation of a committee headed by ex-president Bowman to "restructure" the faculty. In pursuit of this policy, apparently endorsed by the president, all professors were asked to submit their resignations in 1879, and Tingley, Wiley, and Rogers were summarily dismissed. The reasons for removing these particular men, whose service to the university totalled 32, 20, and 18 years respectively, are unknown, but the episode shows clearly the insecure position of the faculty at this time and the forceful role of the trustees and president in university governance.

While President Martin's role in this affair is somewhat unclear, he took the opportunity to build a strong young faculty by filling these and other vacancies. John M. Mansfield was brought in from Iowa Wesleyan to replace Tingley but had to resign in 1883 after a mental breakdown. Most of the others appointed to chairs in this period went on to long careers at the university, including Edwin Post, who replaced Rogers in Latin, and Asbury graduate Henry B. Longden, who began as instructor in Greek and science at his alma mater in 1881. Two men who later became presidents of the institution joined the faculty in 1880 and 1882: Asbury graduate Hilary A. Gobin in Greek and theology, and John P.D. John in mathematics. In 1882 Asbury alumna Alma Holman became the first woman named to a full professorship, although Alice Downey (Porter), another alumna, had taught English, history, and mathematics in the preparatory department from 1880 to 1883. Miss Holman was followed by another

JOSEPH TINGLEY

Joseph Tingley, a graduate of Indiana Asbury in the class of 1845 who began his career at his alma mater as tutor in mathematics, held the professorship of natural science for 30 years, from 1849 to 1879. An energetic and enterprising teacher, he dabbled in photography and drawing and campaigned in the classroom and on the lecture platform against the evolutionary theories of Charles Darwin. After 1860 he also served as vice president of the university. One of his students recalled that:

Dr. Tingley was a man to be loved and honored; a man of fine presence, high quality of nature, lofty aspirations, marked dignity of character and of sweet spirit, a person of singular equipoise of faculties, with a genius for scientific investigation and inventive insight, refined in manners, a cultured Christian gentleman, with a warm heart and a deep and broad soul.

Another student, not long before being killed in battle, wrote of him in his diary for June 6, 1862: "I went out from his presence, having found him to be a real honest, sensible, civilized being."

In 1879 Tingley was forced to resign his university posts by President Alexander Martin and the board of trustees under circumstances that remain very mysterious. The faculty extended him a vote of appreciation, however, and some years later a room was named for him in East College, where his portrait hangs today. After leaving Greencastle, Tingley served as a professor at various normal schools and as a civil engineer for the Kansas City Cable Railroad. Both a brother and son graduated from Old Asbury, and Tingley himself apparently harbored little or no resentment against the institution.

Upon his death in 1892 his body was brought back to Greencastle and buried in Forest Hill Cemetery, which he had plotted south of the city limits in 1855.

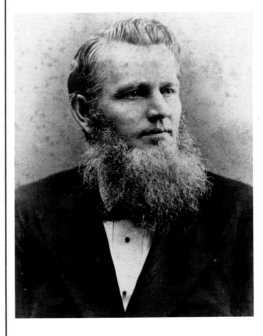

Joseph Tingley, a graduate of Indiana Asbury, was professor of Natural Science at the university from 1847-79.

woman faculty member, Julia Alice Druley, who began a long career as a teacher of piano in 1882.

Over the years the growing Indiana Asbury faculty had become more formally organized with its own secretary and treasurer, holding first weekly meetings and after 1874 bi-monthly meetings. Faculty members also served as university librarian, and from 1881 on, as registrar. Professors continued to be assigned odd jobs. In 1882 Professor De Motte was detailed to visit saloons and gambling halls in town on the lookout for errant students! Professor Alma Holman, of course, was put in charge of floral arrangements for chapel. More importantly, the position of university vice-president was always chosen from faculty ranks, John Clark Ridpath replacing the departing Tingley in that role in 1879.

President Alexander Martin was responsible for the introduction of student military training on campus in 1876. After a year of an informal program led by two former Civil War officers from Indianapolis, in the spring of 1877 the United States Army assigned Captain D.D. Wheeler as commandant of the new-ly organized military department. Upon his arrival on campus Wheeler found four companies already organized and began drilling them with arms supplied by the state of Indiana. Under his successor, Lieu-tenant William R. Hamilton, two artillery pieces were obtained, and in the summer of 1882 the Asbury cadets won honors in both artillery and infantry drill at a military encampment in Indianapolis. Atten-dance was required of freshman and sophomore males as well as senior boys in the preparatory department, but student enthusiam for the pro-gram was so high many others volunteered. From time to time one or more companies of young women were even organized. Though Cap-tain Wheeler tried to raise money for an armory building, the cadets had to be content with using the old chapel in the Edifice, which was equipped as an armory-gymnasium in 1882. Such a program of military

training, while probably owing its great popularity to the recent memories of the Civil War, also cer-tainly served the demands of a grow-ing interest in physical fitness.

A major post-Civil War change came with the expansion of the physical plant. Until the mid '70s the essential college work had been carried on in the Edifice, while preparatory classes were taught in the old county seminary building, which

had become the property of the university. Town landlords provided adequate lodging and board for students; hence little thought was given to building dormitories. In 1870 the cornerstone was laid for the building eventually called East Col-lege, but its construction was long drawn out because of the slow pace of fund raising. Some use could be made of it by 1874 and it was dedicated in 1877. Virtually all col-

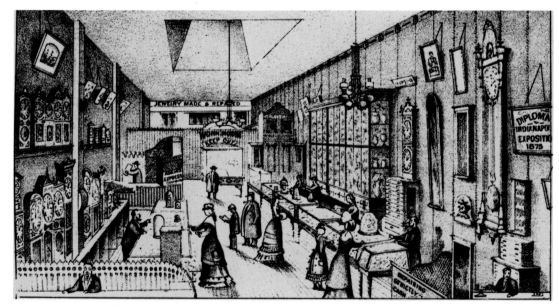

Above: Illustration from the 1879 Putnam County Atlas.

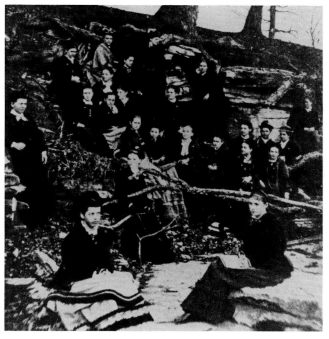

Members of Kappa Alpha Theta picnic in 1875 at Seller's Cave, immediately west of the Indiana Asbury campus.

ALEXANDER MARTIN

Alexander Martin served as the last president of Indiana Asbury from 1875 to 1884 and then five more years as president of the new DePauw University. Born in Nairn, Scotland, of which he wrote a charming description during a visit there while a delegate to the London Ecumenical Conference in 1881, he is said to have retained something of a Scottish burr in his speech to the end of his life.

His early career was varied. Brought as a boy to Jefferson County in Ohio, he spent three years as an apprentice in the tanning and leather dressing trade. He managed to work his way through Allegheny College, graduating at the head of his class in 1847. He took a position as principal of an academy in Virginia and later returned to his alma mater as professor of Greek language and literature. Ordained in the Methodist Episcopal Church, he preached and did hospital work during the Civil War, becoming the first president of West Virginia University in 1865.

Martin turned out to be one of the most effective presidents Indiana Asbury had ever had. His inaugural address revealed some of the ideas for the expansion of the educational program that were implemented in the DePauw period. Gaining the support of Washington C. DePauw, who was president of the board of trustees, Martin became the first of a new breed of university administrators who went beyond the emphasis on piety and scholarship to a new concern for efficiency and growth. His executive decisions were not always popular, as in the case of the dismissal of three senior professors in 1879. Though never adequately explained, this action made way for the introduction of younger and more scholarly faculty members. In 1883 the student paper said of him that he

possesses a sturdy, positive, Scotch character, great natural tact and ability, a broad scholarship, and unusual force; in short, in him unite all elements necessary for a successful college president.

After guiding the university through the transition from the Indiana Asbury era to the new vision of an enlarged and reinvigorated DePauw University, Martin resigned the presidency in 1889 at the age of 65. Until his death in Greencastle in 1893 he continued as professor of mental and moral philosophy, completing a total of 18 years of service to the university during one of its most momentous periods.

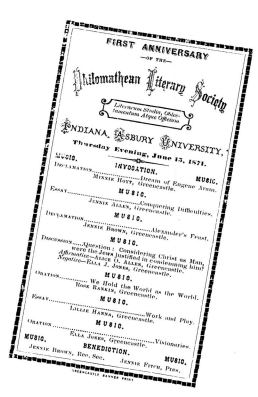

An early program of the Philomathean Literary Society (1871).

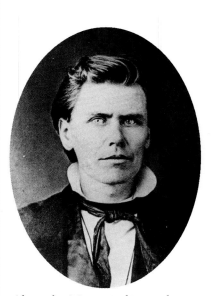

Alexander Martin in his youth, probably during the period when he taught at Allegheny College. He was president of Indiana Asbury from 1875-89.

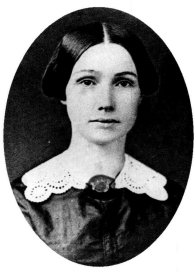

Caroline Hersey Martin, wife of the Indiana Asbury president, as a young woman.

lege classes and administrative offices were moved to East College, while the Edifice continued to house the college library, the armory, and the gymnasium. The preparatory department moved into the Edifice when the old county seminary building was razed to make room for the College Avenue Methodist Church.

In 1879, disaster struck. A fire destroyed virtually all of the Edifice except the outer walls. Plans were quickly formulated to reconstruct the old building, and within eight months it was ready for occupation once more. It had been enlarged by additions on both east and west, with the main entrance now facing east rather than north. While the renovated building lacked the peculiar charm of the old Edifice, the new West College, as it was renamed, gave good service to the university for the next 50 years.

The first foreign students were admitted in 1874, when three Brazilians were recorded in attendance, but little more is known about them. More significant was the arrival of four Japanese students in the summer of 1877. They proved to be the vanguard of a large contingent of Japanese students who studied at the university in subsequent years.

Religion remained an important element in university life in this period, with chapel prayers, church attendance, and Sunday afternoon lectures continuing to be compulsory. Both students and professors often took part in regular revival meetings. In 1847 there were 100 conversions in a 10-day period and about the same number was reported in 1881-82; however, the overall number of Asbury students had grown by then. A shift from faculty initiatives in religious observance can be seen, however, in the formation of a college chapter of the Young Men's Christian Association in 1879, not long after the first such organization appeared at Hanover College. Sponsoring such activities as Sunday school classes and noon prayer meetings as well as evangelistic meetings in nearby communities, the

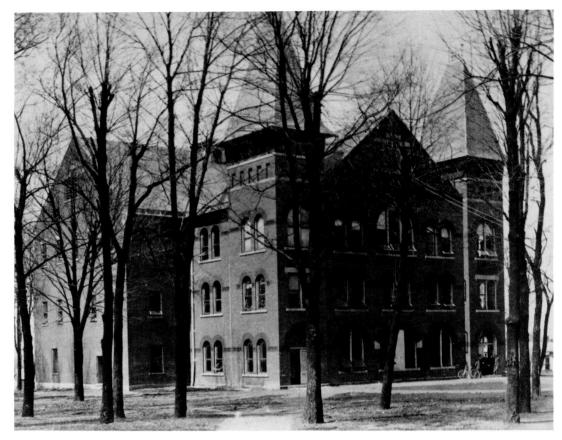

YMCA quickly became a major force on campus. Five years later women students formed their own YWCA chapter, and before long both groups were active participants in the Student Volunteer Movement, which encouraged its members to enter the foreign mission field. The late 19th century saw student piety moving into a more active outward role, as opposed to an emphasis on personal sanctification. While their zenith has now passed, these associations proved to be among the most enduring student organizations the university has known.

Organized sports were slow to develop at Indiana Asbury, though as early as 1866 a baseball team was organized which lost two games to Wabash in November of that year and May of the next, thus inaugurating the long athletic rivalry between the neighboring institutions. There is no record of another engagement until 1875, when Asbury

turned the tables, winning by a score of 39-9. By 1879 an informal program of intramurals had begun, with baseball contests between classes and later between fraternities. On May 20, 1880, the first intercollegiate football game was played in Greencastle between Asbury and Butler University, won by the latter by a margin of four touchdowns. In the afternoon a baseball game between the two institutions ended in a forfeit to Asbury by the score of 9-1 when the Butler team walked off the field for some reason after the sixth inning. In the spring of 1884 Asbury played two baseball games with Indiana University, both won by the state institution, and lost another football match to Butler in Indianapolis. The first "field day" took place on Washington's birthday in 1881, when the military department sponsored a two-mile go-as-you-please race, a wrestling match, a dumb-bell contest,

After the Edifice burned in 1879, it was quickly rebuilt with additions to the east and west sides of the building. The "new" building, called West College, faced east (while the Edifice had originally faced north).

Indiana Asbury students pose on the front steps of East College, in the 1870s. Professor Philander Wiley (man holding a cane) left Indiana Asbury in 1879.

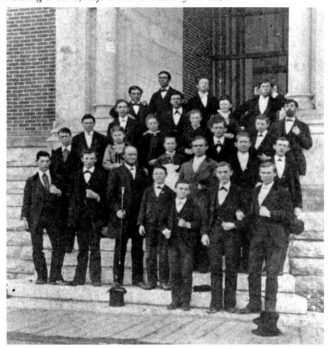

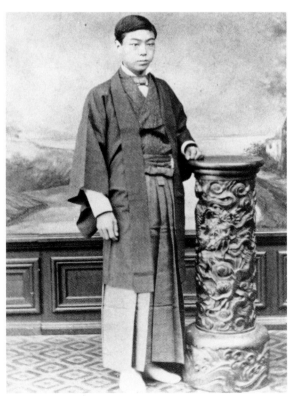

Izumy Nasu was one of the four Japanese students who came to Asbury in 1877, when he enrolled in the preparatory department. Before his death in 1885 he translated parts of the Iliad into Japanese.

THE EDIFICE FIRE

Dramatically, at midday on February 12, 1879, a fire destroyed most of the Edifice except for its outer walls. Greencastle had experienced two major town fires in 1874 and 1875, which had virtually wiped out the south and east sides of the public square and much of downtown, including many fraternity halls. Hence the city fathers had been wrestling with the problem of an adequate water supply and a fire company, which had not been yet resolved. The Edifice fire climaxed this series of disasters.

The fire began at noon, and the fire company arrived about a half hour after its discovery because of a delay in getting the horses that pulled the equipment from the livery stable. Almost immediately water from the nearest cistern was used up; the fire lasted about four hours. The students tried to rescue what they could, and thanks to Captain Wheeler and his cadets there was some system to it all, though later generations might fault the Captain for spending more effort rescuing his cannons than saving books from the library. All the explosives were removed and some of the books were salvaged, many remaining to this day in the library's Whitcomb Collection. Also saved were some specimens from the scientific cabinet and a few odd articles. A student cut the head from the large full-length painting of Bishop Roberts, which hangs reframed today in the hallway outside Meharry Hall. But most of the furniture was gone, the clock destroyed, the charming college bell known for its beautiful tone melted down. To the chagrin of later historians all the records of the preparatory department disappeared.

In two weeks the trustees met, hired an architect, and began rebuilding. The cost was $17,000 and the renamed West College was open for use by the following October. Additions were made on both east and west. The main entrance now faced east rather than north, as originally constructed. The first floor contained a gymnasium and armory with quarters for the military department; the second, an assembly hall and classrooms for the preparatory department; the third, rooms for the university library, the museum, and an alumni hall.

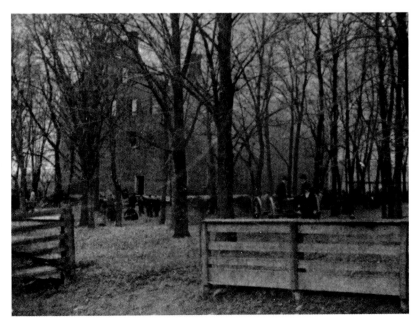

The rear of the Edifice at the time of its destruction by fire in February 1879.

GREENCASTLE

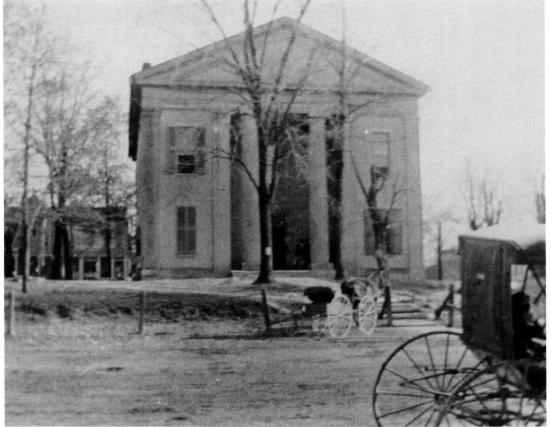

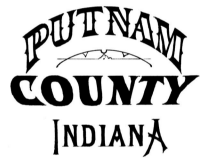

The Putnam County Courthouse, 1848-1905. The building faced the north side of the square, the major site of Greencastle business activity in the 19th century. Elisha Braman was the architect (Putnam County Historical Society).

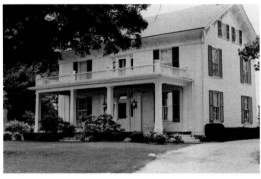

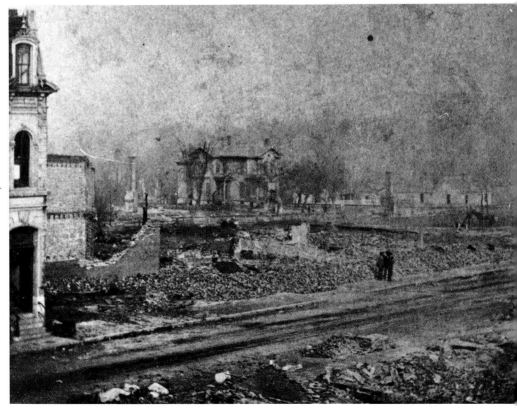

Above: The family farm home of Dr. Alexander C. Stevenson, first president of the Indiana Asbury Board of Trustees. Located on Indianapolis Road east of Greencastle, it still stands as the home of Mrs. Walter Ballard.
At right: Downtown Greencastle following the major fire on October 28, 1874. This view looks north from Washington Street; the building standing on the left is the present First Citizens Bank (Putnam County Historical Society).

Right: A map of Greencastle Township from the 1879 Putnam County Atlas. Below: Engravings like this one of a booming Greencastle business illustrated the atlas.

Bottom: Renick, Curtis and Company Carriage Factory, a leading 19th century Greencastle industry on the southwest corner of Washington and Spring streets. The current St. Paul's Catholic Church is shown at right (Putnam County Historical Society).

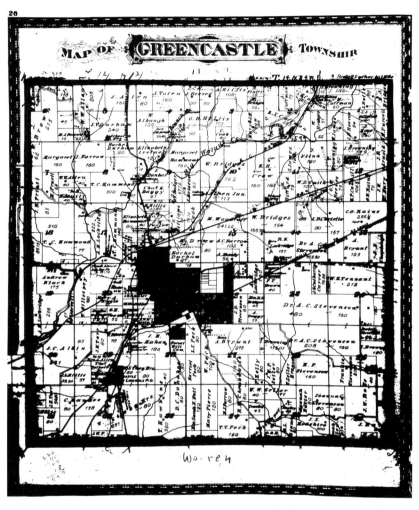

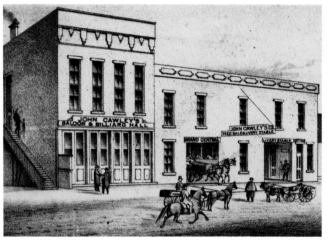

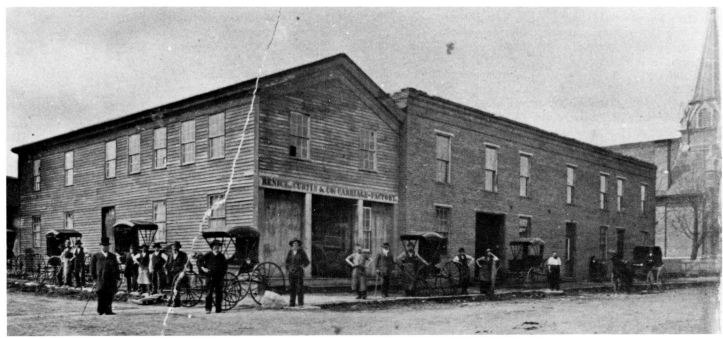

a 200-yard dash, a standing and running broad jump, a wheelbarrow race, and a tug-of-war between classes (won by the freshmen), as well as a ladies walking match. In the meantime the gymnasium in West College was equipped for use by students on a fee basis under the direction of the military department. The 1881-82 catalogue listed its equipment, which included horizontal and parallel bars, a rowing machine, a single and double trapeze, along with boxing gloves, fencing foils, and Indian clubs.

The beginning of the decline in importance of the student literary societies may be dated from the late '70s, when their intellectual and forensic aspect yielded to a more social orientation, perhaps partly as a result of the introduction of coeducation. After 1877 they sponsored three evenings a term which were devoted to music and socializing, with only "short" speeches. Regular meetings were often marked by violent political squabbles between the various fraternities and between fraternity members and "barbs," as non-fraternity men and women were labelled. The faculty finally ordered the selection of a sergeant-at-arms to keep order, even in the all-female Philomathean Society.

A major factor in the decline of the literary societies was undoubtedly the growth of the social fraternities. By 1884 slightly more than three-fourths of the male students were members of the seven fraternities on campus: Beta Theta Pi (1845), Phi Gamma Delta (1856), Sigma Chi (1859), Phi Kappa Psi (1865), Delta Kappa Epsilon (1866), Phi Delta Theta (1868), and Delta Tau Delta (1871). A smaller proportion of women belonged to the two sororities, Kappa Alpha Theta (1870) and Kappa Kappa Gamma (1875). There was also a small association of "organized barbs." The fraternities rented meeting halls, usually second or third floors of downtown Greencastle buildings, and furnished them like the literary societies, quite luxurious for that day. Here they had regular meetings, social activities,

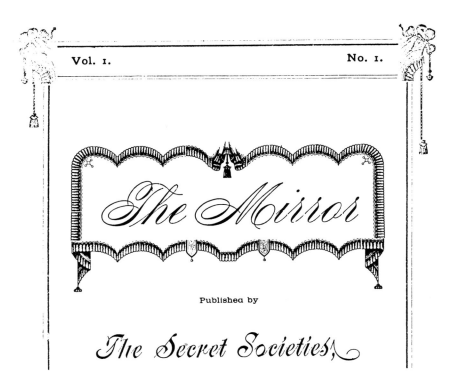

Vol. I.   No. I.

The Mirror

Published by

The Secret Societies

The Mirror *was the forerunner of the yearbook. Some 72 pages in length, it was published in 1877 by five of the seven fraternities and the two sororities, and sold for 30¢. It preceded the* Mirage *by a decade.*

receptions. On Commencement they would have reunions and special meetings.

Historian George Manhart, in his *DePauw Through the Years*, reports a Delta Kappa Epsilon activity in 1883.

About 6:30 a.m. the boys with the ladies started a "jolly drive" of about two and a half hours to Raccoon, a distance of sixteen miles. The morning was given to swings, croquet, and exploration of the surrounding country. Food was served by a Greencastle caterer, and then followed "cool rest in the leafy shades...strolls along the 'forest aisles'" and finally the "trip home more delightful, if possible, than the ride out" enjoying a royal sunset, and reaching Greencastle "long after the moon had risen, lending a tinge of romance to the scene."

The literary societies, however, played a significant role in some of the first student publications. During 1847-48 the *Platonean and Philologian* appeared as a joint enterprise of the literary societies. In 1873 the two male societies were joined by the Philomathean in reviving the *Asbury Review*, which had begun publication in 1866 but ceased to exist two years later, after a confrontation with the faculty and administration over letters and editorials criticizing the introduction of coeducation and other

matters. It halted publication again in 1876.

Then in September 1878, the university sponsored a new journal, the *Asbury Monthly*, with Professor Thomas J. Bassett as editorial director of a staff of five students. The next year the three literary societies took over its management, but by 1880 Philomathean dropped out, apparently because of dissatisfaction with the minor role assigned its members by the male editors. Despite this unfortunate disagreement and continuing conflict with the faculty and administration, the *Asbury Monthly* was relatively successful and continued publication longer than any previous paper.

Besides such legitimate campus publications, from time to time rather scurrilous sheets were put out by students, usually under the title *Bogus*. The first effort at producing a yearbook was made by five of the fraternities which issued the *Mirror* in 1877. It featured names of fraternity members, faculty, students, and trustees as well as information about the literary societies, athletics, and other campus activities. Not until 1884 was another *Mirror* issued, this time as a private enterprise of two

BETTIE LOCKE (HAMILTON)

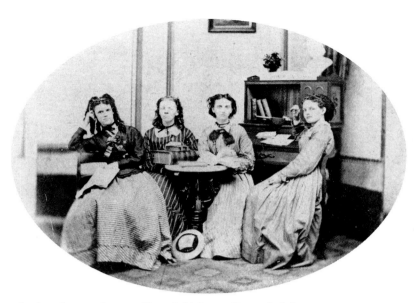

The first four coeds were (from left) Laura Beswick, Mary Simmons, Alice Allen, and Bettie Locke.

Student rooming house on South College Avenue in Greencastle of coeds Alice O. Allen and Hannah Fitch, and where Kappa Alpha Theta was founded.

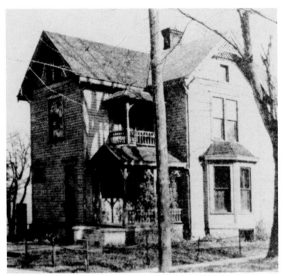

Shady Nook in Greencastle on the corner of South Locust and East Walnut was the 20th century home of Bettie Locke Hamilton, one of Indiana Asbury's first coeds and founder of Kappa Alpha Theta. Still standing, it was the site of a recent gory murder.

Bettie Locke, one of the first coeds and the chief founder of Kappa Alpha Theta, America's first college sorority, was born in 1850 in New Albany, Ind. She grew up in Brookville, where her father, Dr. John W. Locke, was president of Brookville College. He came to Greencastle in 1860 to be professor of mathematics, moved to Baldwin, Kan. in 1865 to be president of Baker University, and then returned to Indiana Asbury in 1866. In 1872 he became president of McKendrie College.

With one year in the preparatory department at Baker and tutored by her father and another college professor, Bettie Locke entered Indiana Asbury in 1867 at the age of 17. When she and the other young women entered chapel that fall, one suggested that they sit in the rear. Bettie Locke replied "What, women take a back seat? Never." So they marched to the front while the men stamped their feet. Bettie herself recalled:

We were not especially good looking. It might have been easier for us if we had been. But we were all refined, good girls from good families, and we realized somehow that we weren't going to college just for ourselves, but for all the girls who would follow after us — if we could just win out.

A male student in her own class of 1871 wrote:

...she was highly regarded as well as duly respected by the men of the class. She did good, solid work as a student and was one of the best. In daily classroom appearance she occupied a front seat, consistently ready for recitation, attentive, alert, interested in all that might be presented by professor or said by the person reciting; ready and clear of statement in her own recitition. She was of sober mien, with a pleasant manner. She was of medium height, possibly slightly below the average, not of slender bodily build, but not inclined to stoutness; her step was elastic, her bearing erect.

According to Bettie Locke's own recollections, the founding of Kappa Alpha Theta came from a suggestion made by her father after her brother's fraternity rejected her request to become a member. As a result four young women met secretly on January 27, 1870 to organize their own social fraternity, or sorority. As historian George Manhart narrated it,

Bettie Locke, standing in front of a mirror, initiated herself, and then the three other girls. The four appeared in chapel on March 14, wearing their kite-shaped pins, larger than the pins of any of the fraternities.... Thus was born what is generally considered the first college...sorority in the country.

Bettie Locke taught school for four years before marrying E.A. Hamilton, a Lawrence College graduate, in 1876. After living in Illinois and Kansas, they settled in Greencastle, where Hamilton died in 1922. Bettie Locke Hamilton lived here until her death in 1939 at the age of 89, the oldest living graduate of Indiana Asbury. Her two daughters both graduated from DePauw University.

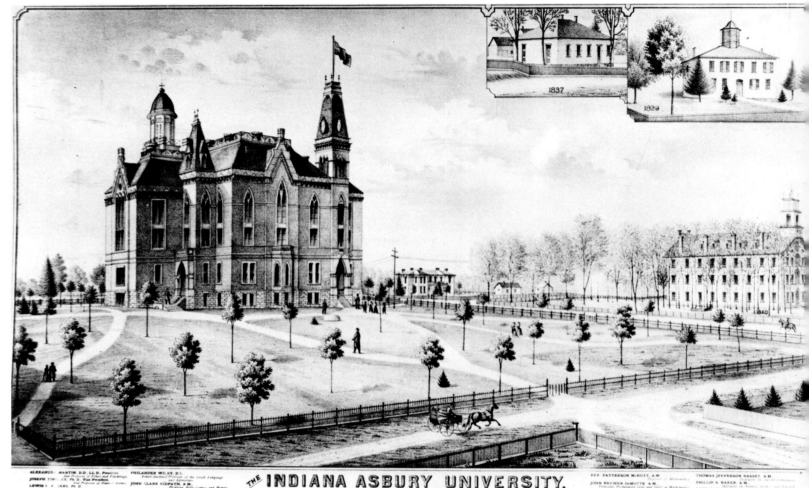

THE INDIANA ASBURY UNIVERSITY,
GREENCASTLE, IND.

members of the senior class, complete with commercial advertisements. Neither contained photographs, the main staple of such publications in a later era.

By the late '70s important innovations in teaching methods and content were appearing which foreshadowed the breakdown of the prescribed curriculum and the textbook recitations. There were more faculty lectures in certain fields, and students began to use laboratories in both the physical and biological sciences. A rudimentary chemistry laboratory was equipped in the basement of East College. The Latin department introduced an "honors" program in 1879 and the 1882-83 catalogue announced first- and

second-class honors in all departments, requiring additional work beyond the regular course of study. The university also moved in the direction of an elective system in 1879 by permitting some choice among subjects in both the Classical and Philosophical curriculum. Apparently the first departmental club was a chapter of the Indiana Scientific Association which was founded in 1875. Six years later the Social Science and Political Club appeared, choosing for its first topic of discussion the question of women's suffrage.

The fine arts had no place in the early Asbury curriculum, though informal musical organizations made their appearance from time to time. The first formal arrangements for instruction in music and art were

made in 1877. The university contracted with Emanuel Marquis, a German immigrant who operated a music store in Greencastle, to furnish instruments and offer lessons in piano and organ. It also engaged a local artist Elizabeth Adelaide Clark, to teach drawing and painting. All these were offered on an individual fee basis. By 1880 a Mozart Society and a college choir had been established. The next year Asbury graduate Minnie Langdon was authorized to teach piano and organ and registered five students. Finally, in June 1882, the trustees voted to establish a Department of Music, which opened the following January under the director of mathematics professor John P.D. John. He was assisted by Professor De Motte, who

A romanticized view of the campus in the late 1870s, as depicted in a lithograph of the period. At far right is the Edifice (before its fire); in the upper right are the buildings where Asbury's first classes and preparatory department met.

Early view of Meharry Hall in East College.

Below, Jesse Meharry, prosperous Methodist farmer from near Lafayette, who was a major donor for the construction of East College. Meharry Hall was named after his wife, Jane.

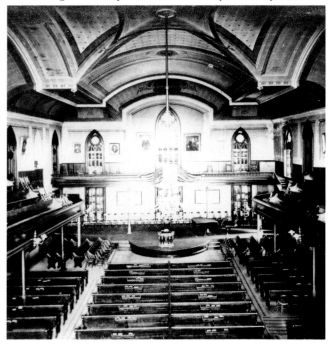

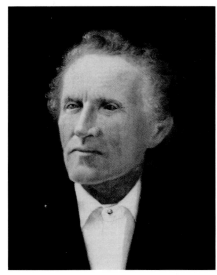

conducted the orchestra, and by Minnie Langdon and two faculty wives, Ora John and Ella Earp, teaching piano and voice.

The instruction in art offered by Elizabeth Clark had come to an end, but in September 1883, another artist, John Western, was granted permission to use a college room for a class in drawing. By the closing years of the Asbury period its educational program was slowly but surely gaining greater breadth and flexibility.

Financial troubles continued to beset the university. Having intro-

EAST COLLEGE

As early as 1861 President Thomas Bowman had proposed that Greencastle and the Indiana Methodist Conferences raise $60,000 for a new college building, but the outbreak of war forced postponement of the project. In 1865, however, Professor Tingley began contacting architects, and the next year the trustees asked Greencastle and Putnam County residents to contribute $30,000, to which they themselves would add another $30,000. A Belgian-born architect, Josse A. Vrydagh of Terre Haute, was chosen to design the structure, which was estimated to cost $80,000.

After considerable discussion the decision was made to build on the vacant lot east of the Edifice across Ephraim Street—now College Avenue—and to proceed with construction as funds became available. On October 20, 1870, the cornerstone was laid in the presence of about 3,000 people, many of whom came from a state Methodist convention in Indianapolis on eight special coaches, courtesy of the Vandalia and St. Louis Railroad. Former Professor Cyrus Nutt led in prayer, and President Bowman and pioneer Methodist preacher Aaron Wood both spoke on the occasion.

It took a year to complete the unenclosed first story. The slow pace of construction, which was dependent upon the availability of funds, was a source of general discouragement. Eventually help came in the form of a contribution of $10,000 from Jesse Meharry (who had once proposed that the university be moved to a location on his Tippecanoe County farm) and a subsequent pledge from Washington C. DePauw to complete the exterior, furnish the chapel, and landscape the grounds. By June 1874 the building was far enough along to hold Commencement ceremonies in the chapel. In the fall of 1875 college classes met for the first time in the new structure, though the basement was still unfinished and the chapel and classrooms lacked suitable furnishings. The building was officially dedicated at Commencement in 1877, with an address by President Martin and prayers by former presidents Curry and Andrus; Simpson and Bowman sent regrets. A temporary system of arc-lights was set up in the chapel for the occasion, but they proved so noisy that they were later replaced by coal-oil lamps. Five more years were to pass before the building's heating problems were finally solved and the basement completed.

The name East College came from a resolution found in the faculty minutes for 1879 offered by professor Edwin Post, who also proposed that the Edifice be called West College. The completed East College was a truly monumental structure, with its Gothic arches, French mansard roof, and Italianate columns. A large tower contained a clock donated by Greencastle citizens and a great bell given by the graduating class of 1879. In the smaller tower a refracting telescope for celestial observation was installed. Inside the main feature was the spacious second-floor Meharry Chapel, named for Jesse Meharry's wife Jane. Beside it was the president's office, the only room furnished with a fireplace. Each professor had his own classroom, and some departments had attached library rooms, while the chemistry laboratory occupied the basement. Almost everywhere, on classroom doors and in the hallways, were the names of important donors.

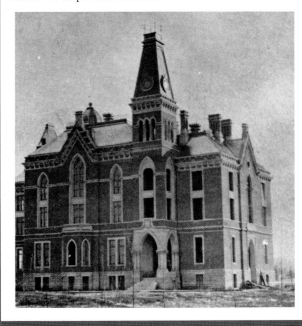

East College under construction in the late 1870s. It was dedicated at Commencement in 1877.

47

The class of 1882 poses for a group photo on the steps of East College. Professor John C. Ridpath is fourth from the right in the back row.

Below: A military unit parades on the southeast lawn in front of the newly constructed East College.

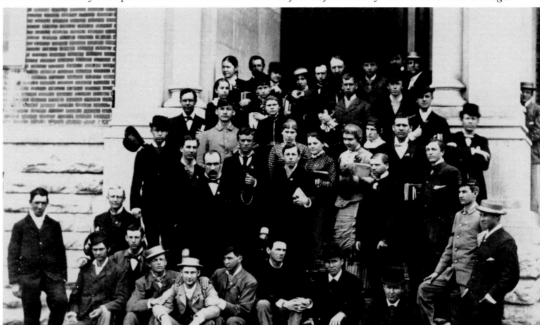

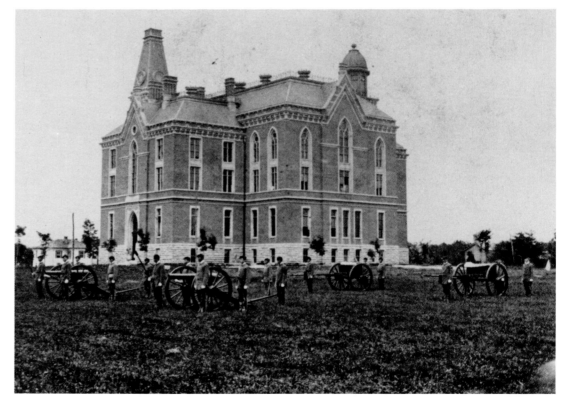

duced a system of free tuition in 1873, the trustees had nullified the many scholarships that had been sold to finance the institution in earlier years. An increased but still modest student contingency fee of $15 per year, together with income from the small endowment, proved insufficient to meet annual expenses. The depression of the 1870s meant default and decreased interest on railroad and other bonds held by the university. In 1876-77 the annual deficit was over $10,000, and it reached $11,000 in 1883-84. No wonder President Andrus was discouraged enough to resign!

Indiana Asbury came close to going under and might have closed as similar institutions were forced to do at this time, had not a financial savior appeared in the person of New Albany industrialist Washington C. DePauw, president of the board of trustees. After long and complicated negotiations between DePauw and the trustees and officers of the university, he agreed to make a substantial contribution to the institution. In return Indiana Asbury was to be renamed DePauw University and to embark upon an ambitious program of expansion of its facilities and educational programs. By May 1884 Old Asbury had passed into history, though mourned by many of its alumni. In its place arose a new and greater DePauw University, which was to carry on the old traditions while at the same time extending the scope and reach of the much-loved institution.

David Graham Phillips, who attended Indiana Asbury in its closing years, wrote a novel entitled *The Cost.* Its central character resembled his college roommate, Albert J. Beveridge, who later became a distinguished U.S. senator. In the book, the novelist penned a vivid description of his fellow students at thinly disguised "Battle Field University," which may serve as an appropriate epitaph for the institution:

Most ... came from the farms of that western country, the young men with bodies and brains that were strong but awkward. Almost all were working their way through — as were not a few of the women. They felt that life was a large, serious business impatiently waiting for them to come and attend to it in a large, serious way better than it had ever been attended to before. They studied hard; they practiced oratory and debating. Their talk was of history and philosophy, religion and politics. They slept little; they thought—or tried to think—even more than they talked.

THE FIRST JAPANESE STUDENTS

In the summer of 1877 four Japanese young men arrived in Greencastle, sent to study at the university by Asbury alumnus John Ing, who directed a mission school in Hirosaki, Japan. All were professed Christians of the samurai class with little financial resources, but willing to work. They were given rooms in the attic of the Edifice, hoisting coal for heating and cooking to their rooms by block and tackle. (They managed to escape the burning building during the great fire but without their cooking stove, which one of them explained afterwards "was too hot!") Fluent in English from their training under Ing, they also earned some of their expenses by lecturing and preaching in the neighborhood. They found general acceptance in the college and the community, and were pledged by social fraternities. A fifth Japanese arrived a little later but became ill and died in Greencastle in 1878 and was buried in Forest Hill Cemetery.

Two who attained international distinction were Sutemi Chinda and Aimaro Sato, who also became brothers-in-law when Chinda married the latter's sister after graduation. In the best Asbury oratorical tradition, Sato was making an impassioned speech in Meharry Hall advocating the election of James Garfield to the American presidency in the fall of 1880, when President Martin interrupted him to halt the proceedings as inappropriate to the occasion! Both Chinda and Sato entered the Japanese foreign service, and both served as ambassadors to the United States as well as in other important posts. Another, Izumy Nasu, translated the *Iliad* into Japanese.

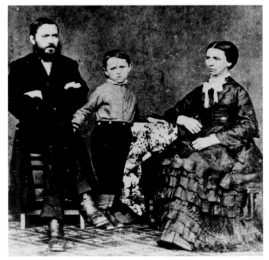

John Ing, Johnny, Lucy Hawley Ing, a missionary family in Japan in 1875. Shortly after this, Ing, an Indiana Asbury graduate, encouraged the first Japanese students to enroll in the university.

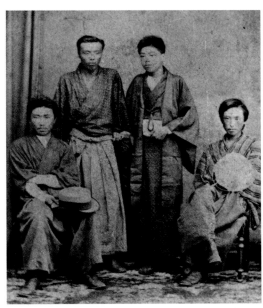

From left: Sutemi Chinda '81, Keizo Kawamura '81, Izumy Nasu '83, and Aimaro Sato '81.

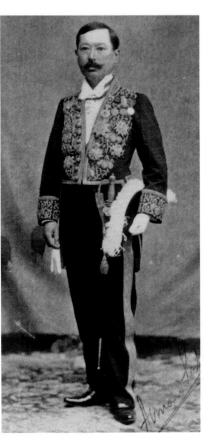

Aimaro Sato served as Japanese ambassador to Austria-Hungary and the U.S., and at the League of Nations, and in the treaty making at Portsmouth ending the Russo-Japanese war.

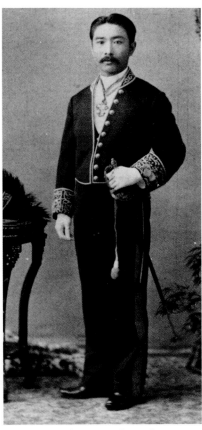

Sutemi Chinda was ambassador to Germany, the United States, and Great Britain. He served as Privy Counselor and Grand Chamberlain to the Japanese Emperor.

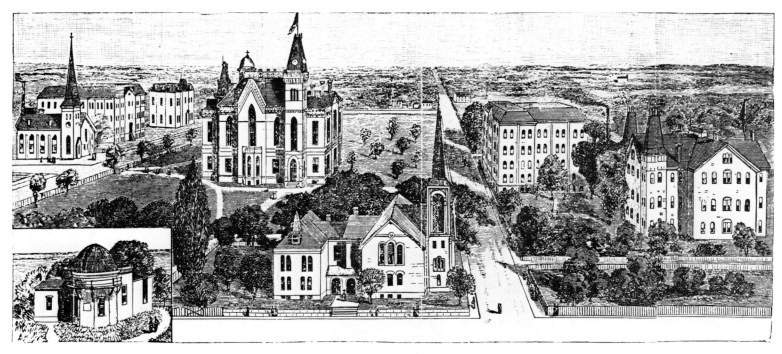

DePauw University,
GREENCASTLE, IND.

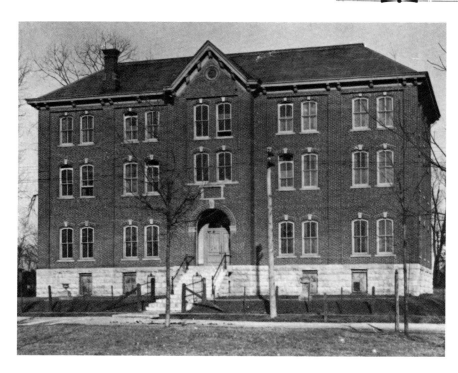

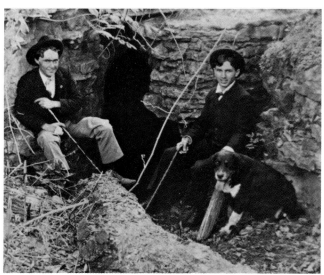

Chapter 2

DEPAUW UNIVERSITY, 1884-1918

In a mood of high optimism inspired by both the actual and prospective financial contributions of Washington C. DePauw, the reinvigorated and renamed university opened the 1884-85 academic year with elaborate – not to say grandiose – plans for an expanding educational program. A 308-page catalogue with a portrait of the benefactor himself on the front cover described them in detail. Despite brief experiments with attached law and medical schools, Indiana Asbury had been a university in name only. The new DePauw University sought to become a genuine university offering graduate and professional instruction in several fields, in addition to undergraduate and preparatory work.

Perpetuating the memory of the man for whom the institution was originally named was the Asbury College of Liberal Arts with its four divisions: the Classical Course, Philosophical Course, Scientific Course, and a new Course in Literature and Art, each with its own curriculum and baccalaureate degree. The ambitious new scheme of organization included separate schools for the three learned professions – law, medicine, and the ministry – along with special schools for music, art, pedagogy, horticulture and "mechanical industries." The School of Military Science and Tactics was also listed in the catalogue among the latter, but was in actuality simply the program of military training required of all underclassmen since 1876. Rounding out the organizational structure was the Greencastle Preparatory School, which continued the work of the preparatory department dating back to the founding of the university.

This expansive vision of a revitalized university called for a new physical plant and a more spacious campus. Citizens of Greencastle and Putnam County had already met one of Washington C. DePauw's conditions for his benefactions by raising funds to purchase large pieces of property adjacent to the old Asbury campus. DePauw himself provided the purchase price for the 120-acre Jacob Durham farm located on the northeast edge of the city, which was visualized as the potential site for an ideal campus of the future. These enlarged grounds were often described as being composed of five "parks" as follows: West Park, a grove of trees where the old Edifice, rebuilt after the 1879 fire and renamed West College, was located; Center Park, a freshly landscaped area surrounding recently completed East College; East Park, a somewhat smaller plot bounded on the north by Anderson and south by Hanna Street and containing the Locust Street Methodist Church and the university-owned home of former president Matthew Simpson; South Park, several acres of land stretching south of Hanna Street, where the most notable structure was Professor William Larrabee's former home and garden known as "Rosabower"; and finally University Park, the huge tract of rolling farmland almost a mile from the main campus with only the Durham home and some outbuildings near its western end.

As chief donor and president of the board of trustees, W.C. DePauw took a personal interest in the planning and construction of additional physical plant to house the enlarged university. He spent considerable time on the scene in Greencastle helping to direct the work. Of the five structures originally planned by the trustees' building committee chaired by DePauw, four were actually erected, and extensive additions were made to West College, including an annex to provide more space for the library. The supervising architect for all this construction was Joseph Marshall, whose designs were plain and utilitarian.

The first building to be ready for occupancy was Ladies' Hall, a three-story dormitory located in East Park on the present site of Mason Hall. It contained rooms for 80 women, a large reception hall, and dining facilities for 250 students of both sexes. This represented a striking innovation for an institution that had never before assumed responsibility for housing students. It was partly inspired by DePauw's recent European tour, during which he observed with interest the residential colleges of British universities. Across campus in West Park on the present site of Harrison Hall was erected

Photos on opposite page, clockwise from top:

The DePauw campus after the new construction of the 1880s. From left to right are Locust Street Methodist Church, Ladies' Hall, the Music School, East College, College Avenue Methodist Church, Middle College, and West College. In the distance, quite small in this picture, is McKim Observatory. On the dormitories, note the two smokestacks for heating.

Two students sit with Jack the Dog at the mouth of Sellers Cave, west of Greencastle, in 1896. Jack the Dog was a stray that appeared on campus in 1892, living on the grounds by eating handouts from dormitory back doors and hanging around downtown groceries waiting for a student to pass by. He joined all student groups, attended classes, football games and morning chapel. He was once "dognapped" by men from a neighboring institution, but was recovered by some disguised hobos from DePauw. Allegedly poisoned in 1896, he had a funeral service in Meharry Hall. The university band played while Jack was buried on the East College south lawn.

The female dormitory, later called Ladies' Hall and after 1918 Mansfield Hall, was completed in 1885 and used until it burned in 1933. On the site of the present Mason Hall, it faced Locust Street. In the right rear is a partial view of the Matthew Simpson home, at this time used for instruction in music and as a boarding hall.

Below: McKim Observatory, on the east end of University Park, was finished in 1884. It was financed by a special gift from Robert McKim of Madison, Indiana. McKim has been used for teaching astronomy for over 100 years and was recently put on the National Register of Historic Places. The original 17' diameter dome was made of iron and activated by a hand pull. In 1975 a new dome with an electric motor was installed. It is one of only 15 American observatories equipped with meridian transits.

Gentlemen's Hall, a somewhat larger, four-story structure of otherwise identical design. It was built on a field that had been used by students for baseball games. Small outbuildings with tall smokestacks located in the rear of each dormitory furnished steam heat, the first central heating system on the campus.

The university was now able to require that all women students live in Ladies' Hall, where they came under strict parietal rules and the watchful eye of a resident preceptress. An unmarried faculty member also lived in Men's Hall to act as proctor, the first of whom testified that "only once were cannon balls rolled down the stairs!" Most men apparently preferred to live out in town, however, and the dormitory was soon converted into a classroom building and renamed Middle College.

The third building planned and financed by DePauw himself was a more elaborate structure, boasting a mansard roof and a small central tower. Erected in East Park on the present site of Lucy Rowland Hall and originally intended for the schools of law and theology, it instead became Music Hall, the longtime home of the School of Music. For a year or two the School of Art also utilized its facilities before moving to nearby Simpson Hall, the former residence of President Simpson and most recently used as a university dining hall. For a time classes in law and theology were conducted in rooms in the Locust Street and College Avenue Methodist churches, both located conveniently close by and virtually integral parts of the DePauw campus.

Finally, the last construction project of this period was completed in 1885 – an observatory erected on a knoll in the eastern part of University Park. This small, two-story building, was the gift of Robert McKim of Madison, Ind. Furnished with a revolving dome made of iron, an equatorial telescope and other

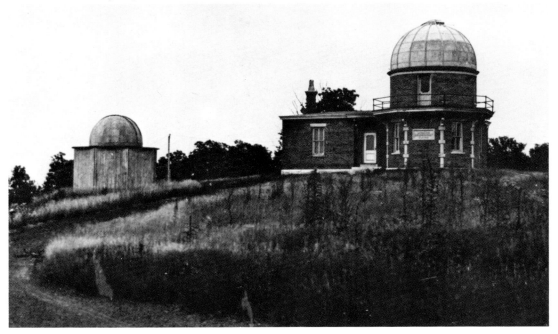

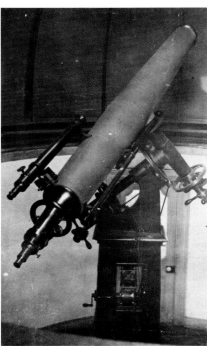

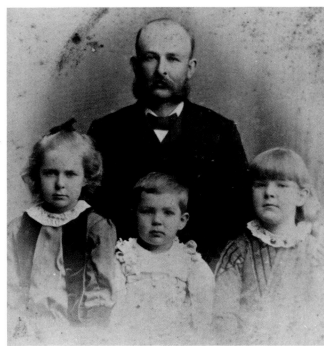

Left: The 9.53" clear aperature refracting telescope was made by Alvan Clark & Sons of Cambridge, Massachusetts, in 1885 and has been used by DePauw students for over a century. In U.S. Observatories: A Directory and Travel Guide, H. T. Kirby-Smith notes, "Since (the observatory) has not been continually modernized, it seems to furnish the outstanding example in the country of an excellent 19th century observatory.... Used for visual observing, such instruments as the Clark refractor are superior to any other telescope for views of the plants and the moon under adverse conditions of light and air pollution."

Right: Felix T. McWhirter was the first of four ever to receive a Ph.D. from DePauw — his being awarded in chemistry in 1886. He left to become a founder of the Peoples Bank and Trust Company of Indianapolis. The children in this 1888 photo are Luella, Felix M., and Ethel, all of whom went on to become DePauw graduates.

WASHINGTON C. DEPAUW

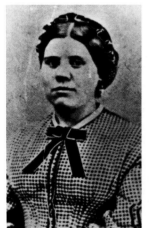

Manufacturer, entrepreneur and philanthropist Washington C. DePauw (1822-87) rescued Indiana Asbury University in 1884 from financial difficulties and the university changed its name to his.

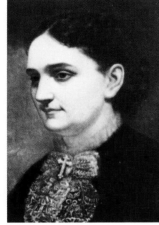

Left: Catherine Newland DePauw, second wife of Washington and mother of his two sons, Newland T. and Charles W., who both graduated from Indiana Asbury. Right: Frances Leyden DePauw, third wife of Washington C. DePauw, who provided the major donation for the construction of Florence Hall.

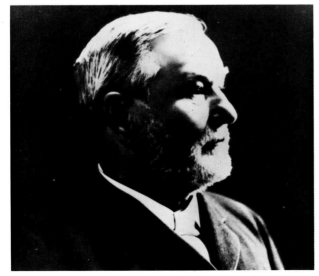

DePauw in his later years, when he became Indiana Asbury's most generous benefactor.

DePauw University's great benefactor was born in Salem, Ind. in 1822, the son of a pioneer lawyer, surveyor, and judge. His father's early death left him on his own resources at the age of 16, but the young Washington C. DePauw soon became a successful merchant, dealing in farms, flour mills, wholesale grain, and, during the Civil War, government supplies. By 1864 he was reputed to have an annual income over $300,000. His investments in banks, railroads, iron factories, a woolen mill, and a chemical plant helped to make him one of the wealthiest men in the state. Moving his headquarters to New Albany, he opened there his American Plate Glass Works, which at one time produced about two-thirds of all such products manufactured in the United States.

DePauw was also a devout Methodist and generous philanthropist who had given so much financial assistance to a New Albany female seminary that it changed its name to the DePauw College for Young Ladies. He had shown great interest in Indiana Asbury University as well, contributing funds to enable East College to be completed in the 1870s and making smaller gifts to the literary societies, the library, and student loan funds. Two sons graduated from Asbury, and he himself served on the board of trustees, becoming president in 1881.

Just before leaving for a European tour as a delegate to the Methodist Ecumenical Conference in London, DePauw drew up a will bequeathing a substantial part of his estate for the establishment of a Methodist university to be located in Indianapolis, New Albany, or perhaps Washington D.C., and named for him, just as Vanderbilt University had been created earlier. When the existence of this will came to the attention of friends of Indiana Asbury, the trustees called an informal meeting in Indianapolis to discuss the matter. In the absence of President Martin, who was at the London conference along with DePauw, Professor and Vice President John C. Ridpath attended the meeting and proposed that the New Albany industrialist be asked to divert his bequest to Indiana Asbury, which would then take the name DePauw University and greatly expand its facilities and educational programs. The trustees concurring in this plan, Ridpath and others conducted a long transatlantic correspondence with DePauw which eventuated in the latter's agreeing to make substantial contributions, provided that Indiana Methodists would raise $150,000 for the endowment and that Greencastle and Putnam County residents would secure $60,000 to purchase land for enlargement of the campus. Though the Methodists came up $30,000 short in their campaign, DePauw matched each dollar contributed with two of his own and signed documents effecting the transaction in October 1883. The board of trustees voted to approve the name change in January 1884, and on May 5 it was made official by the Putnam County Court.

As president of the board of trustees, DePauw took an active part in planning and overseeing the construction of new buildings on campus. He even had built on his own account four frame houses on Hanna Street for rent to the parents of potential students. He died suddenly while on a business trip to Chicago in 1887 but his memory lives on in the name of the university in whose rebirth he played so important a role.

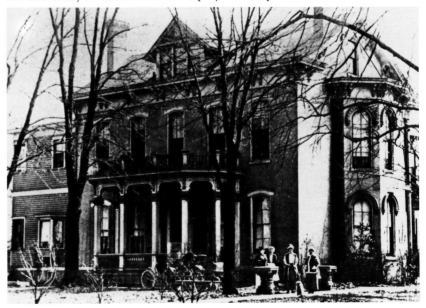

DePauw's residence on Charlestown Road in New Albany, Indiana.

GREENCASTLE

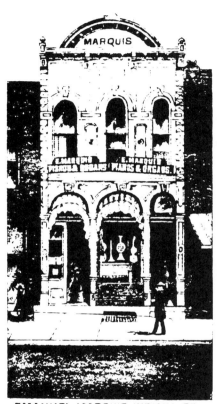

EMANUEL MARQUIS, INDIANA ST.

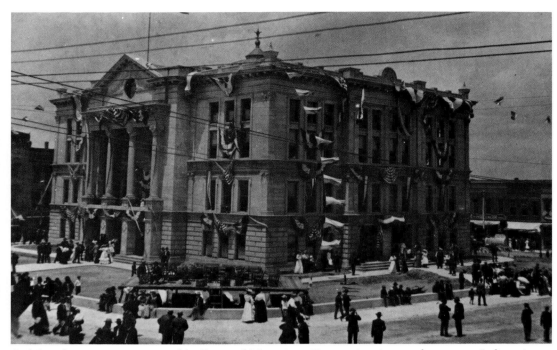

At left is the music store operated by Emanuel Marquis, a German immigrant who came to Indiana in 1852. He taught foreign language at Asbury and gave private lessons on musical instruments, and in 1877 agreed to provide instruction on piano and organ and "to furnish instruments of good quality" in a private room furnished by the university — the first recognized music instruction on campus. Above, the new Putnam County Courthouse, a Neo-classic four-story Indiana limestone building dedicated in July 1905. It remains a hub of county activity today.

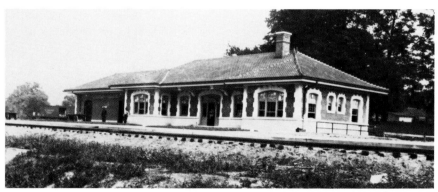

Above: The New York Central Railroad Station was built in 1908 at the north end of Madison Street. The building, which still stands but no longer offers passenger service, was Greencastle's most elegant station.

Right: The Greencastle Banner has been the city newspaper since 1852. It became the Banner Graphic in the 1960s when it merged with the Putnam County Graphic. This was the Banner's office in the 1880s. The paper's motto, "It Waves for All," has continued to the present.

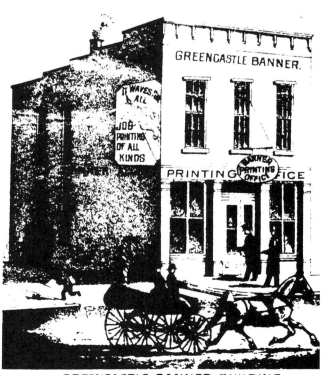

GREENCASTLE BANNER BUILDING.

The Greencastle Fire Department was ensconced in this magnificent fire hall with a bell heard throughout the downtown area about 1918. The building is still used for city offices, including the police department. In the left rear is a corner of the Post Office, finished in 1912.

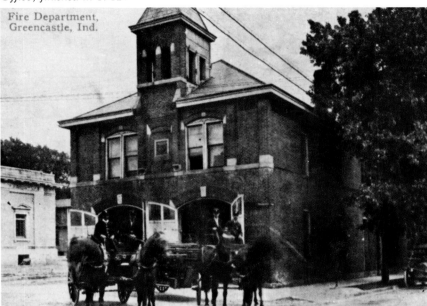

Fire Department, Greencastle, Ind.

At right, the store operated by longtime Greencastle jeweler A. R. Brattin on the south side of the square was a landmark for DePauw students in the last half of the 19th century.

A. R. BRATTIN, JEWELER, S SIDE PUBLIC SQUARE.

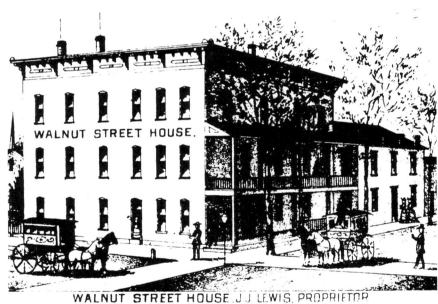

WALNUT STREET HOUSE.

WALNUT STREET HOUSE, J. J. LEWIS, PROPRIETOR

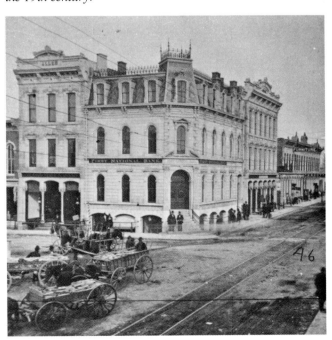

Left: This view of downtown Greencastle shows the Allens' Block and the First National Bank at Washington and Indiana streets, now remodeled into the First Citizens Bank. Note the tracks for the Greencastle Street Railway. (J. W. Hasher)

Above: The Walnut Street Hotel was a major Greencastle hotel for about a century, known to more recent generations as the Commercial Hotel. It was torn down in 1986.

astronomical equipment, it remained the solitary occupant for many years of that remote section of the expanded campus.

Like the two older structures, West and East Colleges, all the new buildings were of solid masonry construction, chiefly red brick with foundations, door and window frames, and some other details of Indiana limestone. A diversity of architectural styles was easily observable in the Gothic arches of East College, the odd-shaped turrets of West College, the high steeples of the Locust Street and College Avenue churches, and the staid utilitarian shapes of the recently erected buildings. Still the campus as a whole, with its predominant red-brick surfaces, simple geometric lines, and central focus presented a harmonious, unified scene.

For various reasons, the plan to reorganize and expand university educational programs proved over-ambitious and was never fully implemented. The Medical School, which like its Asbury predecessor was to be located in Indianapolis, failed to materialize, largely for lack of sufficient financial backing. Instruction in horticulture was offered for only one year under the direction of William H. Ragan, a Putnam County native and well-known horticulturist, who also acted as superintendent of parks. Study in mechanical industries was not offered at all. Presumably there was little student demand for either. In 1885 the School of Pedagogy was renamed the Normal School and placed in charge was Samuel Parr from the State Normal School in Terre Haute. Five years later the trustees, acting on the recom-mendation of President John, eliminated the school because of its low academic standards, despite large enrollments.

The School of Theology came into existence with perhaps the highest expectations of any of the new branches. Designed to prepare men for the Methodist ministry, it offered theological and Biblical courses for upperclass preministerial students in the Asbury College of Liberal

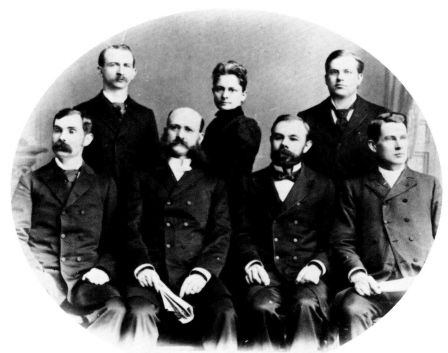

The School of Theology's class of 1893. Anna Downey had graduated from Asbury in 1877 and was the daughter of Professor Charles G. Downey. She became a minister and evangelist.

Arts, graduates of DePauw and other four-year colleges and universities, and also men with little or no background in higher education. The first dean, Shadrach L. Bowman, a cousin of former President Thomas Bowman, was succeeded in 1890 by Asbury graduate Hillary A. Gobin, who was later elevated to the DePauw presidency. Among those serving as professors were John Poucher, George L. Curtiss, and Harry L. Beals. Of the 35 bachelor of sacred theology degrees awarded by the school in its 14 years' existence, the first went to William O. Shepard, who eventually became a Methodist bishop.

The School of Law, directed first by Alexander C. Downey, former Asbury law professor and longtime university trustee, offered a two-year course of study based chiefly on lectures by local lawyers. Downey was succeeded by two Asbury graduates: Augustus L. Mason in 1890 and Charles F. Coffin in 1893.

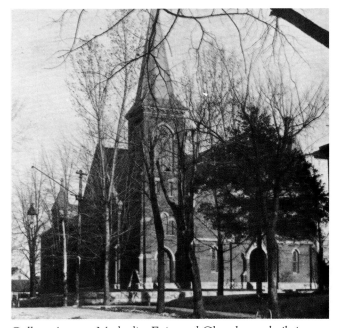

College Avenue Methodist Episcopal Church was built in 1879 on the site of the county seminary used by Asbury's preparatory department. The church stood on the southeast corner of College Avenue and Seminary Street. It merged with Locust Street Methodist Episcopal Church in 1924. Later, the building was acquired by the university, its steeple removed, and it became Speech Hall.

During the school's 10-year existence, 133 persons were granted the LL.B. degree, including three women. One of them, Merta Mitchell, became the first woman to practice law in Indiana.

Much more enduring was the School of Art, which opened in 1885 under the leadership of Dean Henry A. Mills, a landscape and portrait painter who had studied at the National Academy of Design and headed the art department at Albion College. One of the early instructors was Homer G. Davisson, who later became a minor member of the Hoosier Salon and founder of the Fort Wayne Art School. An elaborate four-year program leading to the degree of bachelor of painting was set forth in the college catalogues, but few such degrees were ever awarded. Most students were content to obtain certificates for

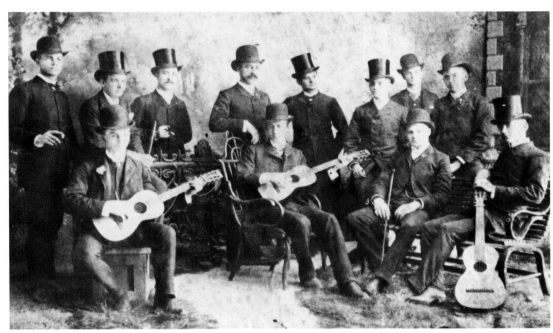

The Men's Glee Club, sometimes called the Apollo Club, around 1885.

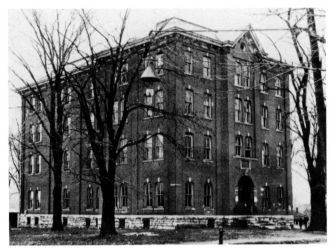

Above: Middle College was constructed in 1885 on the northwest corner of Larrabee Street and College Avenue.

Right: A handwritten letter on university letterhead signed by President Alexander Martin indicates the program for the cornerstone laying of Middle College.

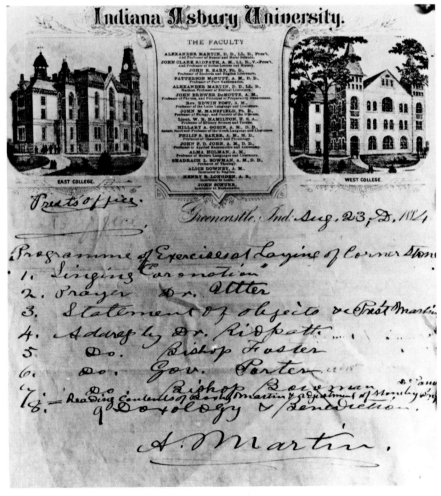

completing briefer periods of study in such fields as painting, wood carving, and repoussé, or hammered brass. Mills himself resigned in 1893 to paint landscapes in the Hudson River valley, but the school continued on for two more decades.

Longest-lasting of all the new institutions was the School of Music, which evolved from a small department begun in 1882 by Professor of Mathematics John P.D. John. Dean for the first 10 years was James H. Howe, a graduate of the College of Music of Boston University, who had been teaching at the New England Conservatory of Music. Among the early instructors were pianist Julia Druley, who remained on the faculty for 50 years; Greencastle violinist Rosa A. Marquis; and cellist Adolph Schellschmidt. There were programs for three classes of students: candidates for the new degree of Bachelor of Music; liberal arts students seeking the Bachelor of Literature degree; and others who simply wished to "pursue music to a greater or lesser extent," as the catalogue stated.

Dean Howe set about energetically to organize the musical activities on campus in a more systematic fashion, helping to form a host of new and old choral groups, instrumental ensembles, and an orchestra. Beginning with the 1885 commencement he arranged an annual musical festival, with large choirs presenting such works as Haydn's *Creation* or Handel's *Messiah*. He was disappointed, however, when the faculty refused permission to stage the *Mikado* – Methodists were not yet ready for opera!

In the fall of 1885 Dean Howe encouraged a group of women students enrolled in the School of Music, not then admitted into any of the existing social fraternities, to establish their own sorority, Alpha Chi Omega. Eventually accepting liberal arts students as well, this organization became the Alpha chapter of a new national social fraternity, the second such founded at DePauw.

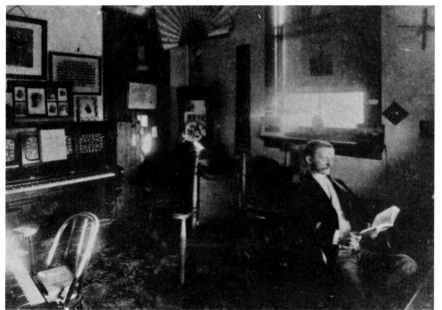

James Hamilton Howe is shown in his office in the School of Music, where he was dean from 1884-94. He inaugurated many music activities and recitals, but was checked by the faculty when his exuberance included preparing the light opera Mikado.

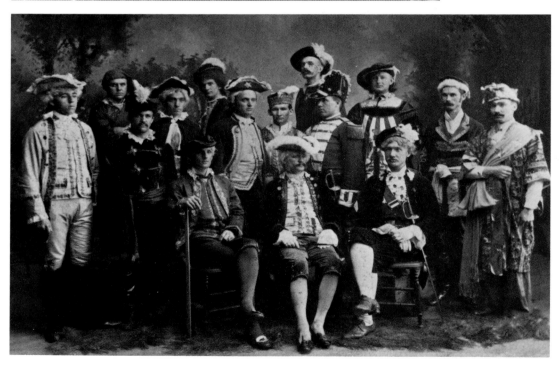

A music school group around 1890. Dean James H. Howe is seated in the center.

Asbury alumnus Thomas Jefferson Bassett directed the Greencastle Preparatory School, successor to the preparatory department which had existed since the founding of Indiana Asbury in 1837. Originally the school was projected as only one of a network of similar institutions intended to feed into the collegiate branches of DePauw University, but the others never materialized. The Preparatory School flourished for many years before the public high school movement reached full tide in Indiana. Its rigorous three-year course of study comprised Greek, Latin, mathematics, English, history,

Music Hall, erected in 1884 on the northeast corner of Locust and Hanna streets, faced Locust. In 1927 it was moved to the southwest corner. The building served as headquarters for the Music School for 92 years, until it was torn down in 1976.

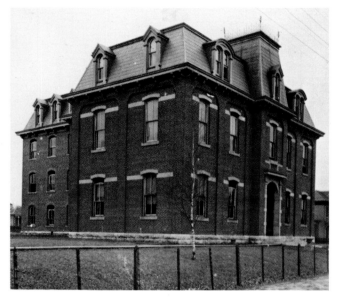

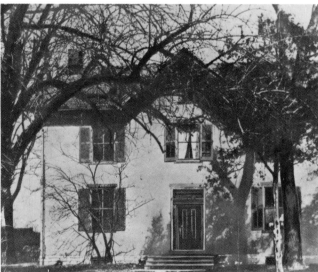

The Simpson home housed the School of Art from 1887-1913.

MEMOIRS OF JOSEPH E. NEFF

With our trunk packed we boarded the train at LaFontaine for Greencastle on a hot September day in 1884. Father went with us. We changed cars in the bewildering city of Indianapolis and reached Greencastle in mid-afternoon. When we landed from the Vandalia train the job was to find our way to the college. A horse-drawn street car was leaving and it was a reasonable conclusion that we should follow in its track. That was somewhat roundabout and we were sweaty and dusty when at last we reached the public square. The sidewalks were well occupied with farmers, it being a Saturday afternoon ... Few if any students had yet arrived. In a book store we were given directions to the Campus. We found the office that was open for matriculation. Father explained that he wanted his sons to have a good room and good boarding place. A local student who was present volunteered to conduct us. He took us to the home of widow McGee who boarded students and had a room to rent. We did not know it but it was the most select and expensive boarding place among students. The other boarders turned out to be Seniors and Juniors. One was Albert J. Beveridge and another James Watson. This was the year of the Cleveland-Blaine campaign and both these youngsters were making campaign speeches for Blaine. They did not return to college till after the election...

By the end of the year two dormitories built by DePauw were furnished and we took a room in the men's and boarded at the women's which furnished meals for both boys and girls. During our years we had rooms in various private homes but always boarded at this dormitory.

Since we had no high school education we were enrolled in junior preparatory .... A strong class spirit soon developed and there was much healthy social intercourse. The boys outnumbered the girls almost two to one. With the middle preps, drill by the Cadet Corps was compulsory. I was especially interested and continued active up to and through my Junior college year and ending up as Captain of one of the four companies and Commander of an artillery squad ....

Greek letter fraternities and sororities had a big play in student life. Prep students were not eligible but the fraternity men kept a close eye on preps with a view of capturing the better students or more prominent ones by pledging them. So we preps were much interested in these fraternities. In our middle prep year four of us were pledged to the Phi Delta Theta fraternity. While in prep we looked upon the graduating seniors as mounted atop of Mt. Olympus and to reach it seemed a long hard steep climb ....

The Pettibone Uniform Manufacturing Company of Cincinnati furnished most of the cadet uniforms and had a student agent at the college. At the beginning of my junior year this agency became vacant. I went after it and got it. Commissions as such agent were remunerative. I bought a bicycle – a high front wheel and a small rear wheel. It took some skill to mount and ride it. On my first attempt I took a header and fractured a bone in my right wrist. This wheel gave me much prominence. There were only two others on the campus. My income provided indulgences very few other students possess ....

I was a livery stable's best customer. One stable had a handsome four-passenger open runabout. I would have shafts attached and hitch the horses tandem, drive up on the campus, load up with girls and sweep about the campus and city streets and sometimes long runs in the country. This was a great treat for the girls. The tables at the dormitory had seats for twelve. Several of them were organized. Ours was. We adopted a Greek name Epsilon Beta Chi and when a member dropped out and a successor elected we had an initiation. Tennis was popular those days and several pairs of boys would take campus space and build courts. A Mr. Herman Ritter and I had one. A small sapling interfered with our space. At one or two o'clock at night that obstruction disappeared. All the men had girl partners and there were tournaments ....

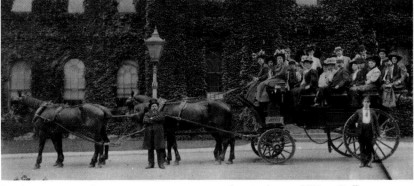

Students prepare for an excursion in an omnibus in front of West College. (Indiana State Library)

59

and natural science, taught by its own corps of instructors, often including recent graduates of DePauw. Preparatory students participated in military drill along with college students, fielded athletic teams, and even published their own school paper from time to time.

Finally, the university proposed to inaugurate post-graduate work leading to both the M.A. and the Ph.D. degrees. Various honorary degrees had long been awarded, as well as the M.A. *in cursu* to graduates who presented evidence after three years of their intellectual growth and good moral character. Under the new program five Ph.D.s were actually conferred between 1886 and 1893 before the faculty wisely voted to halt the practice on the grounds of inadequate resources. The M.A. *in cursu* was itself eliminated by 1894, but the university maintained a modest program of earned master's degrees that has continued to the present time.

Vice President John Clark Ridpath, who had been one of those most responsible for obtaining the assistance of W.C. DePauw and for planning the reorganization of the university, resigned suddenly in 1885 at the age of 45. Already the author of several textbooks, he gave up his university post in order to devote himself fully to literary endeavors. Working in his home on East Washington Street – now the Bittles and Hurt Funeral Home – he set out upon a prolific publishing career that made his name a household word in many parts of the country and Greencastle a minor Hoosier literary center. Writing not for a scholarly audience but for "the practical man of the shop, counter, and the plow," he produced scores of volumes bearing such titles as *Popular History of the United States, Cyclopaedia of University History,* and *Great Races of Mankind.* They were sold by subscription in small towns and villages by travelling book agents such as young Huey Long, who peddled them in rural Louisiana to earn money for his education.

In 1896 Ridpath interrupted his literary labors briefly to run for

Congress from his home district on the Populist-Democratic fusion ticket. Losing the election, he moved to Boston to edit a muckraking journal, *The Arena,* and two years later went to New York to edit the literary department of his publisher. He died there in 1900. A contemporary journalist described the former DePauw professor and administrator as not only a "popular historian ... but also a profound thinker, a man of deep convictions, and a political and social reformer of absolute courage."

One of Ridpath's former students, Jesse W. Weik, was a Greencastle native who added to the literary luster of his hometown at this time by gathering materials from Abraham Lincoln's onetime law partner, William Herndon, and collaborating with him in publishing *Herndon's Lincoln* in 1888. Written largely in Greencastle while Herndon was visiting Weik in August 1887, the volume was the first to describe in detail Lincoln's early life in Indiana and Illinois. After Herndon's death Weik kept the manuscripts in his Greencastle home, where he utilized them in several articles and another book on Lincoln and made them available to Lincoln biographers such as his fellow Asbury alumnus Albert J. Beveridge and Ida Tarbell.

Alexander Martin, whose presidential term spanned the last decade of Indiana Asbury and the opening years of DePauw University, resigned his administrative duties in 1889 but remained professor of mental and moral philosophy for another five years. He had been a strong executive who had worked closely with Washington C. DePauw in successfully effecting the transition to the new, expanded university. But the times called for a different, more modern type of leader.

The trustees chose as his successor Professor of Mathematics John P.D. John, who had also been vice president since 1885. The first member of the faculty to be elevated to the presidency, John was immensely popular with students, as

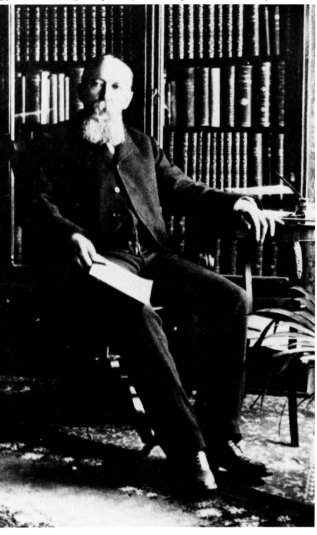

John Clark Ridpath, professor at Indiana Asbury from 1869-85, taught English literature, normal instruction, belles lettres, history and political philosophy. He was vice president from 1879-85 and was instrumental in acquiring the DePauw gift and making the plans for the expanded university.

evidenced by a petition signed by a majority of them and sent to the trustees urging his appointment. Despite his lack of academic credentials – he had no earned degree – he was a man of wide-ranging intellectual prowess. He was familiar with the ideas of such educational reformers as Charles W. Eliot of Harvard and Daniel C. Gilman of Johns Hopkins and had thought deeply about the aims and methods of higher education. His relatively short tenure as DePauw's president was to witness significant change in the university's academic program as part of the general movement that was transforming

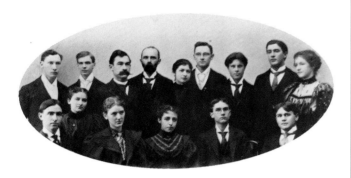

Professor Henry B. Longden (with the beard) and the DePauw German Club around 1895.

American colleges and universities of that time from rather narrow, pedantic seminaries into more open, intellectually freer institutions of learning.

President John set forth his ideas in an inaugural address entitled "The New Education," perhaps the most important ever delivered at the university. Turning away from the rigidities of the prescribed curriculum, he advocated a wider choice of elective studies to provide "freedom for the pupil, freedom for the teacher, and freedom in the subject." No iconoclast, John was not ready to abandon completely the older emphasis on classical languages and mathematics; instead he opted for broadening the variety of disciplines through which students might experience the "process" of intellectual growth.

The university had already begun to move cautiously in the direction of electives, especially for students in their junior and senior years. Now the movement was accelerated, culminating in a program based on a core of basic requirements with the rest of the curriculum more or less open to free choice. To provide greater intellectual depth in particular fields, students were required to elect "majors" and "minors" for the first time. Depending upon the choice of major and of a classical or modern foreign language, graduates were awarded the degree of bachelor of arts, bachelor of philosophy, or bachelor of science. The bachelor of literature degree, which accepted credits in music and art, was eliminated.

The departmental structure of the university also expanded to reflect

JOHN P.D. JOHN

The first of only two presidents to be appointed from the teaching faculty, John Price Durbin John was one of DePauw's most popular teachers and administrators. He was born in southeastern Indiana and attended Brookville College but did not graduate. Later he went back as first professor and then president of that institution before moving on to become president of Moore's Hill College – now the University of Evansville. After further study in Europe he was invited to join Indiana Asbury in 1882 as professor of Hebrew and adjunct professor of Latin. The largely self-taught John showed his versatility, however, by instead accepting the chair of applied mathematics and astronomy. In addition he was briefly director of the department of music and conductor of the college chorus. His wife Orra John taught piano and voice from 1883 to 1890, making them the first married couple on the university faculty.

John was the favored candidate of the student body for the presidency when Alexander Martin resigned in 1889, as evidenced by a petition to the trustees signed by 800 undergraduates. When the news reached Greencastle of his election to that post on December 12, the college bell was rung for three hours and a holiday from classes declared. A large throng went to the Vandalia railroad station to meet the new president, the cadets marching in full uniform with the Greencastle Brass Band. Students pulled his carriage to East College for speeches and general festivities in Meharry Hall.

While John played a major role in creating an elective system at DePauw replacing the rigid classical curriculum as part of his advocacy of the "New Education," he was less successful as an administrator dealing with the board of trustees during a time of financial retrenchment. In 1895, after a bungled attempt by the board to name a chancellor in charge of financial affairs to share authority with John, the latter submitted his resignation as president. Although there seemed to be considerable support for the embattled president among students, faculty, and the whole university constituency, the resignation was accepted. John continued to reside in Greencastle for the remaining 21 years of his life, earning a living as a visiting Methodist preacher and on the traveling lecturer circuit. As a main opponent of the famed agnostic orator Robert Ingersoll, he delivered a lecture entitled "Did Man make God, or did God make Man?" 500 times in three years. He was also in demand for his stereopticon-slide talks on his travels in Alaska and the Yukon. He is chiefly remembered at DePauw for the professorship of mathematics endowed in his name.

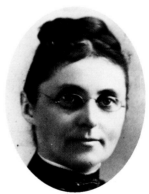

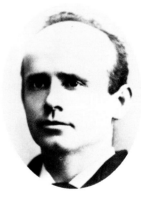

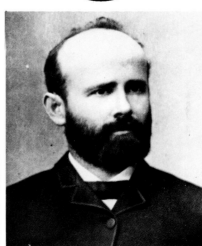

Top left: Orra P. John, wife of President John, joined the faculty from 1883-90 as a voice and piano teacher. The Johns were one of the first couples who both held teaching appointments at the university.
Above: President John Price Durbin John came to Indiana Asbury in 1882. He was professor of mathematics about the time this picture was made.
Left: John served as president from 1889-95. Most popular and innovative as an administrator, he was forced to make serious reductions as a consequence of the financial panic of 1893.

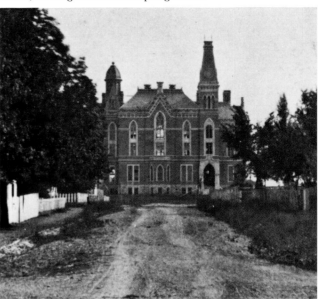

the widening body of knowledge and more specialized subjects in the modern curriculum. Latin and Greek remained important departments, but modern languages were divided into departments of German and the Romance languages. Separate departments emerged for oratory and for rhetoric and English literature. Mental and moral philosophy became simply philosophy, and Biblical literature was renamed the English Bible, which was required of all students. Joining chemistry and physics as independent departments were botany and zoology, formerly united in the department of biology. Astronomy was separated from mathematics and history from political science, though the latter still included work in sociology and economics.

Concomitant with these changes was the tendency toward increasing professionalization and specialization of the faculty. The first DePauw professors with earned doctorates were Wilbur V. Brown in mathematics and Oliver P. Jenkins in biology. Both received their degrees in the late 1880s, Brown from Stevens Institute and Jenkins from Indiana University. President John added three more men with Ph.D.s – Eugene W. Manning in Romance languages, Lucien M. Underwood in botany, and Andrew Stephenson in history – as well as several others with advanced training short of the doctorate. Among the latter were Joseph P. Naylor in physics, William E. Smyser in English, and Jesse F. Brumbaugh in rhetoric.

There was also a continuing secularization of the faculty. Except for the president himself and holders of the chairs in philosophy and Bible, DePauw professors were no longer expected to be ordained clergymen, though most were presumably Methodist church-goers. After long student agitation against the compulsory Sunday afternoon faculty lectures, the John administration first reduced their frequency and finally eliminated them altogether.

A revolution in teaching methods took place at this time with the disappearance of the daily class recitations, so long a fixture in American college education. Their place was taken by classroom lectures, laboratory exercises, and library research assignments. Professors Edwin Post in Latin, James R. Weaver in political science, and Andrew Stephenson in history conducted German-style seminars for advanced students, and the latter two established departmental library-laboratories funded by student fees. The chemistry laboratory in the East College basement and the physics and biological laboratories in Middle College began to be furnished with increased amounts of equipment, enabling

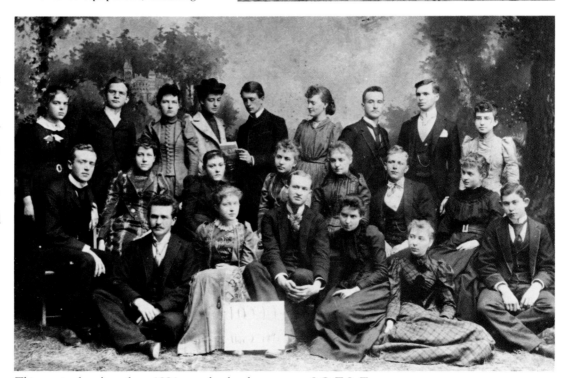

This group of students from 1891 went by the obscure name I.O.T.L.T.

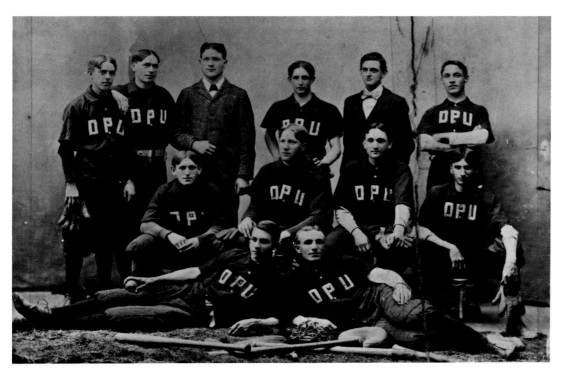

The 1896 DePauw baseball team is shown here with the manager and umpire.

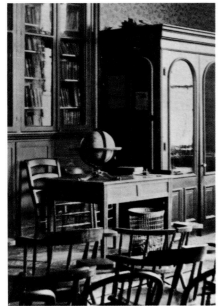

Richard Biddle Hall of Mathematics on the first floor of East College, as it looked in 1895. It is now used as the faculty lounge and reception room.

them to play a much larger role in education in the natural sciences.

Organized sports were beginning to find an accepted place in the early DePauw years, though with little official encouragement. In 1890 students organized an athletic association with the help of a few faculty members to support varsity teams in baseball and football. At the same time DePauw joined with Indiana, Purdue, Butler, Wabash, and Rose Polytechnic to form the Indiana Intercollegiate Athletic Association under the auspices of the state YMCA. The next year the faculty voted strict eligibility rules for participating athletes and appointed a special committee to oversee intercollegiate competition.

At first the lack of a suitable playing field hampered all such efforts. Banned from the campus proper by the administration, varsity teams resorted to a rough field west of the city beyond the Monon

Railroad tracks. After a long campaign by students and faculty to obtain better facilities closer to campus, land was purchased on West Hanna Street in 1895 for McKeen Field, named for the president of the Vandalia Railroad, W.R. McKeen, who made the first major contribution to the project. It was formally dedicated in October of that year with a football victory over Indiana University.

Basketball was introduced in the mid-1890s as a "mild form of work for the winter months," as the college catalogue put it, and was apparently played chiefly by coeds at first. The lack of adequate indoor court facilities slowed its development as an intercollegiate sport. Annual field days were held from an early period and time records kept for DePauw athletes as early as 1893. In that year the first black athlete at DePauw, James U. Turner, held the college record for both the 100 and 220 yard dash. Both men and women played tennis on improvised grass courts on the East College lawn.

The DePauw chapter of Phi Beta Kappa, the national honorary society for scholarship founded at the College of William and Mary in 1776, was granted a charter in 1889, largely through the efforts of Dean Shadrach Bowman of the School of Theology. Bowman, a Phi Beta Kappa from Dickinson College, organized DePauw's Indiana Alpha chapter in his classroom in Middle College with the assistance of two other initiates from Terre Haute.

The first members elected were Professors James R. Weaver, William F. Swahlen, and George L. Curtiss, former Professor John C. Ridpath, local Methodist minister Salem B. Town, and two DePauw trustees. Within a few days nine more were added: President John P.D. John, ex-President Thomas Bowman, the two sons of Washington C. DePauw, and five trustees. In June Professors Edwin Post and Philip S. Baker were elected along with two additional trustees. Only then did the chapter get around to its original purpose by initiating five men of the

SPORTS

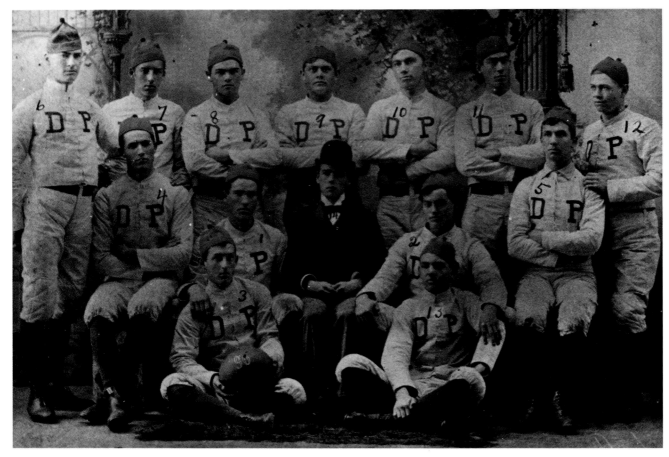

The first DePauw football team was organized in 1889 by Guy Morrison Walker, seated in the second row, second from the left. The team wore stocking caps instead of helmets.

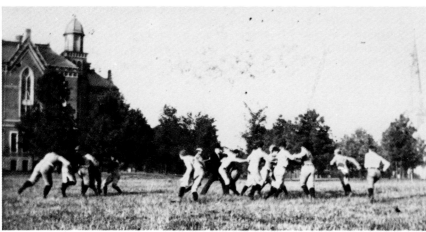

An early scrimmage takes place on the East College lawn.

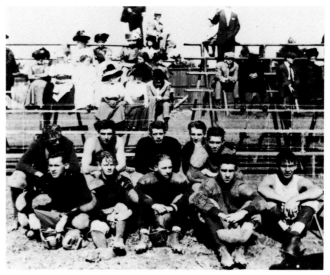

In time, DePauw created suitable athletic facilities. Here, spectators sit behind the players along the sidelines during a football game on McKeen Field about 1910.

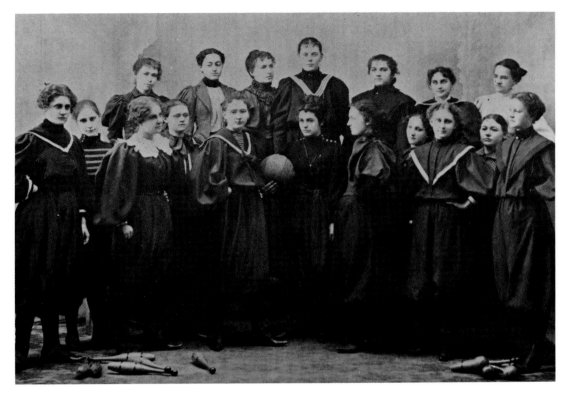

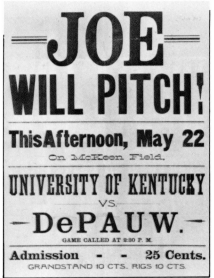

JOE WILL PITCH!

This Afternoon, May 22

On McKeen Field.

UNIVERSITY OF KENTUCKY
VS.
— DePAUW. —

GAME CALLED AT 2:30 P. M.

Admission - - 25 Cents.

GRANDSTAND 10 CTS. RIGS 10 CTS.

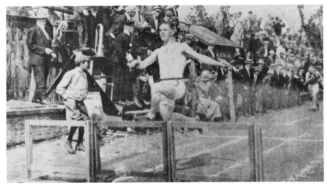

A DePauw hurdler in an intercollegiate track meet in 1914.

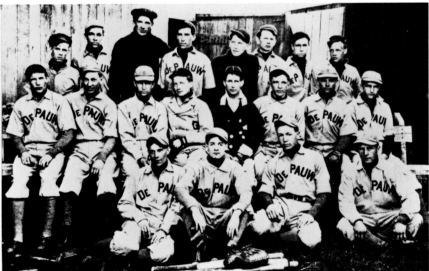

The 1905 baseball team

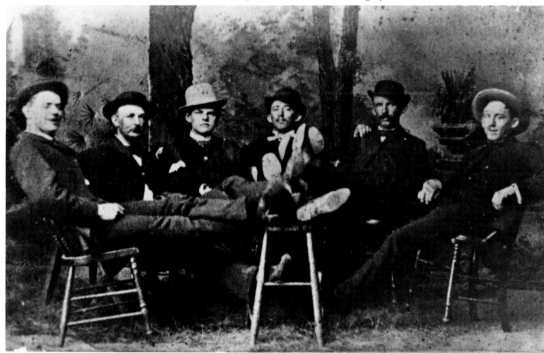

senior class. (Women were not elected to membership until 1898, but at the chapter's 50th anniversary in 1939 amends were made by belatedly adding the names of all surviving female graduates who would have been eligible between the founding and 1897.)

Weaver served as president and Swahlen as vice president for the first 20 years. Most meetings were held during this time at the Weaver home on South College Avenue. Tradition has it that strawberries were always served. In its early years the DePauw chapter of Phi Beta Kappa elected distinguished former students such as Governor Albert G. Porter and Senator Albert J. Beveridge, as well as Hoosier luminaries who had never attended the institution, including James Whitcomb Riley and Edward Eggleston.

In his drive to modernize the university and raise academic standards, President John closed the Normal School with its large number of below-college level pupils and sought in vain to acquire improved library and laboratory facilities. The only addition to the physical plant during his tenure was Florence Hall, a dormitory erected in South Park on the present site of Bishop Roberts Hall in 1891, through the generosity of Washington C. DePauw's widow and daughter. Designed primarily for the use of students in the School of Theology, it later became a general rooming and dining hall for men.

DePauw's death in 1887 and subsequent litigation of his will along with the reduction in the value of the estate's assets caused by the Panic of 1893 brought about lowered estimates of the financial assistance the university might expect to receive from that quarter. In fact, by the time the estate was settled in 1895, the total amount of the DePauw benefactions, including gifts from other members of the family, came to approximately $300,000, far below the anticipated $1 million, but still a munificent sum for that time.

At any rate the John administration faced a financial crisis less than a decade after the refounding of the institution as DePauw University. Faculty salaries were reduced and educational programs reorganized. When Dean Mills resigned from his post in the Art School in 1893 and Dean Howe from the School of Music the following year, the administration decided to economize by appointing Professor Belle Mansfield to head both institutions, receiving a portion of the proceeds from student fees in lieu of salary. Mansfield, who had been preceptress of Ladies Hall as well as professor of both history and aesthetics at DePauw, brought the two schools to a measure of prosperity by efficient management. The Law School, however, experiencing falling enrollments, was allowed to expire by the spring of 1895, while the School of Theology limped on for another few years.

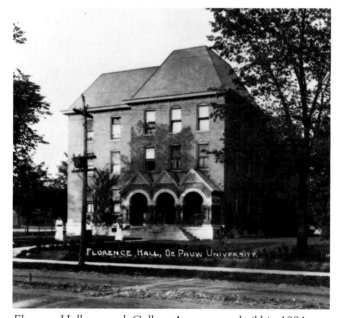

Florence Hall on south College Avenue was build in 1891 as a rooming and boarding dormitory for the theological students. It was a gift of Mrs. Frances DePauw, widow of the university benefactor, and named for their daughter. After 65 years of use as both a men's and women's dormitory, it was demolished to make room for Roberts Hall.

One of the early customs at DePauw was for each class to adopt a special form of clothing, usually a hat. Pictured here are men of Sigma Chi posing for a formal picture in their top hats.

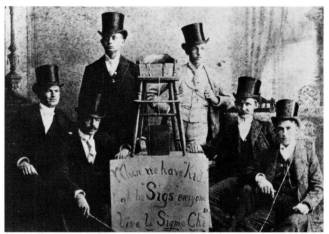

In the crisis President John found little support among the trustees, divided and virtually leaderless since W.C DePauw's death. The aging Bishop Bowman, who served as both university chancellor and president of the board of trustees, proved unable to control the infighting among various factions, such as the one led by Evansville businessman J.D. Iglehart. Finally, discontent with John's leadership rose to the point where an attempt was made to replace Bowman with an active chancellor charged with managing the university's financial affairs.

The person chosen for this task was Charles N. Sims, an Asbury alumnus and prominent Methodist minister who as chancellor of Syracuse University had rescued that institution from financial distress. After Sims and John had tried but failed to reach agreement on a plan to share administrative responsibilities, John retaining the educational initiative and Sims handling the financial side, the latter withdrew his name from consideration. John, feeling he had lost the board's confidence, submitted his resignation, which was reluctantly accepted. The retired mathematics professor and president spent the rest of his life in Greencastle, sallying forth frequently to propound his views from the lecture platform around the country.

Once again the trustees turned to the ranks of the faculty in their search for a president, naming Hillary A.

EARLY DEPAUW CUSTOMS

According to Irving F. Brown, author of *Indiana Asbury-DePauw University*, the custom of each class adopting its own special garb originated in the early 1880s, when the sophomore class donned plug hats. Shortly afterwards, the juniors adopted the "Oxford hat." His 1914 historical account goes on:

This custom lasted for several years, and since then, from time to time, there have been many different garbs.

The cap and gown was not introduced into DePauw until 1894. On May 29, of that year, the seniors wore them to a reception given by Dr. John. The next day they appeared in them at chapel for the first time. Tradition gives it, that on their first appearance, the juniors undertook to confiscate them. No year has passed without this attempt in a more or less violent form.

His description of other early DePauw customs follows:

The first class numerals to be put on the standpipe were placed there in February, 1889. A member of the class of 1892 put up his numerals in orange letters seven feet in length .... Since that time no class has failed to carry out this custom.

Old Gold was first used as the college color at the DePauw-Wabash football game in the fall of 1890. Previous to that time the color had been blue, although the college papers, up to that time, do not speak of a college color. In fact, until within recent years, blue remained a semi-official color, since it was always used on the diploma.

The present DePauw yell was given for the first time at the DePauw-Butler football game in Indianapolis, on November 1, 1890. It is an outgrowth of an earlier attempt at a college yell,

> *Zip Rah Hoo*
> *D.P.U.*
> *Rip Saw! Boom Baw!*
> *DePauw*
> *Ah-h-h-there!!!!*

"In Praise of Old DePauw" was sung for the first time, at chapel on April 4, 1893, by the DePauw Glee Club. The words and music were both taken from the Princeton song, "In Praise of Old Nassau."

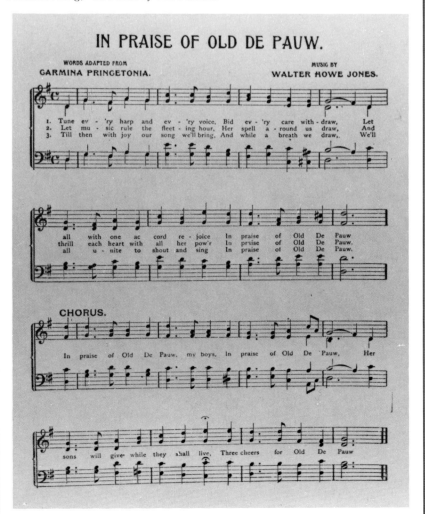

Gobin to that position in 1896. Terre Haute-born Gobin was an Indiana Asbury graduate and Civil War veteran who had taught briefly at his alma mater before becoming president of Baker University in Kansas. Returning to DePauw in 1890 as dean of the School of Theology, he was appointed vice president in 1894 and was acting president in 1895-96. The quiet, self-effacing Gobin was a good choice to guide the university through the less strenuous years that followed the rather tumultuous, innovative first decade of the reorganized institution. It was a time of partial retrenchment and of rethinking the shape and goals of the university.

One of the new president's first major decisions was to dismantle his own School of Theology in 1898 after several years of declining enrollments. Undergraduate interests were also shifting rapidly, as indicated in a survey of alumni occupations made at the turn of the century and published in the annual college catalogues. It showed that the

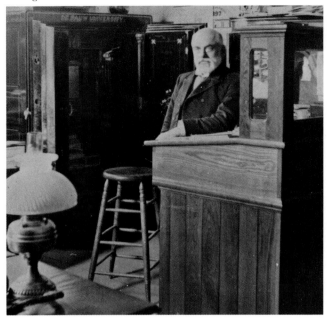

ministry had slipped to third place after education and the law. The next three professions listed in order of their numerical representation among DePauw graduates were business, medicine, and journalism.

Unlike the Civil War, the Spanish-American War of 1898 brought little disruption to the campus. A group of cadets traveled to Indianapolis to volunteer their services but returned to Greencastle after being informed that their services were not needed at the moment. The campus newspaper, the *Palladium*, congratulated the student body on the "absence of the cheap patriotism and jingoism which have been so prevalent at many other institutions." Falling victim to the crisis, however, was the military department of the university when the U.S. War Department recalled its commandant along with all the federally supplied armament, including two artillery pieces so often wheeled out and fired off to celebrate grand academic occasions. The next year, after failing to regain

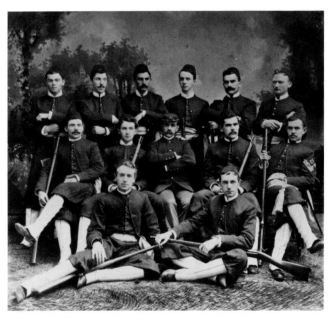

Above: Drill team of the Zouaves, part of the DePauw Cadet Corps in the 1890s.

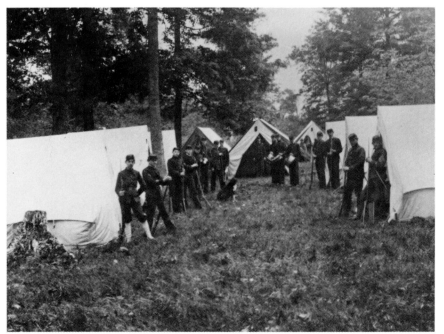

Left: In 1894, the DePauw Cadet Corps, including Jack the Dog, bivouacked at "Camp Alexander Martin," a mile and a half northwest of Fern. (A. Carl Andrews)

STUDENT PUBLICATIONS

In the early DePauw period campus publications continued to serve as an outlet for the expression of student opinion and literary creativity. The *Asbury Monthly* became the *DePauw Monthly* in 1884 and lasted four more years under the sponsorship of the fading literary societies. Its successor was the biweekly *Adz*, published by the short-lived DePauw Literary Society from 1888 to 1890, when factionalism brought about a split in the editorial staff resulting in two separate papers, both called the *Adz*. These soon became the *Bema* and the *Record*, each controlled by a combination of social fraternities and published weekly. Finally in the fall of 1893 they were replaced by a single *DePauw Weekly*. When Charles A. Beard became editor in 1897 he changed its name to the *Palladium*, which continued until 1904, becoming then simply *The DePauw*. Three years later, under the auspices of the newly organized DePauw Press Club and its sponsor, Professor Nathaniel W. Barnes, appeared the *DePauw Daily*, an ambitious enterprise that endured until 1920.

These student papers were generally four-page sheets each printed in four columns, with a great deal of space devoted to local advertisements to help pay the printer. Printed on the press of the *Greencastle Herald* or another local daily, with headlines set by hand, the papers frequently contained typographical and other errors. A limited number of photographs and line drawings were employed. Particularly outstanding were the drawings of Paul "Pete" Willis, later a cartoonist for the *Indianapolis Star*, whose work also appeared in the college yearbook. Under the guidance of Professor Barnes, who taught a course on reporting and editorial work, student journalism at DePauw became more and more professional. Among the staff on the *DePauw Daily* were such men as Kenneth C. Hogate, W. Don Maxwell, and Eugene C. Pulliam, who later headed the mastheads of the *Wall Street Journal*, the *Chicago Tribune*, and the *Indianapolis Star*, respectively.

Successor to the Press Club was Sigma Delta Chi, organized in 1909 as a journalistic honorary fraternity by DePauw students Gilbert C. Clippinger, Charles A. Fisher, William M. Glenn, Marion H. Hedges, L. Aldis Hutchens, Edward H. Lockwood, LeRoy H. Millikan, Eugene B. Pulliam, Paul M. Riddick, and Lawrence H. Sloan. Within a few years it had spread to a dozen other campuses and eventually became a national institution and an influential voice in American journalism.

Two yearbooks called the *Mirror* were published by the social fraternities during the Asbury era. Their successors in the DePauw period were the annual *Mirages* put out by the junior class, the first of which appeared in 1886. Several times during the next decade and a half the junior class failed to produce a yearbook, however, and the 1908 publication was given the name *Sombrero*, from the hat worn with a red neckerchief as the class garb of that year. From 1909 on the *Mirage* made an annual appearance. The early yearbooks contain not only the names and sometimes the pictures of faculty and students but also literary pieces, including humor, verse, essays, songs, and occasionally even plays. Later they concentrated on portraying campus life and student activities by photographs, sketches, and words, providing this volume with many of its best illustrations.

The DePauw Daily *began publication in October 1907 and continued until 1920. DePauw was the smallest college in the country to have a daily newspaper. This picture shows the editorial staff in 1908, which includes men who founded the Sigma Delta Chi journalism fraternity in 1909.*

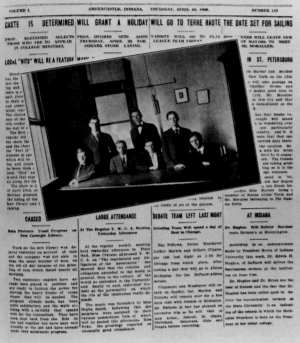

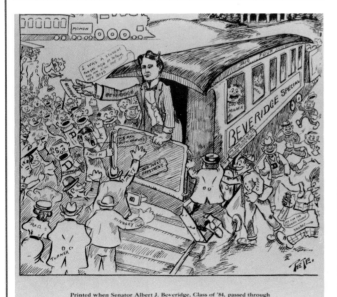

Above: This cartoon, from the 1907 Mirage, recalled the day when Senator Albert J. Beveridge, class of 1884, passed through Greencastle and addressed the students. Right: The editorial staff of the Bema, *a weekly school newspaper published between 1890 and 1893. It was controlled by Sigma Chi, Beta, Phi Psi, Phi Delt, Sigma Nu, and non-fraternity men. The women in the photo were the literary editor and the poetry editor. A rival paper, The Record, was published by other Greek organizations. After 1893 they were combined into the* Weekly.

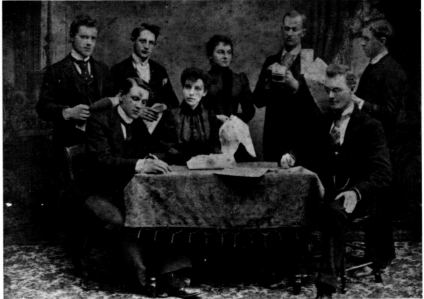

government support for the program, the board of trustees voted to abolish the department, thus ending 20 proud years of student military training at Indiana Asbury-DePauw University.

While the national economy experienced a gradual recovery from the financial panic of 1893, the university itself continued to post small annual deficits for a time. The board of trustees, now headed by Newland T. DePauw, decided to revert to the earlier scheme of naming a special administrator to organize efforts to raise money both for current expenses and endowment. Accordingly William H. Hickman, an Asbury graduate and Methodist minister with a successful record as a fund-raiser for Clark College in Georgia, was appointed to the post of vice chancellor in 1897 and was made chancellor two years later when Bishop Bowman assumed the honorific title of chancellor emeritus.

Hickman, who seems to have worked harmoniously with President Gobin, managed to raise nearly $100,000 for an endowment fund before launching in 1899 a more ambitious campaign to add $550,000 to that amount. The first major gift came from South Bend buggy

manufacturer and DePauw trustee Clement Studebaker, whose $5,000 "saved the university," Hickman gratefully acknowledged. In December 1901 the new chancellor resigned suddenly, however, leaving the campaign far from complete and relations with the trustees strained.

While Hickman never fulfilled all the hopes engendered by his appointment, he was able to strengthen the university's endowment considerably and to announce a gift of $50,000 from Terre Haute industrialist D.W. Minshall for the construction of much-needed laboratory facilities for the physical sciences. Minshall Laboratory, designed by D.A. Bohlen and Sons of Indianapolis, was erected in 1901-02 on Center Campus near East College but facing College Avenue. The three-story, U-shaped, red brick and limestone structure departed from the utilitarian style hitherto employed, chiefly in its rather ornate doorway, flanked by classical columns.

Minshall's children later added $26,000 for an endowment for the building. The chemistry department occupied its northern wing, while the physics department shared the

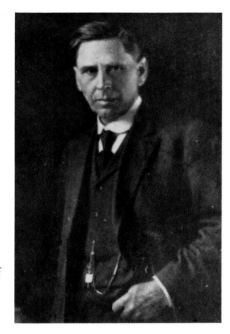

William H. Hickman, Asbury graduate of 1873, was chancellor of the university from 1897 to 1903. His major responsibility was raising funds for the endowment and current expenses.

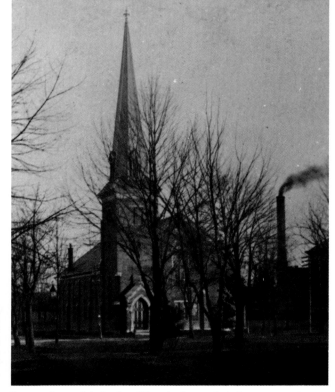

Locust Street Methodist Church, located at the corner of Anderson and Locust streets. The church was built in 1876 and always had a vigorous congregation of students, faculty and townspeople. After it merged with College Avenue Methodist Episcopal Church in 1924, the university acquired the property, removed the steeple, and used it as an armory until it was demolished in 1934.

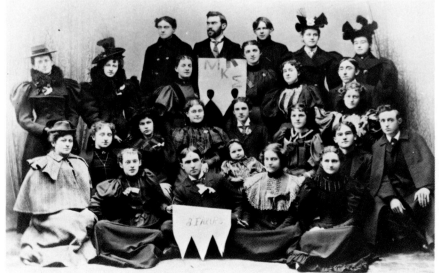

These students boarded at Coopers in 1895. The child in the first row was not then attending DePauw. (A. Carl Andrews)

"The Old Stock," as this group of students was known in 1892-93, posed for this photo while breaking the university rules of that time for moral conduct.

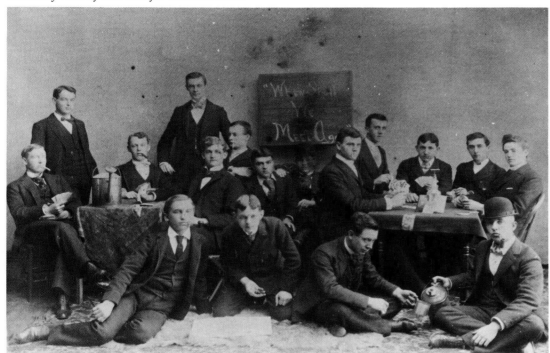

southern wing with mathematics. Professor of Chemistry Philip S. Baker, an Asbury graduate who had taught at his alma mater since 1874 and helped plan the construction of the laboratory, did not live to see the building completed, dying in 1901. A chemistry library in Minshall Laboratory was named in his memory.

The Gobin administration proved to be a transitional one in many respects. It was the last administration to make a serious effort to enforce the traditional compulsory attendance at daily chapel and Sunday morning church services, though students were still "expected" to attend these functions for some time to come. Hillary Gobin himself was also the last president to make his presence felt in the classroom on a regular basis, continuing to carry on the old-time presidential responsibility for the teaching of philosophy and religion. Most appropriately, upon leaving the presidency in 1903, he returned to teaching as professor of the English Bible as well as vice president of the university, holding both positions until his final retirement in 1922.

A new breed of Methodist ministers was called to the DePauw presidency in the early 20th century, equally devout but equipped with more advanced theological education than their predecessors. The three who followed Gobin in rather rapid succession were Edwin Holt Hughes (1903-09), Francis J. McConnell (1909-12), and George R. Grose (1912-24), all graduates of the Boston University School of Theology. There they had come under the influence of Professor Borden Parke Bowne, who expounded a Christian philosophy called Personalism, which soon became a powerful school of thought among Methodist academics. This philosophy, which was to have an especially long-lasting influence at DePauw, stressed the unique worth of the human personality and the working of the "divine will" in all of life.

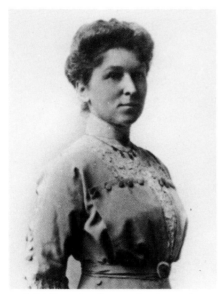

Isabel Elbert Hughes, wife of President Edwin H. Hughes (1903-09) came from Atlanta. "Hers was a charm and grace and a friendliness which endeared her to all who came within the sphere of her motherly heart," noted a pastoral friend.

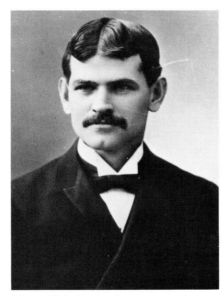

Edwin Holt Hughes became president in 1903 after studying at Ohio Wesleyan and Boston University, and serving a pastorate in Malden, Massachusetts. He left DePauw in 1909 after his election as bishop, but maintained a strong interest in the university until his death in 1950.

STUDENTS

The East College bell was a gift of the graduating class of 1879 and originally cost $350. It was hand rung on all special college occasions, to celebrate athletic victories, and as a result of student hijinks. It also rang to announce class hours. In recent years its mechanisms have been updated so that the bell is now controlled electrically.

The "Skulls" club, founded in 1890, consisted of two senior men from each fraternity. Its major activities were banquets, picnics, and looking tough for Mirage pictures. The group disbanded in 1916 after their nightly "horsing around" was condemned by the faculty and Greencastle citizens.

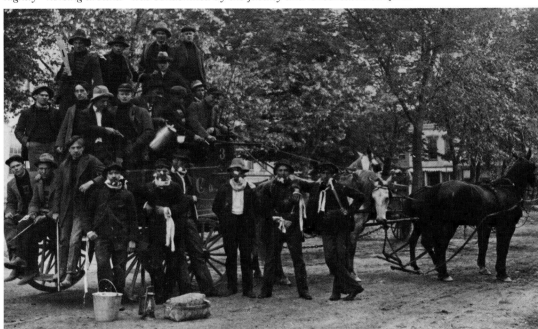

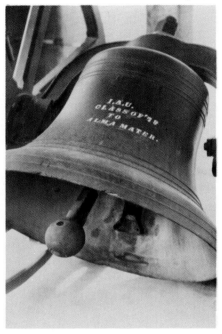

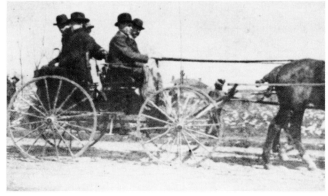

Above: The debate team heads for the Vandalia station in April 1897 to take the train for a debate with Earlham College in Richmond, Indiana. One of the team members is historian Charles A. Beard.

Right: The histological laboratory in Middle College about 1895.

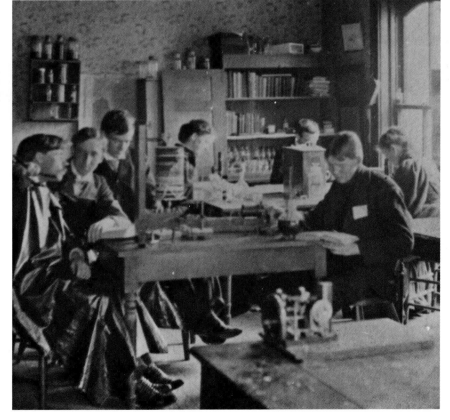

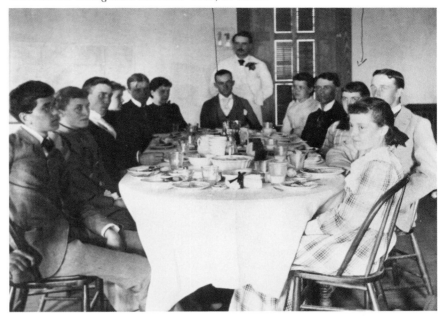

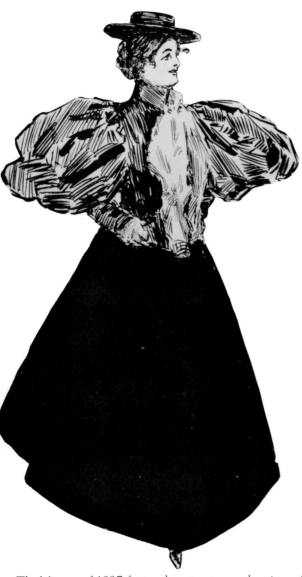

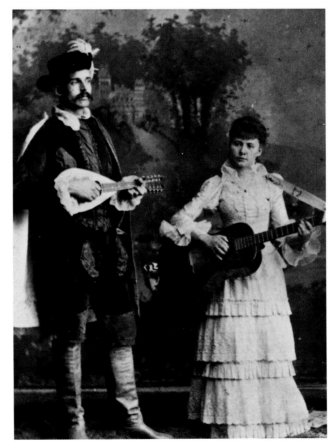

The Mirage of 1897 featured contemporary drawings of the pretty girls of the era in period dress.

Even though student drama and operettas were frowned upon by the university, this picture of a student group in the early 1890s suggests there were ways to get around the ban.

With presidents now out of the classroom for the most part, the person responsible for introducing this point of view into the curriculum was William G. Seaman, a DePauw graduate with a doctorate from Boston University who came in with Hughes in 1903 as professor of philosophy. He and his immediate successor, Lisgar R. Eckardt, who had also studied with Bowne at Boston University, established Personalism as a major force in the mental and spiritual life of the university.

The most troublesome problem facing Hughes at the outset of his presidency was student indiscipline, which had apparently been growing at DePauw since the 1890s. Mild-mannered President Gobin, for example, found it necessary to suspend several sorority women for attending an off-campus party involving social dancing, a form of recreation strictly forbidden by university regulations, together with such activities as card playing and the consumption of alcoholic beverages. Fraternity and class rivalries burgeoned in this period, while students also began to display a heightened interest in intercollegiate athletics.

Partly accounting for all this may have been the rapid rise in university enrollments, which almost doubled during Hughes' presidency, reaching 1000 by 1909, along with putative changes in the social and economic backgrounds of the students. Formerly recruited in large part from families of modest means and rural or small-town origins, the student body now included a growing number of more affluent, city-bred youth, many of whom were ready to rebel against what was perceived as a repressive social and religious atmosphere.

At any rate the young president took firm measures to restore campus order, even going as far as to patrol the local saloons from time to time on the lookout for students breaking the anti-drinking rule! He halted the practice of declaring frequent holidays from classes to celebrate athletic victories or similar events. Using his personal popularity with students to promote campus religious observance without resorting to the former emphasis on compulsory attendance, he initiated a monthly Sunday afternoon university service which attracted a large attendance.

Hughes also spoke out strongly against the practice of celebrating Washington's birthday on February 22 each year by the traditional freshman-sophomore class scrap. These battles over possession of the opponents' flag or the Columbian Boulder in front of East College had grown increasingly violent in recent years, often causing serious injuries to students taking part in them. He used his presidential authority to call off the 1907 scrap and in its place in the fall substituted a new all-campus celebration featuring a morning chapel service, a milder version of the freshman-sophomore

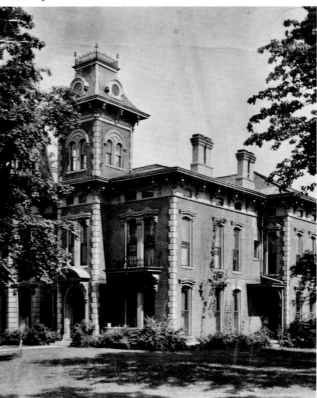

The Towers, on the northwest corner of Seminary and Arlington streets, was built in 1875. It was the first president's home, purchased by the university for President Hughes and used as well by presidents McConnell and Grose. It was later made into apartments for faculty, until sold by the university in the 1970s.

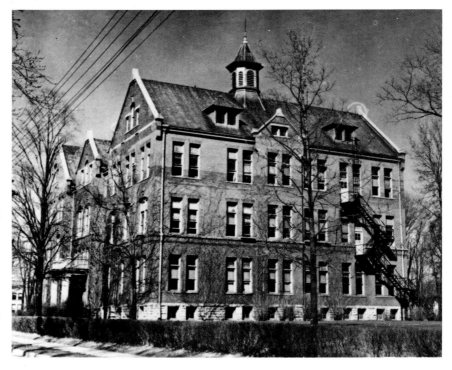

Minshall Laboratory on College Avenue was the gift of D. W. Minshall of Terre Haute and cost about $56,000. It opened in 1902. Minshall served the chemistry and physics departments until being razed in 1973.

The university library, Newkirk Hall, was located on the third floor of West College from its reconstruction in 1879 until the collection moved to the new Carnegie Library in 1908.

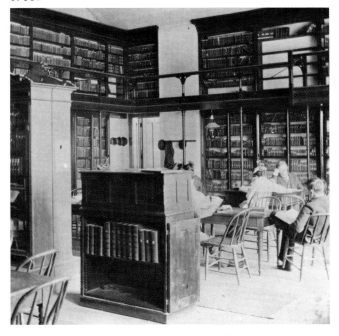

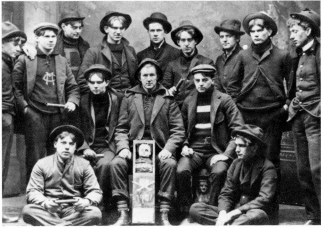

This picture of DePauw students is labeled T.N.E., apparently a men's club of 1901. The tradition of appearing tough continues — note the sticks of dynamite or large firecrackers the students hold. (McWhirter family photo)

ORATORY AND DEBATE AT EARLY DEPAUW

Oratory and debate at DePauw is founded upon a long forensic tradition reaching back into the Indiana Asbury period, with its emphasis on public speaking in the literary societies and its graduates' inclination toward such vocations as the ministry, law, and teaching. As early as 1875 a branch of the Indiana Oratorical Association was founded at Asbury, and in 1881 Charles Coffin won both the state and interstate oratorical contests.

The next student to achieve that same double honor was Albert J. Beveridge, later the distinguished U.S. Senator and historian. His victory in 1885 set off an explosion of excitement on the DePauw campus. On his return from the contest held in Columbus, Ohio, he received an artillery salute at the railroad station and was escorted to Meharry Hall by a brass band and military company. The faculty declared a holiday from classes. During the next several years DePauw won many state and a few interstate contests, all celebrated in similar fashion, the victors accorded honors usually granted only to heroes of the gridiron or baseball diamond. Few women participated, but there was a special celebration when coed Jean Nelson won both the state and interstate in 1892, defeating in the latter contest the representatives of 62 colleges from 10 states.

By 1918 DePauw had won 19 out of 37 oratorical contests but only five interstate contests, the last in 1905. David E. Lilienthal won the last state contest in 1918 with a speech on "The Mission of the Jew." There were other oratorical victories as well: DePauw won 10 of 15 contests sponsored by the State Prohibition League and four of seven in the state Peace oratorical contests and two interstate contests.

DePauw also took an active part in intercollegiate debate in this period, beginning with three consecutive victories over Indiana University in 1894, 1895 and 1896. Student interest remained high in this form of public speaking throughout the period, when DePauw teams debated Earlham, Butler, Wabash, Notre Dame, and other colleges to the accompaniment of campus enthusiasm similar to that shown for intercollegiate sports.

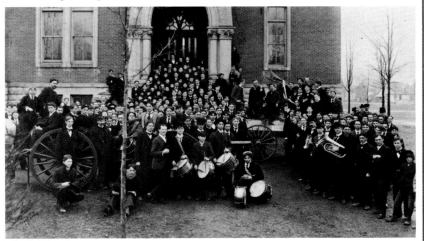

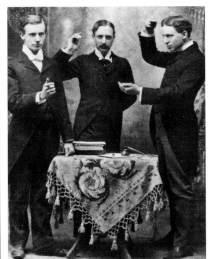

Above: DePauw students in front of East College celebrate the defeat of Indiana University in Intercollegiate Debate in the spring of 1896.

At left: The DePauw debate team of 1897 displays the favorite attitude of each speaker when debating. From left to right are Thomas W. Nadal, who later became president of Olivet and Drury colleges; Thomas P. Woodson, a prominent Indianapolis minister, businessman, and son-in-law of President John P. D. John; and Charles A. Beard, historian.

confrontation, several interclass athletic contests, and in the afternoon the Earlham-DePauw football game. The newly organized university band played, a great bonfire was lit after the football victory, and Hughes himself presided over an evening of "jollification" in Meharry Hall on this first Old Gold Day. Not long afterwards, the women students, feeling left out of much of the Old Gold Day activities, organized their own May Day festivities, with elaborately costumed dancing around a May pole, the election of a Queen of the May, tennis matches on the East College lawn, and theatrical entertainments in the evening. Both became annual campus events, May Day eventually giving way to Mothers' Day Weekend and Old Gold Day surviving to the present as alumni homecoming.

On the financial side, President Hughes managed to end the annual deficits. In effecting this he had the help of Salem B. Town, an Asbury alumnus and former minister of the College Avenue Methodist Church whom he persuaded to become the university's first full-time financial officer in 1905. Town not only put the institution's books in order but proved to be an energetic fund-raiser. Methodist businessman Melvin Campbell of South Bend also played an important role in bringing the university back to financial stability by creating a sustaining fund from contributions of alumni and others that brought in about $45,000 over five years. Another $35,000 was added to the endowment with the final settlement of the affairs of the defunct DePauw College for Women in New Albany in 1907. During the Hughes administration the university's total endowment more than doubled, rising from $231,000 to $530,000.

The crowning achievement of the Hughes administration was the acquisition in 1908 of the Carnegie Library, replacing the long-obsolete facilities in West College. Shortly after his appointment as financial secretary, Salem Town reopened negotiations, hitherto unavailing, with the steelmaker-philanthropist

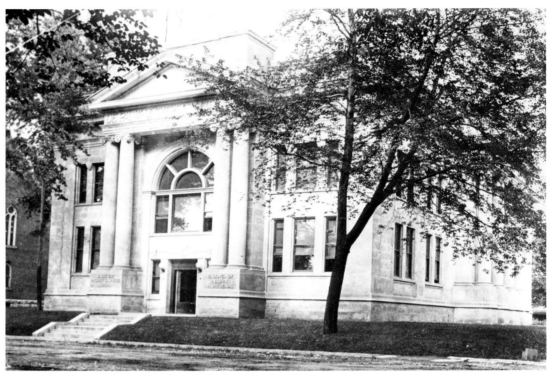

In 1908 the Andrew Carnegie Library was built with a grant from the industrialist of $50,000, plus a subscription from donors of $57,000 for maintenance. On the ground floor were a large reading room and stacks with seminars and departmental libraries on the second floor. After nearly 50 years as the DePauw main library, it was converted into what is now the Emison Art Center.

Andrew Carnegie, who eventually agreed to contribute $50,000 for the construction of a library building if the university raised an equal amount for its endowment. When that condition was finally met, the new library was erected on a lot next to the College Avenue Methodist Church.

Designed by Indianapolis architect Oscar Bohlen, it was constructed entirely of Bedford limestone in a neo-Greek style, with four great columns of the Ionic order adorning both the front entrance and the south side facing East College. Contrasting strikingly with the predominantly red-brick surfaces of the rest of the physical plant, the Carnegie Library was described at the time as the "most beautiful building on campus." Inside, the main floor contained the book stacks and a spacious reading room, its ceiling supported by massive pillars echoing the classical columns on the

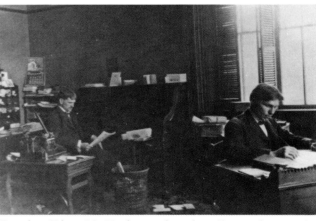

President Edwin H. Hughes works in his office on the second floor of East College, with his secretary. His typewriter introduced the university to a new era of bureaucracy and record keeping. (Indiana State Library)

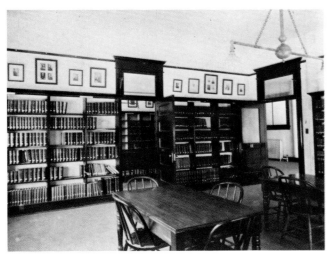

The reading room of the new Carnegie Library in 1908 featured closed stacks behind the glass partitions. On the left of the main desk were the current periodicals. The grandfather clock along the left wall is still in the main library, but has not run for many decades. In later years, male students studied on the left side of the reading room and the coeds on the right. Today this room is the main gallery of the Emison Art Center.

Political science seminars were held in this room on the second floor of the Carnegie Library. This photo was taken around 1910.

DEPAUW FOOTBALL AT THE TURN OF THE CENTURY

In a letter to the DePauw archivist in 1966, Charles A. Robbins of the class of 1904 described his experiences as a member of the varsity football team:

I began turning out for football .... Football suits were not too elaborate, certainly not like today. The coach gave each man a pair of cleated shoes, stockings, pants with some padding on the front of the legs, and a jersey. For protection he gave us four pieces of canvas, and some cotton padding, and we were expected to sew these on the point of each shoulder and elbow. Not much as compared to the harness of today. We also had a head gear made of padded strips of leather, which of course gave little head protection, nothing like the helmets of today. Some wore shin and nose guards – but believe it or not we played Indiana University, Wabash, Purdue, Notre Dame, Michigan State, Ohio Wesleyan, Illinois and other schools. It is fair to say that we did not win every time, and got some bumps and bruises. One game with Washington University in St. Louis we came back, after winning, with one man with a broken leg, Pat, and another, Albert Reep, knocked silly and had to be cared for for several days before recovery .... Our field was not turfed, and perhaps one Saturday it would turn cold and the water and edges of the holes freeze. We hated to fall on it but naturally did. ... The type of play was entirely different then than now. We depended much on power, a V forming and the ball carrier inside. There was no forward passing then – we did skirt the ends or play off tackle but usually someone pushing behind the carrier. Flying tackling was legal and one player, Parker Wise, was especially good at this although he was not large or heavy, but he would get his man.

Football players were also in strong demand for the annual scraps around the Boulder on Washington's Birthday. Robbins recalled that *it was not uncommon for one class to kidnap some of the bigger men of the other class to keep them out of the fray. In my sophomore year another football player and I were kidnapped and taken to a farm house near Putnamville and locked in an upstairs room. However, we opened a window, opening on a porch roof, slid down the roof and to the ground. We walked to a railway station, caught a train and got back to Greencastle in time to walk into chapel service and to participate in the scrap.*

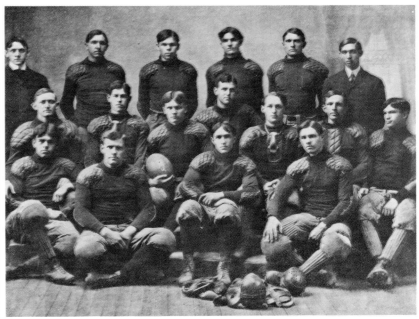

Charles A. Robbins played on the football team of 1904. He is the second from the right on the top row.

exterior of the building. Second-floor seminar rooms provided housing for several of the departmental libraries formerly located elsewhere. Unfortunately, the Greek temple-like structure proved less than adequate for the expanding functions of the university library long before it was finally replaced.

The only other addition to the physical plant in this period was an official residence for the president. In 1906 the trustees authorized the purchase for that purpose of the F.P. Nelson home on the corner of Seminary and Arlington Street. Known as "The Towers," this handsome Italianate structure became the Greencastle home of President Hughes and his two immediate successors, furnishing a gracious setting for formal receptions, trustee sessions, and an occasional faculty meeting.

President Hughes was elected a bishop of the Methodist Episcopal Church in 1909, the third Asbury-DePauw president to receive that honor, and went on in the prime of life to a long and notable career in ecclesiastical leadership.

To succeed him the trustees turned to another graduate of Ohio Wesleyan and the Boston University School of Theology, Francis J. McConnell, who was serving as pastor of a large Methodist church in Brooklyn, New York. Though he remained only three years in the DePauw presidency before following his predecessor into the Methodist espiscopacy, McConnell took a special interest in the university's financial condition and led the institution's first major fund drive.

Directed by financial secretary Salem Town and endowment secretary Cyrus U. Wade, the campaign for the Seventy-Fifth Anniversary Fund, as it was called, was extraordinarily successful, producing a total subscription of $550,546 by mid-1912. This included $100,000 provided by the Rocke-

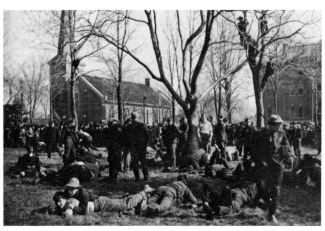

Class Scrap Day in either 1908 or 1909 on the East College lawn. In the rear are the Locust Avenue Methodist Church and part of Ladies' Hall.

feller-funded General Education Board as well as substantial individual gifts from Washington C. DePauw's widow, Clement Studebaker, and Asbury alumnus Jay H. Neff and smaller sums donated by trustees, faculty, students, and Methodist clergy.

In his later career as a leading Methodist bishop, McConnell was able to exert a wider influence and achieve a national reputation as a religious thinker and social reformer. He was the author of numerous books, including biographies of his Personalist mentor Borden Parke Bowne and Methodist founder John Wesley. As did his predecessor Hughes, McConnell published an auto-biography which devoted an appreciative chapter to his DePauw years.

The Hughes-McConnell era witnessed significant growth in the administrative organization of the university. One of President Hughes' first steps was to name Edwin Post, who had been professor of Latin language and literature since 1879 and vice president since 1896, to the office of dean of the College of Liberal Arts, an office he held until 1930. At the same time the

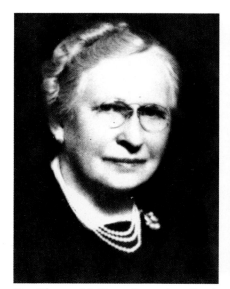

Eva Thomas McConnell was the wife of Francis J. McConnell, who served as DePauw's president from 1909-12. She was active in Methodist circles, particularly after her husband became bishop.

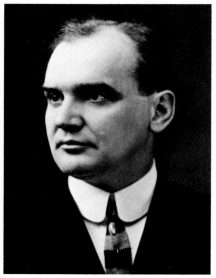

Francis J. McConnell, like his presidential predecessor Edwin Hughes, was a graduate of Ohio Wesleyan and Boston School of Theology. A pastor in Brooklyn before his appointment to the DePauw presidency, he came to DePauw in 1909 and was elected bishop in 1912. He died in 1952 at the age of 82.

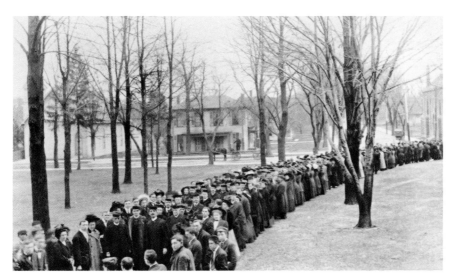

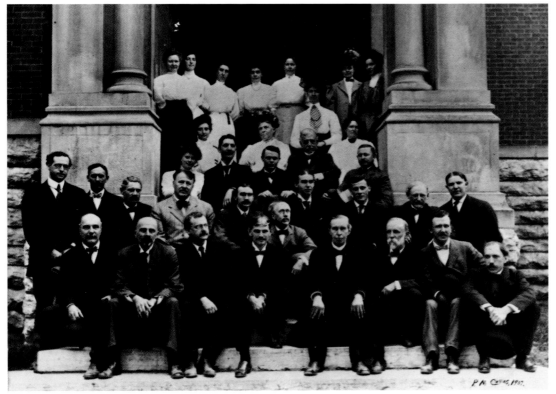

Most of the DePauw faculty gathers on the steps of East College in 1907. Front row, from left: J. Dobell, H. B. Longden, H. J. Banker, E. H. Hughes, H. A. Gobin, J. P. Naylor, W. M. Blanchard, A. Schellschmidt; second row: H. B. Gough, W. T. Ayres, W. V. Brown, A. Stephenson, F. E. Watson, E. Post, N. W. Barnes, A. M. Brown, W. G. Seaman, W. M. Hudson. Third row: A. V. McCoy, R. B. von KleinSmid, R. Baker, J. R. Weaver, A. F. Caldwell. Fourth row: Margaret Overbeck, Belle Mansfield, B. N. Smith, M. M. Kern. Fifth row: R. M. Rutledge, M. M. Zabriskie, D. B. Shearer, R. Laitem, unidentified, E. P. Sawyers, and J. Druley.

administration replaced the former position of preceptress of Ladies' Hall with that of dean of women, assigned on a part-time basis first to Rose F. Laitem of the department of Romance languages and then to Bessie M. Smith of the School of Art.

The two women's dormitories, Ladies' Hall, usually known simply as "The Dorm," and Florence Hall, converted from a rooming and boarding facility for men, were placed under the management of Lucy Black, who may be considered the first director of residence halls. Men continued to live out in town, either in rooming houses or fraternity chapter houses, but many of them joined the women students at the coeducational dining tables in the halls. Other non-residence diners in the dormitories included single faculty members and sorority women living in chapter houses.

The faculty still took on a variety of non-teaching tasks, despite the general tendency toward specialization. For example, the titular librarian was usually a professor, even though most of the actual operation of the library was carried on by an assistant engaged for that purpose, the first of whom was Martha B. Longden. Margaret Gilmore began her long career in that role in 1908, just in time to help organize the move to the new Carnegie Library on College Avenue. The office of the registrar grew in importance in these years, its duties assigned to Joseph T. Dobell, an instructor in mathematics at the Academy, the new name of the preparatory school after 1896.

Some professors took on a wide variety of chores outside the classroom. A striking case is that of Rufus B. von KleinSmid, the colorful professor of education and principal of the Academy who coached fencing, directed the men's glee club, and put on an annual minstrel show and other stage performances! Moreover, most members of the faculty carried heavy teaching loads, with little opportunity for scholarly production.

FACULTY

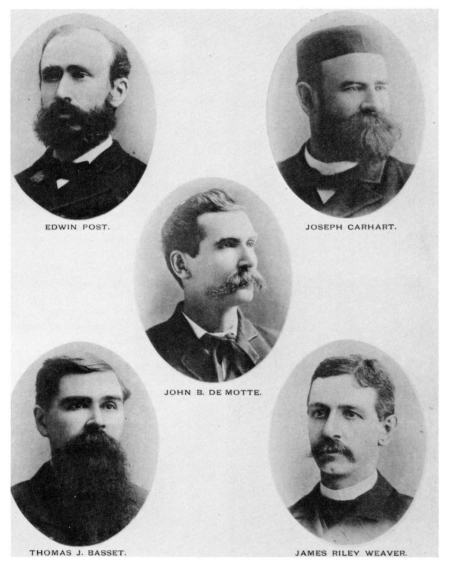

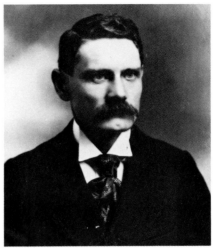

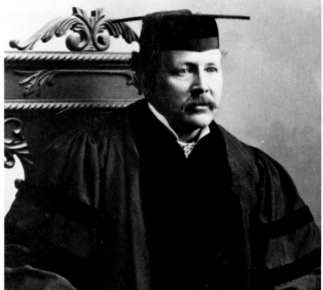

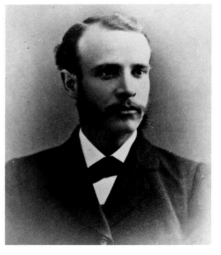

EDWIN POST.

JOSEPH CARHART.

JOHN B. DE MOTTE.

THOMAS J. BASSET.

JAMES RILEY WEAVER.

Above, a faculty composite from the period.

Right hand column, from top: Wilbur Vincent Brown taught mathematics, astronomy, and was director of the observatory from 1885-1928. He was one of the very first faculty to have an earned Ph.D.

Middle: Andrew Stephenson, a DePauw alumnus who was a Ph.D. from Johns Hopkins, taught history from 1894 to 1913. Remaining popular with students such as Charles A. Beard, "Stevie" introduced the rigorous seminar method for undergraduate social science students at DePauw.

Bottom: Philip S. Baker taught natural science, English, chemistry and physiology from 1875-1901. The founder of the modern chemistry department, he died while Minshall Laboratory, which he virtually designed, was under construction. It is suspected his premature death was due to poisonous fumes from the poorly ventilated laboratory in the basement of East College.

Rose Adelaide Marquis, a graduate of DePauw, taught stringed instruments from 1886-94. Her father, Emanuel Marquis, a Greencastle music store operator, was a private instructor in music in 1877 at Indiana Asbury.

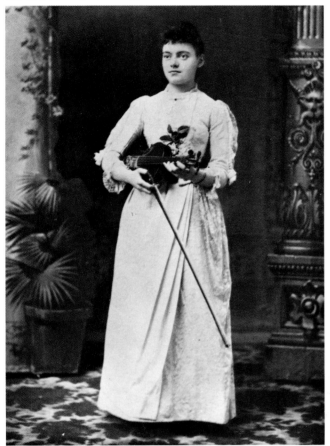

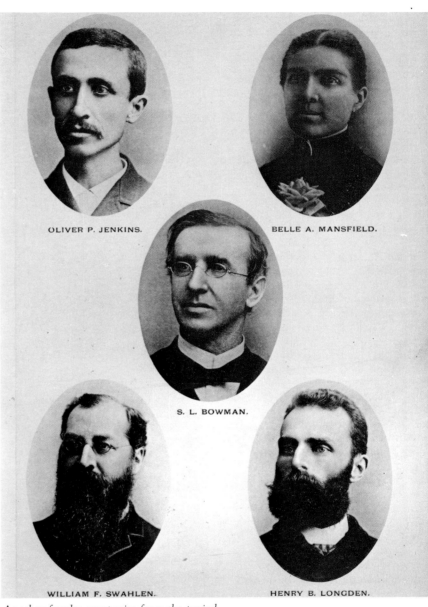

OLIVER P. JENKINS.

BELLE A. MANSFIELD.

S. L. BOWMAN.

WILLIAM F. SWAHLEN.

HENRY B. LONGDEN.

Another faculty composite from the period.

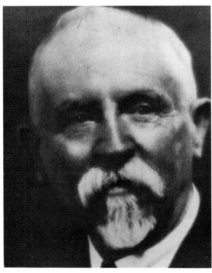

Joseph P. Naylor became professor of physics in 1891 and remained until retirement in 1925. He was not only a popular teacher, but also an inventive one; some of his innovative laboratory equipment, which he personally built, is still in use.

President McConnell, who showed a special concern for the faculty, did initiate a rudimentary system of sabbaticals in 1910, but they did not become a general institutional practice for many years.

Most academic departments remained the domain of a single full professor, often with an instructor or assistant professor added in these years to help with the increased student enrollments. The growth in subject areas within an elective-system curriculum also brought about expansion of the departmental organization. Separate departments of English composition and rhetoric, English literature, comparative literature, and public speaking and debate came into existence, headed respectively by Nathaniel W. Barnes, Adelbert F. Caldwell, Francis C. Tilden, and Harry B. Gough.

In 1906 the indefatigable KleinSmid expanded the department of education to the department of education and psychology, which began to offer specialized training for careers in secondary teaching and administration. The social sciences finally came into their own, with the separation of sociology from Colonel James R. Weaver's political science department in 1908 and economics in 1912, made possible by the appointment to the faculty of Cecil C. North and Frank H. Streightoff.

The curriculum also underwent considerable reorganization at this time. In 1903 the course was replaced by the credit hour as the basic unit of study, meaning one hour of class work per week for each of the three terms into which the academic calendar was then divided. A minimum of 180 hours, or an average of 15 hours per week for each of the 12 terms, was required for graduation. The major consisted of 36 hours in one department, and the minor was dropped.

Graduation requirements, divided into four groups, included 24 hours in a foreign language, 12 in science, six in mathematics, three in rhetoric,

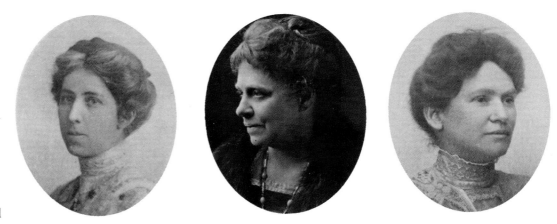

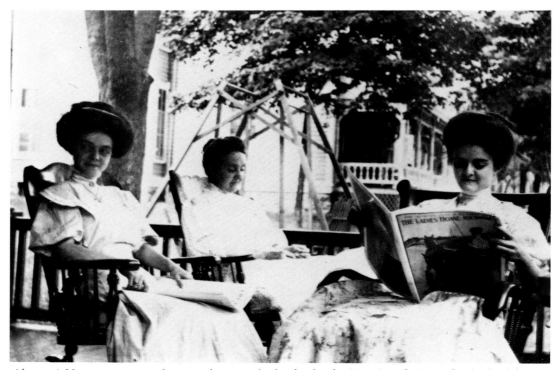

Above: A Victorian summer front porch scene of a faculty family: Mrs. Joseph P. Naylor (wife of the physics professor) and her daughters Elsie and Mamie.

Top of the page, from left: Dade Bee Shearer, a graduate of the University of Chicago, came to DePauw as a Latin instructor in 1907. A Phi Beta Kappa who received her M.A. at DePauw in 1910, she became head of the Latin Language and Literature Department in 1934. She retired in 1942.
Middle: Julia Anne Druley taught piano at Indiana Asbury and then at DePauw from 1883-1933 — a record span of time that will probably never be challenged by a woman faculty member.
Right: Minna May Kern came to DePauw in 1895 to assist Professor Henry B. Longden in German. Popular with the students, she had the yearbook Sombrero dedicated to her in 1907. She retired as associate professor in 1932 after 37 years on the faculty.

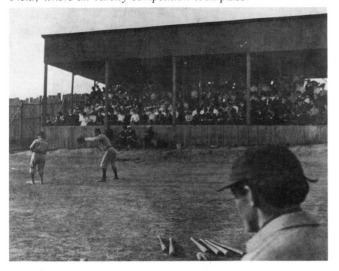

When DePauw played Notre Dame in baseball around 1925, the competition filled the grandstand at McKeen Field, where all varsity competition took place.

three in Bible, and six in physical education. For the first time there was no absolute requirement in philosophy, but students had to choose 12 hours in either history, political science, or philosophy. Two years later the faculty voted to eliminate the bachelor of philosophy and science degrees as no longer applicable to the new set of graduation requirements, and in future years to offer only a bachelor of arts degree in the College of Liberal Arts. In 1910 a major shift was made from the three-term to a two-semester plan, with 120 semester hours now required for graduation and 24 hours for a major.

The growing importance of organized sports at DePauw was signalled in 1903 by the creation of an Athletic Board consisting of the University president, three faculty members, and three students. Financial support derived from student fees and an annual fund-raising carnival. The first athletic letter "Ds" were awarded in 1905 and a "D" Association formed two years later.

The joint board of trustees and visitors in which the original Indiana Asbury charter had vested the general oversight of the University

EDWIN POST

Edwin Post, who held the chair of Latin language and literature from 1879 to 1932, the longest continuous period of service as a full professor of anyone teaching at the university before or since, was born in Woodbury, N.J. in 1851. He received an A.B. in 1872 from Dickinson College, which granted him an A.M. in 1875 and honorary degrees of Ph.D. in 1884 and LL.D. in 1927. Before coming to Greencastle he was a teacher and administrator at a private seminary and held a Methodist pastorate in New Jersey. He took two years' leave from DePauw in 1886-88 for advanced study in Berlin and Bonn and became one of the most scholarly members of the faculty. He was awarded one of the first sabbaticals in 1910. He found time during his busy career to publish scholarly articles as well as two books, *Latin at Sight* and *Epigrams of Martial*.

His diaries, which he kept from the age of 10 to his mid-30s reveal his scholarly concern and his distaste with the heavy emphasis on the physical expansion of the university in the early DePauw period: *The policy by which the future is to be determined seems to be the "big show policy," big buildings, crowds of matriculates, while scholarship, through tests of work are to be subordinate.*

From 1880 to 1896 he was librarian, reorganizing the books saved from the West College fire and personally cataloging them and for the first time establishing regular library hours. Vice president from 1896 to 1903, he was then named the first dean of the college. As professor of Latin he initiated a "seminarium" for advanced students memorialized in a series of annual photographs. A member of Phi Beta Kappa and the social fraternity Phi Kappa Psi, Post was a popular teacher who in 1924 received the first leather medal for service to the university.

He died in Greencastle a few months after his retirement in 1932 at the age of 81, leaving behind him a memorable heritage of scholarship and devotion to teaching.

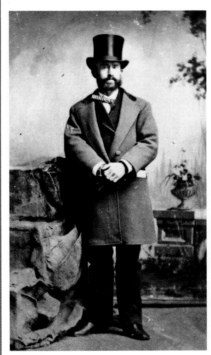

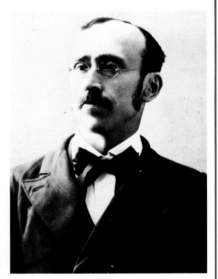

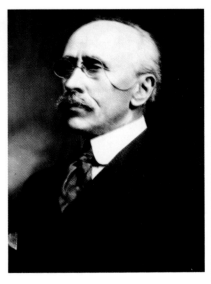

Above: Professor Edwin Post came to Indiana Asbury as professor of Latin in 1876. This picture was made from a tin-type made about 1886.
Top right: Post at the end of the 19th century, when he had been promoted to librarian and vice president.
Right: Post near the end of his career, after he had served as the first dean of the college. He retired in 1932, having served 53 years continuously as professor of Latin, a record probably never to be broken.

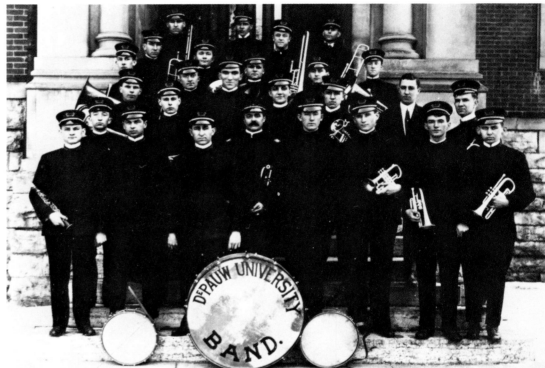

The DePauw University Band on the steps of East College in 1910.

promulgated an important change in its membership in 1909. Taking advantage of a 1907 enactment by the Indiana General Assembly, the board amended the charter to increase the number of trustees from 25 to 35, of which 21 were elected by the three Indiana conferences of the Methodist Episcopal Church, 10 by the board itself, and four by the Society of the Alumni. The nine visitors named by the Indiana Methodist conferences remained, though their role had been declining for some time. The chief significance of this change was to provide for representation on the board by DePauw alumni, a measure long sought by many of their number. But the effect was also to modify slightly the institution's affiliation to the Indiana Methodist conferences, which had hitherto named all members of the board.

President McConnell had to deal with the problems of the Schools of

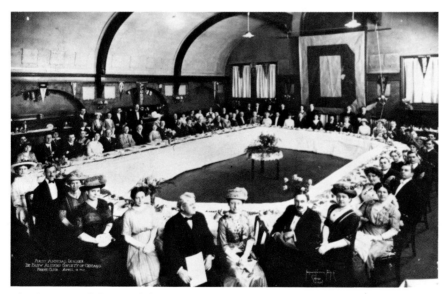

The first annual dinner of the DePauw Alumni Society of Chicago was held at the Press Club in 1913.

Art and of Music, both suffering enrollment declines under the leadership of the aging and ailing Belle Mansfield. In January 1911 Robert G. McCutchan was appointed the new dean of the School of Music, which experienced a renaissance under his vigorous direction. It remained on the traditional proprietary basis whereby instructors received a proportion of the student fees in lieu of a regular salary. Soon joining McCutchan's staff were accomplished musicians Van Denman Thompson in organ and piano and Howard J. Barnum in violin, the latter of whom also became the conductor of the university orchestra.

No such recovery proved possible in the case of the School of Art. After the death in 1911 of both Dean Mansfield and the talented art instructor Margaret Overbeck, Bessie M. Smith, who had taught in the school since 1897, presided over the

HILLARY A. GOBIN

Like his predecessor, John P.D. John, President Hillary A. Gobin was a native Hoosier, a member of the DePauw faculty, and a very popular figure on campus. Born in Terre Haute, he served in the Union Army during the Civil War and graduated from Indiana Asbury in 1870. After 10 years in the Methodist ministry he returned to his alma mater as professor of Greek and then became president of Baker University in Kansas in 1886. Four years later DePauw recalled him to become dean of the School of Theology. Gobin was also named university vice president in 1894 and served as acting president for a year following John's resignation. In 1896 he succeeded to the presidency, an office he filled with quiet competence for the next seven years.

The mild-mannered, highly respected Gobin gave the university the conservative, conciliatory leadership it needed after the turbulence and innovation of the John years. He had to decree the closing of his own School of Theology in 1898 as part of a general retrenchment and to preside over the demise of the popular military department the next year, when the federal government ended its support for the program during the Spanish-American War. President Gobin gracefully accepted the appointment of William H. Hickman as university chancellor in charge of fund raising and worked closely and harmoniously with him in sharing administrative authority.

In his memoir *Past Perfect*, Jerome Hixon recalls a story about Gobin's presidential style told him by the latter's widow:

It happened while Dr. Gobin was president, that after a particularly important football victory, some exuberant students placed a donkey in the tower of East College, its distressed braying could be heard all over campus. Everyone wondered what punishment would be meted out to the offenders. The air in Meharry Chapel the next day was tense.

Dr. Gobin delivered appropriate remarks about the significance of the victory of the day before. "There was," he said, "only one unfortunate incident connected with the occasion. In the rejoicing, some of the students climbed up into the tower, but forgot and left their little brother there. I would suggest that they rescue him as soon as convenient, for he is in considerable distress."

In 1903 Gobin resigned the presidency but remained on the faculty as professor of theology and English Bible until his retirement in 1922 at the age of 81. He died in Greencastle the following year. A few years after his death, plans were made for the erection of a building bearing his name to be used by both the Methodist Church and DePauw classes in philosophy and religion, but this project did not materialize. Instead the neo-Gothic church constructed on Locust Street in 1929 was named for him and remains today his chief monument as the Gobin Memorial United Methodist Church.

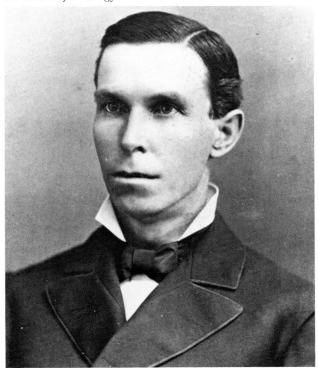

After graduating from Indiana Asbury in 1870, Hillary Asbury Gobin joined the faculty in 1880 as professor of Greek. He left in 1886, but returned in 1890 as Dean of the School of Theology.

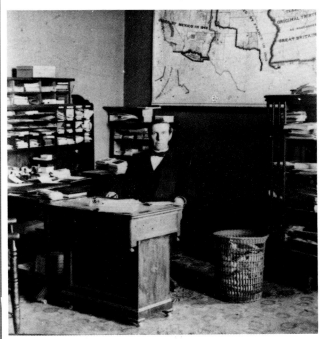

President Hillary A. Gobin at his desk in the president's office on the west end of the second floor of East College. His trash basket is prominent.

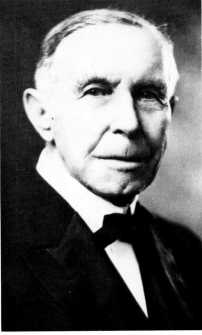

Former President and Professor of Bible Hillary A. Gobin at the close of his career in 1922.

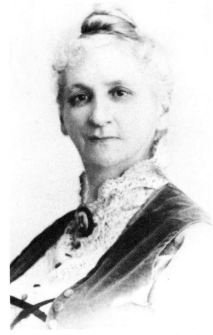

Mrs. Clara Gobin, second wife of Hillary A. Gobin.

fading institution until its close a year and a half later. Now only the School of Music remained of the ambitious program of professional education envisioned at the re-founding of the university under the DePauw name in 1884.

In 1912 the trustees once again chose for the DePauw presidency a graduate of both Ohio Wesleyan and the Boston University School of Theology. He was George R. Grose, minister of a Methodist church in Baltimore and, at 43, six years older than either of his two predecessors at the time of their election to the presidency. His 12-year term as president was to bring stability and financial strength to the university during a period of expansive growth.

He faced serious challenges immediately upon his inauguration.

His first annual report in 1913 mentioned the need for an endowment for faculty chairs, an organ for Meharry chapel, improvement of the physical plant, including overhaul of the campus heating and lighting system, and a new gymnasium to replace the entirely unsuitable facilities in West College formerly used as an armory for the military department. The university basketball team, for example, had resorted to using the second floor of the Greencastle Opera House for both practice sessions and home games. In 1913 the intercollegiate basketball schedule was actually called off for lack of an adequate playing floor. Also high on the list of university needs were an administration building, a student union, and another women's

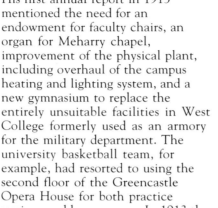

Lucy Dickerson Gross, 1914, wife of President Grose, with daughter Virginia.

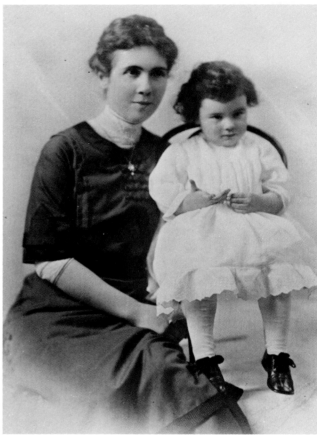

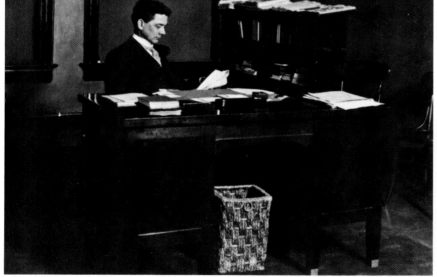

Above: President George R. Grose (1912-1924) works in his new private office in Studebaker Hall. The pigeon hole desk of earlier is gone, but the waste basket remains prominent as in most presidential office pictures.

At right: George R. Grose had been minister in Baltimore when he was called to become president of DePauw in 1912. His 12-year tenure was a progressive period of expansion as well as the first World War. Elected bishop in 1924 he initially served in China. He died in 1953.

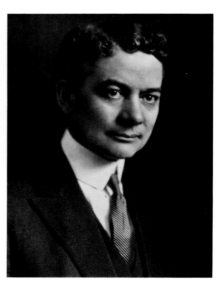

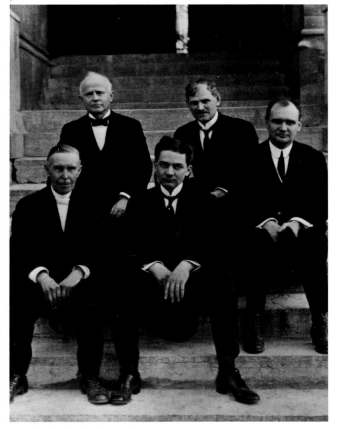

This unusual picture of five DePauw presidents was taken on the steps of East College. Back row, left to right: John P. D. John, Edwin H. Hughes, and Francis J. McConnell. Front row: Hillary A. Gobin, George R. Grose. Their service spanned the years from 1889-1924, a total of 35 years.

dormitory. In the meantime President Grose moved in the direction of partial retrenchment by deciding to close the declining Academy in 1914 in order to permit the university to concentrate its resources on college-level work.

In 1916 the board of trustees launched a new financial drive to raise $1 million, broken down into $600,000 for endowment and $400,000 for buildings. The campaign, led by Grose with the assistance of Cyrus U. Wade and another Methodist minister, Demetrios Tillotson, as field representatives, was hugely successful. Once more the General Education Board came to the aid of the university, contributing $150,000 toward the endowment fund on the condition that the campaign goal was met. At the end of 1916, $602,000 was added to the endowment including $250,000 for five faculty chairs.

THE BEGINNINGS OF DRAMA AND THEATRE AT DEPAUW

The traditional Methodist prejudice against the theatre effectively banned dramatic and other stage performances from the campus during the entire Indiana Asbury period as well as the early DePauw years. Occasional visits by faculty members and students to Indianapolis to view such forbidden entertainments came under the strong disapproval of President Alexander Martin as late as 1881. Nevertheless, the senior class was somehow able to put on a play at the Opera House on the square in the spring of that very year. Entitled "Esmerelda," it was a popular hit with both students and townspeople but apparently so alarmed the university authorities that no similar performance took place for more than two decades. The next recorded presentation of an English-language play at DePauw was in 1905, when Shakespeare's "As You Like It" was performed in Meharry Hall.

In 1906 Professor Rufus B. von KleinSmid organized a Dramatic Club which presented two plays, "His Lordship" and "She Stoops to Conquer." Though this organization proved short-lived, it signalled the onset of a flood of student interest in the theatre. In the next few years there were presented senior class plays, May Day plays performed by coeds, and a dramatized version of Charles Dickens' *Our Mutual Friend* sponsored by the Y.M.C.A. In 1913 students in the Music School presented the first opera seen at DePauw, the "Bells of Corneville," with a 25-piece orchestra and a chorus of 25 voices all directed by Professor Howard Barnum. The next year the operetta "Bohemian Girl" was performed as a part of a May Music Festival. By this time Harry B. Gough, head of the department of public speaking, had begun to bring most campus dramatic activities under departmental control. Duzer Du was organized under his auspices as a dramatic honor society in 1913 and presented its first production, Sheridan's "School for Scandal," on April 28, 1914 on the stage of Meharry Hall. But the installation of the Bowman pipe organ made Meharry Hall practically useless for such stage presentations. With the closing of the Academy in 1914 the administration decided to remodel the assembly room on the second floor of West College into a small auditorium, constructing a stage at the south end of the room and installing a number of old opera chairs and school benches for seating. The theatre opened with Duzer Du's performance of George Bernard Shaw's "Arms and the Man" in the fall of 1914. For 14 years this auditorium served as the home of DePauw's Little Theatre. Before West College was declared unsafe for public accommodation in 1928, 53 full-length plays and 35 one-act plays had been presented on its stage. Theatre had arrived to stay.

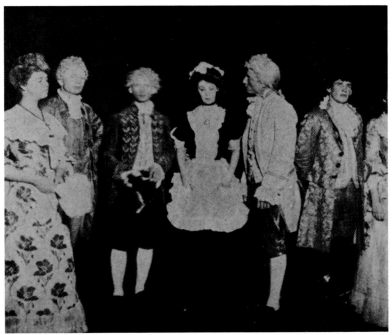

She Stoops to Conquer was performed in 1907 and was one of the first live dramas given by students at DePauw.

In 1916 Bowman Gymnasium was dedicated by Governor Ralston of Indiana and President Thompson of Ohio State University with a later address by former Vice-President Charles Fairbanks. Costing about $127,000 it was a major asset for the physical education program, including a large gymnasium that could be used as an auditorium, swimming pool, bowling alley, lockers, showers (they never really worked and dripped profusely for over a half century), offices, and meeting and social rooms.

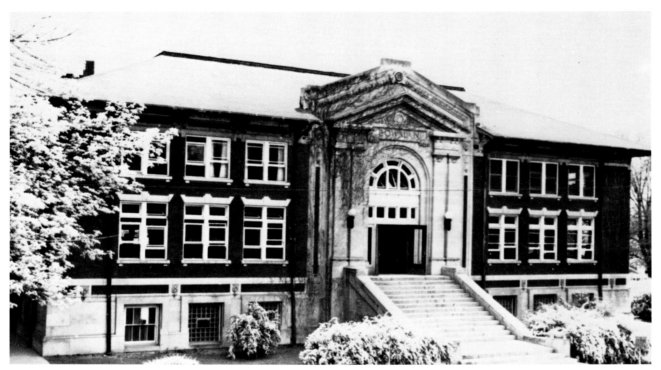

Large individual gifts also made possible the construction of three buildings. The first was the Bowman Memorial Gymnasium, named for the former president and chancellor, Bishop Thomas Bowman, and funded in part by his daughter Sallie Bowman Caldwell and her husband, who had already contributed the large organ installed in Meharry Hall in 1914. Designed by the well known Indianapolis architectural firm of Robert P. Daggett & Company, this imposing structure provided not only much-needed indoor athletic facilities for both men and women, including a swimming pool, but also space that could be used as an auditorium for large university gatherings and meeting rooms for various student activities. The large Hugh Dougherty Room on the main floor, named for the president of the board of

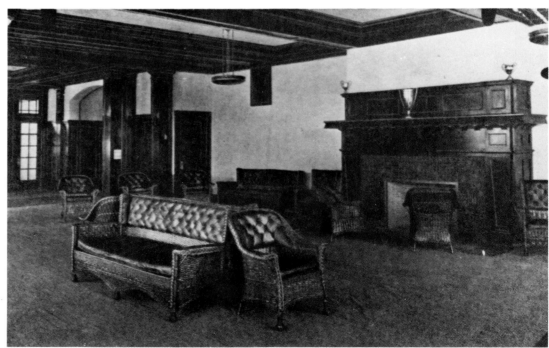

Reception room in the new Bowman Gymnasium, to the right of the main entrance. It was named Dougherty Hall after the chairman of the Board of Trustees from 1904-1924. This was a favorite place for student and faculty gatherings.

SOCIAL FRATERNITIES IN EARLY DEPAUW

Delta Kappa Epsilon bought this residence originally built by prominent Greencastle businessman Thomas Bayne. It stood on the northwest corner of Seminary Street and College Avenue. In later years D. B. Johnson built a series of stores on the frontage, which included a student hamburger "joint", barber shop, watch repair, and miscellaneous shops.

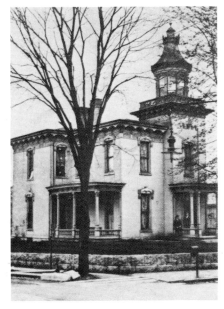

Social fraternities, which had gained a strong foothold in Old Asbury, grew even more important in the new DePauw University. By 1918 seven new fraternities had been organized on the DePauw campus, though only three proved permanent additions. These were Delta Upsilon (1887), Sigma Nu (1890), and Lambda Chi Alpha (1915), the last of which had originated as the Darsee (DePauw Rooming) Club in 1912. Even more sororities were organized at DePauw during these years, six of which have persisted to the present. The first was Alpha Chi Omega (1885), which began as a group of music students but widened to include others; a second musical sorority, Phi Mu Epsilon, was founded at DePauw but disbanded in 1905. Additional permanent sorority chapters appearing on campus before 1918 were Alpha Phi (1888), Alpha Omicron Pi (1907), Alpha Gamma Delta (1908), Delta Delta Delta (1908), and Delta Zeta (1909).

In 1889 Phi Kappa Psi became the first fraternity to rent a whole building as a chapter house rather than simply meet in rented rooms on the courthouse square. The next year Beta Theta Pi took the further step of purchasing the home of a departing professor, which 13 years later was incorporated into a brick fraternity house, the first such on campus. Shortly afterwards Sigma Chi built an entirely new chapter house. By 1918 most fraternities and sororities either owned or rented such residences to house their members.

Although membership in the social fraternities was growing, they still composed only a minority of the student body. Competition for new members was fierce, and the pledging process largely unregulated. Rushing was called "Spiking," and often consisted of active members going to the railroad station with a carriage to meet incoming trains and seizing upon unsuspecting freshmen whom they took back to their chapter houses, where the newcomers were promptly pledged. The attempt to keep spiking under control was one of the factors behind the organization of both men's and women's Panhellenic societies in the 1900s. As early as 1887 a men's Panhellenic banquet was held, and in 1890 there was founded an organization called the Skulls, composed of two senior members of each fraternity and later known as Kappa Phi Omicron Kappa. A similar organization for women was Ribs and Jawbones, also known as Gamma Tau Pi. Both eventually disbanded without having served any very significant purpose. Kappa Tau Kappa, founded in 1902, survived almost to the present as an important interfraternity council.

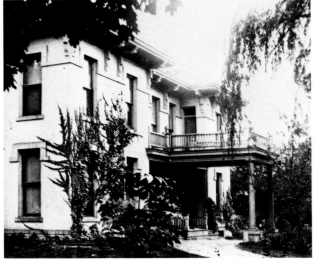

The Phi Kappa Psi fraternity bought this house on the southwest corner of College Avenue and Larrabee Streets. Extensively remodeled several times, the chapter still lived here in 1986.

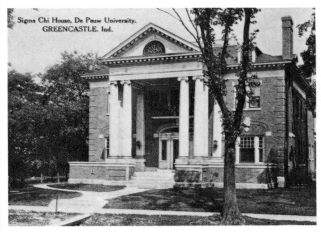

In 1914 the Sigma Chi fraternity built this house on Locust Street facing the campus, site of the present chapter house. It was the first fraternity to build an entirely new house for a fraternity residence.

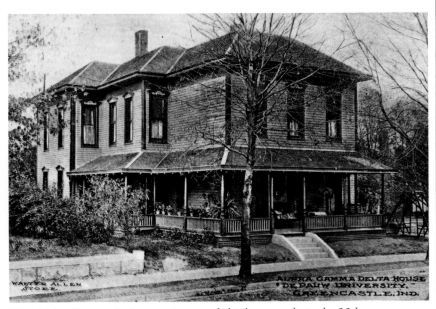

The Alpha Gamma Delta sorority rented this house early in the 20th century.

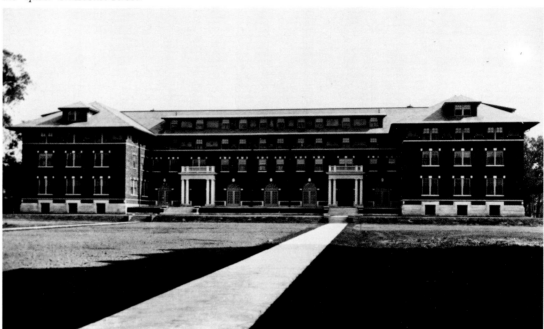

trustees, was set apart especially for the use of the YMCA and YWCA. Bowman Memorial thus served for many years after its erection in 1916 as a student union as well as gymnasium.

One of the major contributors to the building of Bowman Gymnasium was Edward Rector, a wealthy patent attorney whom his friend Roy O. West, a DePauw graduate and fellow member of the Chicago bar, had drawn into an active interest in DePauw affairs. Learning that the university needed an additional dormitory to house the growing number of women students, Rector agreed to provide $100,000 to construct one. The result was the erection in 1917 of Rector Hall on the site of the former Simpson Art Hall.

The new dormitory was named for the donor's father, Isaac Rector, a trustee of Indiana Asbury University at the time of the introduction of coeducation. This handsome and commodious structure was the first of several campus buildings designed by Robert Frost Daggett, son of the founder of the firm which did the architectural work for the gymnasium. Trained at the Ecole des Beaux-Arts in Paris, Daggett mingled elements of the Classical Revival and Italian Renaissance styles to create a dormitory majestic in appearance and at the same time highly functional. Its dark red brick walls, constructed on an H-shaped floor-plan three stories high, enclosed a spacious reception hall and dining facilities as well as both single and double sleeping rooms.

Daggett also designed the Studebaker Memorial Administration Building erected in 1918 on Locust Street to house the offices of the president, dean, registrar, treasurer, and other members of a growing administrative staff. The gift

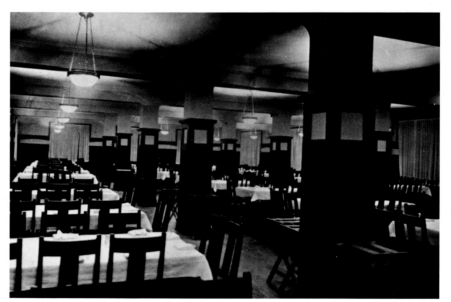

The dining room of Rector Hall, pictured shortly after the completion of the dormitory in 1917, is still in use in 1986.

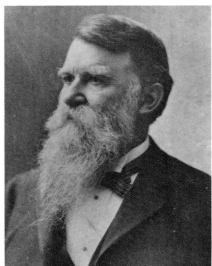

Clem Studebaker, carriage manufacturer of South Bend, was on the Indiana Asbury-DePauw Board of Trustees from 1881 to 1892. He was a major benefactor to the school and was honored by his family with their gift of Studebaker Hall, the DePauw administration building, in 1916.

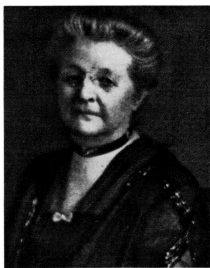

Mrs. Clem Studebaker and her sons provided $58,000 in 1916 for the DePauw Administration Building in honor of her husband, although she did not live to see the building completed. Her first gift to the university was the donation of a grand piano in 1882.

of the family of Clem Studebaker, the recently deceased industrialist and longtime DePauw trustee, the two-story brick and limestone building boasted a large classical-columned entrance. Inside was an ornate marble stairway with busts of Clement and Anne Wilburn Studebaker on the first landing, along with a statuary group of the three Studebaker children as youths in romantic pose. On the second floor of the building was a large, well furnished Trustees' Room, which came also to be used for faculty meetings.

The more sophisticated style and relatively lavish decor of these new structures represent a significant departure from the austere,

THE FLAG POLE INCIDENT

Prominent among the many student hijinks of the time was the disappearance of the university flag pole, the gift of the class of 1908, just before it was to be ceremoniously dedicated. After President Edwin H. Hughes issued a statement that he had the names of the five presumed perpetrators and that stern action would be taken if the pole were not returned, the pole reappeared the next morning just as silently as it had disappeared. The *DePauw Daily* faithfully recorded the incident, including an account of the great difficulties students participating in the escapade encountered in retrieving the 1,200-pound flag pole from the water-filled quarry west of town where they had disposed of it.

Once again a ceremony of dedication was planned, with musical offerings by a band from neighboring Brazil and suitable speakers to solemnize the occasion. But alas, just as the ritual of hoisting the pole into place near Middle College began, it bent under the strain, threatening the safety of the entire throng in attendance. A few weeks later a sturdier pole was installed and the flag finally hoisted to its top with less ceremony and probably far less sense of triumph than originally envisioned.

A year later the *DePauw Daily* noted that the ill-starred pole had suffered further indignity. Its gilded ball on top had fallen during the summer and the upper section, which had been part of the original pole stolen and deposited in the quarry, had become rusted and unsightly. Not long afterwards it was discovered that the pole was leaning severely, as much as 22 inches out of plumb. The student paper's last notice of the matter was to quote the superintendent of grounds as saying he would attempt to draw the pole back to its vertical position by use of steel cables.

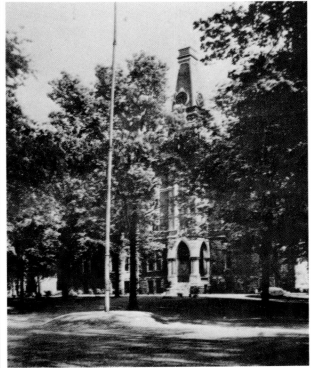

Later flagpole on the northwest corner of the East College lawn (c.1925). The flagpole of the incident narrated above was probably located near Middle College. Today it stands next to the Bookstore on the opposite side of East College.

91

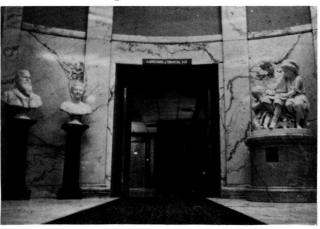

Interior view of the mezzanine landing of the administration building with the statues of Mr. and Mrs. Clem Studebaker and their children, which originally were in the Studebaker home in South Bend. The door is the entrance to a later addition to the building.

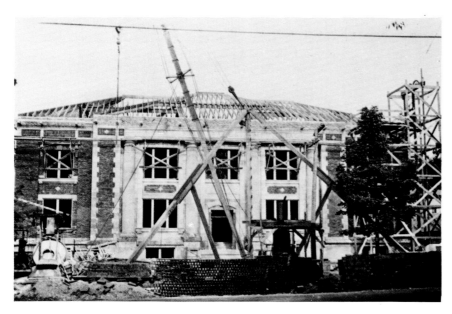

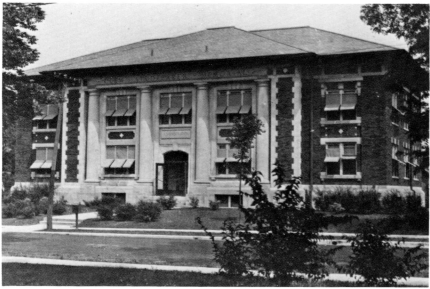

Top left: The Studebaker Administration Building on Locust Street is shown under construction. It was dedicated and completed in 1918 and allowed all the scattered university offices to be centralized.
Above: The completed Studebaker Administration Building. The second floor included the impressive faculty and trustee meeting room paneled with gum.

utilitarian designs of the early DePauw years. The old dream of someday relocating the campus to remote University Park had been long abandoned, and most of the acreage surrounding McKim Observatory originally purchased for that purpose was sold. In 1917 the trustees engaged the services of landscape architect Ralph M. Weinrichter of Rochester, N.Y. to draw up a comprehensive campus plan. His chief contribution turned out to be the planting of 2,500 shrubs in the first systemic landscaping effort at DePauw University.

In 1918, Women's Hall, whose residents now took their meals in the superior dining facilities of Rector Hall, was extensively remodeled and renamed Mansfield Hall in honor of its first preceptress, Belle Mansfield. At the same time Florence Hall, which had housed women since 1904, reverted to its original use as a men's dormitory, with a sleeping porch added for additional space. "Flossie," as its residents more or less affectionately dubbed the hall, was chiefly occupied by non-organization men, for most members of fraternities preferred to live in their chapter houses. The far greater need for dormitory rooms for women than for men arose from the administration's insistence that all freshman women reside in university halls as well as from the fact that sororities claimed a much smaller number of members than did the fraternities.

The DePauw Summer School,

SYMBOLS OF OLD DEPAUW

The Scarritt Fountain on the East College campus was the gift of Winthrop E. Scarritt of the class of 1882 in honor of his brother Alfred, who died while a student on campus. It has rarely been used as a fountain, but the owl on top, representing wisdom, has often been the butt of college pranks.

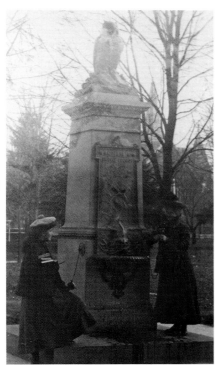

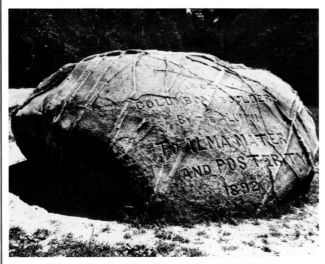

Above: The Columbian Boulder was brought to the East College campus in 1892 as an appropriate marker in honor of the Columbian celebration of that year. It has served ever since as a center of campus activities and traditions.

Right: The ornamental gateway of brick and iron on Locust Street at the foot of Anderson Street and opening onto the East College campus is a gift of the class of 1890, presented in 1910.

East College from its very construction has been surrounded by monuments that have become dear to the hearts of generations of students. Perhaps least known of them all is the first Boulder, a pink-colored stone placed near the front of the building at its dedication in 1877 by the senior class of that year. Weighing 5,000 pounds and bearing the class motto in Greek, "Andrizometha," or "Let us be manly," it was procured from the property of Dr. A.C. Stevenson, the first president of the board of trustees of Old Asbury. When underclassmen attempted to bury the stone two nights before the commencement exercises, the seniors who were guarding it drove them off with stones, firing revolvers as the attackers fled, according to a contemporary newspaper account. It remains today rather inconspicuous beside East College, its inscription barely legible.

The better known Columbian Boulder was placed near the main entrance to the building in 1892 at the instigation of former Professor John C. Ridpath to mark the 400th anniversary of Columbus' first voyage to the New World. This granite rock with prominent ridges of quartz dykes was discovered near Morton about 12 miles northeast of Greencastle. Hiram Thomas moved it to his farm, fenced it in and charged visitors 10 cents apiece to view the "petrified turtle." It was purchased by a few alumni and brought to Greencastle by a 26-horse house-moving wagon and the Monon Railroad. Inscribed and known as the Columbian Boulder, it soon grew to be a favorite meeting place on campus. Many a DePauw couple met for chapel dates "at the Boulder." Honorary societies often held their initiation rituals there, and it was long the scene of annual freshman-sophomore scraps. In recent decades the Boulder seems to have lost its focal position on campus, except for a brief period in the late 1960s and early 1970s when it became the scene of the "Boulder run," which featured freshman pledges of Phi Kappa Psi scrambling around it in the nude and trotting back to the chapter house on the night of the first snow of the season.

On the northern rim of the East College lawn there stands a small stone pedestal which once held a metal sun dial, now long missing. It was presumably placed there around the turn of the century and is today generally overlooked by all and sundry. Much more prominent is the Scarritt Memorial Fountain, erected in 1903 as a gift from alumnus Winthrop E. Scarritt in honor of his brother Alfred, who would have graduated in the class of 1881 had he lived. Sitting atop the fountain, which has lacked water for as long as anyone can remember, is a large bronze owl – the symbol of wisdom. Frequently covered with splotches of paint – as is the Columbian Boulder from time to time – the owl was at one time reputed to hoot when a virgin passed by, but has today lost most of its significance.

The most beautiful monument of all is the ornamental gateway constructed of brick and iron located on Locust Street at the western end of Anderson Street. The gift of the class of 1890 at their 20th reunion in 1910, this gateway has long served as a major entrance to the campus and familiar symbol of the university. Several concrete benches donated by alumni, such as the recent one honoring Fred and Bernice Tucker, lie scattered about the East College lawn but have as yet gathered no special traditions around them. New concrete sidewalks have replaced the originals given by various college classes while the bronze plates with the class numerals remain. The newest monument to grace the front of East College is the modernistic triangular metal shaft placed there in 1967 to memorialize the founding of the journalistic honorary Sigma Delta Chi at DePauw in 1909.

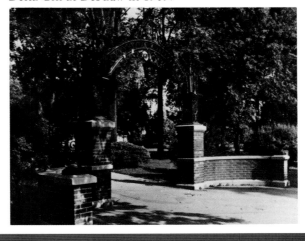

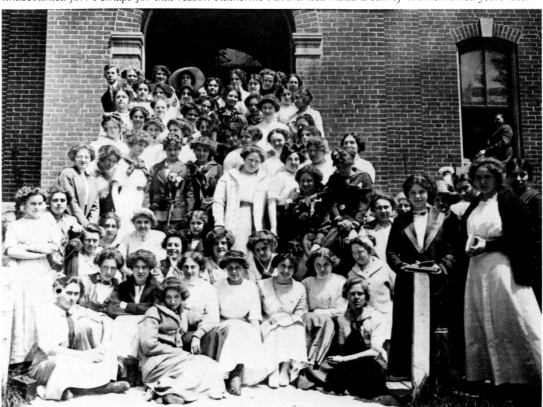

The residents of Mansfield Hall on the steps in 1912. How the man got into the picture on the last row is unaccounted for. Perhaps for that reason Katherine Alvord was made Dean of Women three years later.

which had its origins in the special summer classes first held in 1893, expanded its operations considerably at this time. Courses in domestic science offered in the summer of 1915 for prospective teachers of that subject led to the organization of a regular department of home economics in the fall of that year under the guidance of a series of young women instructors. Classes were held first in Simpson Hall, no longer needed since the demise of the Art School, and later in a house remodeled for that purpose on the corner of Spring Avenue and Simpson Street. Eventually a small student cafeteria was established nearby that was operated by the home economics department for about a decade.

In 1913 the board of trustees shifted control of organized sports at DePauw from the student-faculty board to a committee made up of nine alumni, chiefly residents of Indianapolis. Taking complete charge of the athletic program, this

Alumni Athletic Board ushered in a new era of increased emphasis on intercollegiate competition. Coeds, who were excluded from such activities, organized their own Women's Athletic Association in 1915 to sponsor intramural contests in such sports as basketball, swimming, and tennis. In that same year a women's tennis team played the first recorded intercollegiate match with Butler University. Two years later the W.A.A. awarded letters and numerals to outstanding DePauw women athletes.

While black and gold had recently been adopted as the official school colors, there was yet no generally accepted name for DePauw's varsity athletic teams. "Fighting Parsons" was occasionally applied to the football eleven, but the usual term for the university's representatives in intercollegiate sports competition was simply "Old Gold." The present usage dates from the spring semester of 1917-18, when the "D" Association sponsored a contest to pick an appropriate epithet, one that would reflect varsity

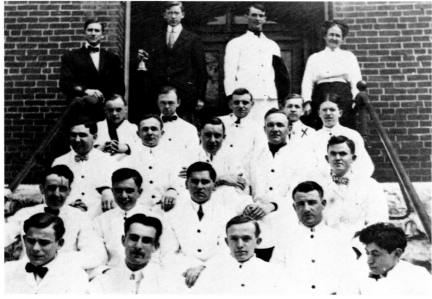

The waiters of Ladies' Hall (Mansfield after 1912) on its steps in 1910. Mrs. Lucy Black was put in charge of the dining room in 1900 and managed it with noteworthy efficiency. Second from the left on the fourth row of this picture is Clyde Wildman, who became president of the university in 1936.

STUDENT HAUNTS

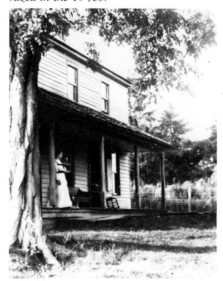

Top: Halfway House on the National Road (Route 40) in Mt. Meridian was a favorite inn for DePauw student dinners and buggy trips from Greencastle. Mrs. J. O. Cammack is standing on the front porch. Originally a stagecoach stop, it was razed in the 1940s.

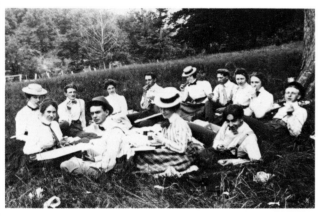

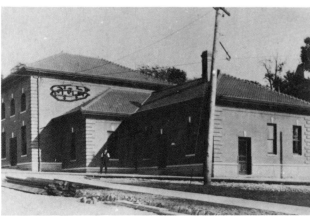

Middle: Picnicking has always been a student favorite. Here is a picture of a group of Phi Kappa Psi men with their dates at the Eel River Falls in south Putnam County in June 1900.

Bottom: In 1907 the Terre Haute, Indianapolis, and Eastern Interurban ran its first electric car into Greencastle. The station stood on Seminary Street and the interurban existed until 1940. The building then became the bus station. The Walden Inn is located on its site.

DePauw students did not spend all their time in classrooms, dormitories, boarding houses, or fraternity and sorority houses. The natural beauty of Putnam County invited excursions into the countryside, normally in this period by horse and carriage rented from a local livery stable. One of the more popular resorts was Cataract, or Eel River, Falls in the southern part of the county. Here two small waterfalls – the Upper Falls and the Lower Falls – were surrounded by a shady glade providing a perfect setting for picnic lunches and sightseeing walks. An equally long and pleasurable ride took one to the Cliffs of Fern, near the Fern Station of the Vandalia Railroad about 12 miles west of Greencastle. The large sandstone cliffs "covered with rare giant ferns and moss with good cold spring water available" along with the virgin hardwood forest, wild flowers, and meandering creek attracted students to the spot for recreation as well as for botany field trips. At one time it became so popular that the railroad ran excursion trains to it from Terre Haute and Indianapolis.

In another direction lay the Halfway House, a former stagecoach stop on the Old National Road in Mt. Meridian, about 12 miles southeast of Greencastle. Taking its name from its location halfway between Indianapolis and Terre Haute, the old inn, built of logs covered by weatherboard remained an important center of student social life until the mid-1920s. Many a romance began en route to or from Halfway House for an evening dinner. Indeed, university regulations expressly forbade couples traveling there in a "single rig," or two-seated buggy. Fraternities and sororities and other congenial college groups held parties there; even the faculty occasionally patronized the hostelry. Within its unpretentious exterior were well-furnished dining facilities. In a low-ceilinged dining room over a long table hung red oil lamps with glass pendants. On the table itself were many refined accoutrements to fine dining such as vinegar castors, stemmed compotes, and butter dishes. The cooking itself followed the native Hoosier tradition, with lots of fried chicken, dumplings, and home baked bread cut lengthwise. For dessert there were mince, pumpkin, and apple pies and the specialty of the house, cherry preserves.

A place students often visited closer to campus was McLean Springs, near Limedale on the Manhattan Road within hiking distance of the campus. The clear springs here were so attractive that plans were formulated to bring in electric lights and make it a summer resort, but nothing came of the idea. A shorter walk south of the city took one to Forest Hill Cemetery with its grassy slopes among the tombstones. To the west was Sunset Hill, along the ridges behind present-day Blackstock Stadium, where student sweethearts could watch the evening star appear. Another place was the "Wall," a stone farm fence along Indianapolis Road at its juncture with Franklin Street about where the McDonald's franchise is today. Pittman's Pond on the site of the Quonset hut used as a university store room was available for boating in summer and skating in winter.

In Greencastle students could ride the Street Railway which operated from 1866 to 1890. Drawn by two horses, or sometimes by mules, wearing bells that tinkled noisily, two small closed cars with side seats and a stove in the center carried mail, baggage, and passengers from the Monon station past the hotels, the courthouse square, through the campus and on to the Vandalia station on the south edge of town.

The city boasted three hotels, where students could hold banquets and house their visitors. One was the Grand Central or Belknap Hotel, a tavern built of logs and weatherboards to which a three-story brick addition had been made. More luxurious was the Commercial Hotel, originally known as the Jones Hotel and from 1880 to 1896 as Walnut Street House. It was famous for its mirrors and chandeliers as well as good dining. Closest to campus was the Crawford House which opened for business in 1908 on Seminary Street across from the interurban station. Its proprietor, "Greasy Fred" Crawford, hired DePauw men as waiters and catered to students and traveling salesmen.

Affording students an escape route to the joys of big city life was the Terre Haute, Indianapolis, and Eastern Interurban Railroad which ran through Greencastle from 1907 to 1940. An hour's trip brought one to the "sin city" of Terre Haute or to Indianapolis for shopping, dining, or the theatre. Whole carloads of students boarded the train at the interurban station located on the present site of the Walden Inn to attend oratorical contests or athletic events.

Professor of Mathematics and Astronomy Wilbur Vincent
Brown is shown with a group of students in a surveying class
around 1914.

fighting spirit as well as the school colors. "Tigers" won out easily over such suggestions as "Yellowjackets," "Wasps," and "Yellow Demons," and quickly attained the popular favor still evident today.

By 1918 President Grose had been able to make significant additions to the teaching faculty. Among those who were to have relatively long careers at DePauw were Lisgar R. Eckardt, another Boston Personalist, in philosophy; Raymond W. Pence, a specialist in writing, along with Edna C. Hayes in English; William W. Sweet, who replaced the popular Andrew Stephenson as head of the history department; William Wallace Carson and Katherine Alvord, also in history; Edwin B. Nichols in Romance languages; Rufus Town Stephenson in Greek language and literature; and Walter N. Hess in biology. Classicist Stephenson also introduced courses in art history in a new department by that name.

Important administrative changes were also made. In addition to her history teaching duties, Katherine Alvord took on the office of dean of women and soon became a powerful influence in the lives of DePauw coeds. Lisgar Eckhardt also was made part-time dean of freshman men. From 1914 to 1916 DePauw alumnus Charles D. Anderson served as the first executive secretary to the president. Another recent graduate, Catherine Tillotson (McCord), began her long service to the university as cashier in the treasurer's office in 1918. The university support staff had grown to include a director of residence halls, superintendent of buildings and grounds, and an engineer.

In the meantime the entry of the United States into the First World War in April 1917 brought disruption to the campus somewhat comparable to that of the Civil War era. Intercollegiate athletic events were called off for the remainder of the semester, and men began drilling each afternoon under the command of the director of physical education. Not to be outdone, women students signed up for Red Cross first-aid classes, and some even practiced military drill themselves.

Before the close of the academic year 62 men had left campus for military service and 42 for farm work. Classes opened in the fall with 140 fewer students enrolled than the previous year, and men continued to withdraw during the next several months. Students and faculty started war gardens, subscribed to relief funds, purchased Liberty Bonds, and sent Christmas boxes to men in the service. In August 1918 DePauw contracted to take part in the belatedly organized Students' Army Training Corps and sent 17 students and two faculty members to a

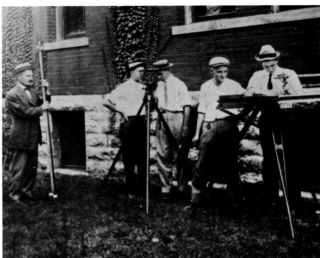

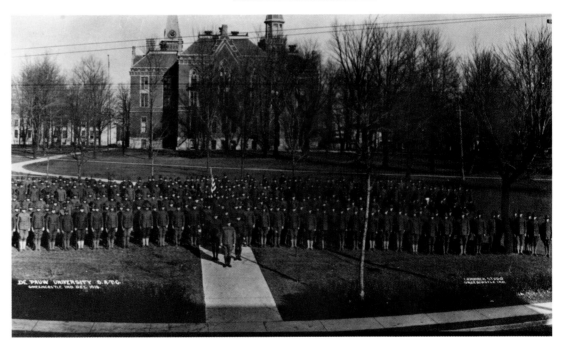

DePauw unit of the Student Army Training Corps (SATC) organized in the fall of 1918.

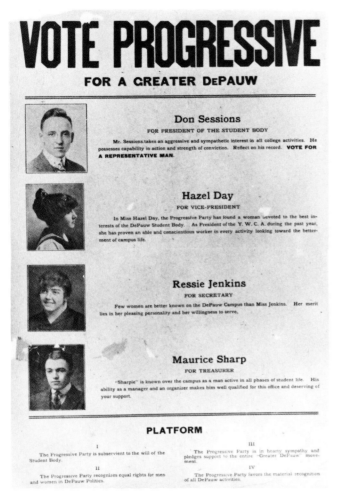

VOTE PROGRESSIVE

FOR A GREATER DePAUW

Don Sessions

FOR PRESIDENT OF THE STUDENT BODY

Mr. Sessions takes an aggressive and sympathetic interest in all college activities. He possesses capability in action and strength of conviction. Reflect on his record. **VOTE FOR A REPRESENTATIVE MAN.**

Hazel Day

FOR VICE-PRESIDENT

In Miss Hazel Day, the Progressive Party has found a woman devoted to the best interests of the DePauw Student Body. As President of the Y. W. C. A. during the past year, she has proven an able and conscientious worker in every activity looking toward the betterment of campus life.

Ressie Jenkins

FOR SECRETARY

Few women are better known on the DePauw Campus than Miss Jenkins. Her merit lies in her pleasing personality and her willingness to serve.

Maurice Sharp

FOR TREASURER

"Sharpie" is known over the campus as a man active in all phases of student life. His ability as a manager and an organizer makes him well qualified for this office and deserving of your support.

PLATFORM

I
The Progressive Party is subservient to the will of the Student Body.

II
The Progressive Party recognizes equal rights for men and women in DePauw Politics.

III
The Progressive Party is in hearty sympathy and pledges support to the entire "Greater DePauw" movement.

IV
The Progressive Party favors the material recognition of all DePauw activities.

Progressive Party campaign poster for student offices. Don Sessions became a successful businessman; Hazel Day, the wife of Grafton Longden and daughter-in-law of Professor Henry B. Longden; and Ressie Jenkins, a homemaker and wife of Julien Fix of Crown Point, Indiana.

summer training program at Camp Sheridan. On October 1, 500 men were inducted into the S.A.T.C. in a ceremony near the Boulder.

The old West College gymnasium became a mess hall and the Little Theater a barracks, along with Florence Hall, while Rosabower was transformed into an infirmary and the East College basement provided space for the post exchange and barber shop. After the Armistice in November 1918 the short-lived military program was phased out, and the campus returned to normal. University buildings reverted to their former uses, and academic life resumed its ordinary pace. Moreover, the university received compensation from the federal government for every dollar expended on conversion to military purposes.

FROM HOBO TO COLLEGE GRADUATE

Two stories of unusual student careers during this period illustrate the opportunities DePauw could provide for needy youth who showed ambition and a capacity for hard work.

A young hobo stopped at the back door of Women's Hall in 1891 to ask for a handout. Learning that he was on a college campus, he found that he could go to school by working at odd jobs. He entered the preparatory department and stayed there three years until he could qualify to enter the college. During summers the old wanderlust would overcome him, and he would roam the land again, returning each autumn to Greencastle. Finally he conquered his nomadism and stayed on campus long enough to graduate in 1898. He was so successful in finding jobs that he developed his own employment agency, finding work for other needy students. He graduated with a bachelor of science in 1898, served in the Spanish-American War, returned to Indiana University where he earned an M.D. degree in 1903, married an Eminence, Ind. girl and moved to China, Texas, where he became a respected and well-to-do-physician, Dr. Nelson Elbert Laidacker.

In the other instance a young man came to town in 1909 and pitched a tent south of Greencastle on the abandoned railroad right-of-way. He was arrested by authorities when suspicious neighbors reported him for a crime he did not commit. He spent some time before he convinced authorities of his real status as a DePauw student. No one knew where he had come from. Having only enough money for his books and tuition, he carried his books and clothing and tent with him when he came to town. Sympathetic citizens, learning of his real identity, let him work for lodging and board in their homes. Four years later John Egbert Frazeur '13 graduated with Phi Beta Kappa honors from DePauw, where he was vice-president of the Preachers' Club.

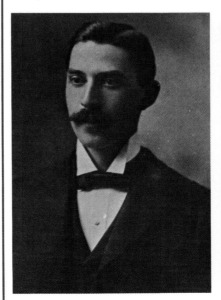

Nelson E. Laidacker

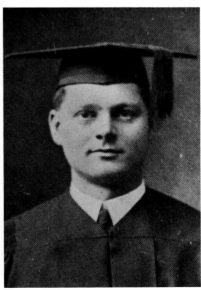

John E. Frazeur

97

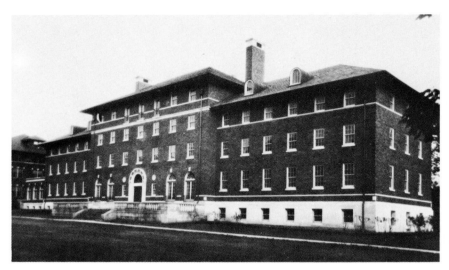

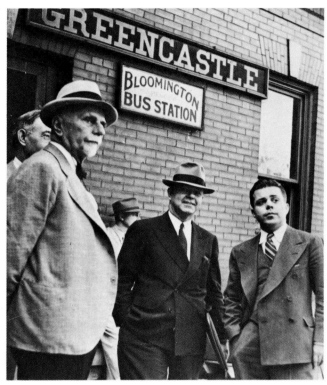

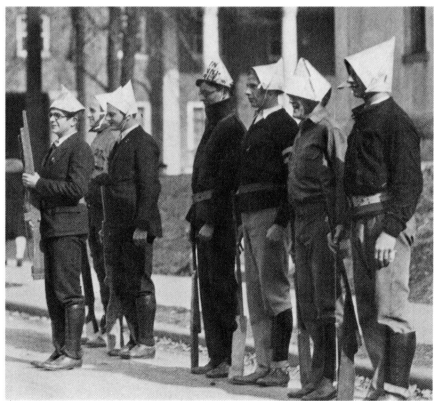

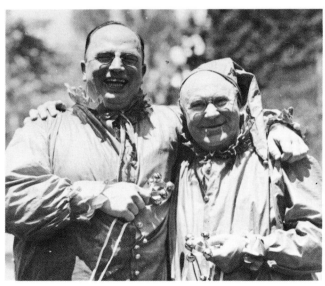

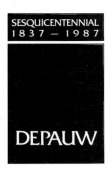

Chapter 3

DEPAUW BETWEEN THE WARS, 1918-1941

The restoration of peace after the First World War ushered in a period of prosperity and growth for the university as for the nation. Not only did annual deficits become a thing of the past, but contributions from generous benefactors swelled the endowment and underwrote the construction of important new facilities. For almost a decade DePauw's student population rose steadily, passing the 1,000 mark in 1919 for the first time since the closing of the Academy and reaching 1,800 in the 1925-26 academic year.

To meet the additional teaching responsibilities, the instructional staff expanded rapidly. In the fall of 1919 the faculty gained a dozen new members, the largest number added in a single year up to that time. Most of them remained long enough—some for over 30 years—to have a major impact on the institution. The group included Walter F. Bundy in Bible; Truman G. Yuncker in botany; A. Virginia Harlow and Lester E. Mitchell in English; George B. Manhart in history; Frank T. Carlton in economics; Anna E. Olmstead (Raphael) in French and German; and Margery Simpson (Hufferd) in physics. Among those arriving in the next few years were John L. Beyl and Oscar H. Williams in education and psychology; Ralph W. Hufferd in chemistry; Catherine F. MacLaggan, Mildred Dimmick, and Percy G. Evans in Romance languages; Andrew Wallace Crandall in history; Herrick E.H. Greenleaf and William Clarke Arnold in mathematics; William R. Sherman in economics; Ernest R. Smith in geology, a new department added in 1921; Robert E. Williams in speech; Lilian B. Brownfield, Elsie D. Taylor, Lloyd B. Gale, Jerome C. Hixson, William A. Huggard, and Judith K. Sollenberger in English; George R. Gage in biology; Ruth E. Robertson in Latin; Cleveland P. Hickman in zoology; Edward R. Bartlett in religious education, a department he created in 1923; and Rheamona Green, Samuel C. Ham, Margaret Pearson (Sage), and Eugene C. Hassell in the Music School.

The administrative staff also expanded to handle the widening sphere of university operations deemed necessary in an institution of higher education in the 20th century. Harrison M. Karr served from 1920 to 1922 as an assistant to the president in carrying out the increasing tasks of that office. His successor, DePauw graduate M. Henry McLean, also undertook the duties of alumni secretary and editor of the *Alumni Bulletin*, in the first systematic attempt to keep in touch with former students. After 1922 the work of keeping track of student records required the efforts of a full-time registrar, Marion Bradford (Crandall), who took the place of a series of faculty members who held that post in addition to their teaching duties.

For lack of a faculty pension plan, many professors continued in active service well into their seventies; former President Gobin did not retire from teaching until he reached the age of 80 in 1922. In that same year, however, the trustees devised DePauw's first systematic pension program, making retirement optional at 65 but compulsory at 72—the latter provision not applying to anyone who had joined the faculty before 1885. Retirees would receive a pension amounting to one-half of their salary at the time of retirement, with widows obtaining two-thirds of that sum. Later a more elaborate system affiliated with the Carnegie Foundation-backed Teachers Insurance and Annuity Association was adopted; pensions were then based on annuities financed by contributions by both the university and individual faculty members.

The demise of the wartime military training program was followed by the establishment in January 1918 of a unit of the Reserve Officers' Training Corps under the command of Captain John L. Frazee, who had directed the former S.A.T.C. on the DePauw campus. He was succeeded within a few months by Captain—later Major—Martyn H. Shute, whose appropriate surname inspired the nickname of "Don't Shoot." In a close vote the trustees decreed that participation in the program should be compulsory for all able-bodied freshman and sophomore males, thus reverting to a practice of the last quarter of the 19th century, when the university's cadet corps was in its heyday. Upperclassmen who took the advanced military classes and

Photos on opposite page, clockwise from upper left:

Lucy Rowland women's dormitory was dedicated in 1928 and, except for World War II, has housed freshman women for 60 years.

Waiting at the Greencastle Interurban Bus station are Professor Henry B. Longden, President Clyde Wildman, and Admissions Secretary Robert Farber.

G. Bromley Oxnam and Robert G. McCutchan.

Lineup of an honorary fraternity hazing in front of the College Church on College Avenue in 1927.

attended a summer training camp were eligible for commissions as second lieutenants in the U.S. Army Reserve upon graduation. DePauw's R.O.T.C. unit frequently won high commendations from military officials, but opposition to its presence on campus gradually mounted in the ensuing years, especially in Methodist and pacifist circles. It was often noted that DePauw was apparently the only Methodist-related college or university to maintain a compulsory military training program of that kind.

Interest in athletics resumed after the war with renewed emphasis on intercollegiate competition. In 1921 alumni, who were primarily responsible for the oversight of the program through the DePauw Athletic Board, formed a new advisory council of 100 men which met annually in Indianapolis and helped to recruit promising athletes. President Grose was moved to remind the university constituency that it "must not yield to the prevalent wild craze over athletics." The next year DePauw joined with other colleges and universities in the state, large and small, in forming the Indiana Intercollegiate Athletic Conference, which adopted the rules and regulations of the Big Ten Conference. DePauw still scheduled football, baseball, and basketball games with such rising athletic powers as Notre Dame, Purdue, and Indiana University for a few years. The need for better outdoor athletic facilities was met by the gift of $25,000 by Ira B. and Mary H. Blackstock in 1921 for that purpose. Two years later Blackstock Field was dedicated in a football game with Franklin College on Old Gold Day, 1923. Comprising a sodded gridiron and baseball diamond as well as a quarter-mile track, it superceded the smaller McKeen Field, which was diverted chiefly to intramural athletics.

The outstanding accomplishment of the immediate postwar years was the creation of the Rector Scholar-

ship Foundation, first proposed in June 1919 by Edward Rector, the Chicago lawyer and philanthropist who had already financed the construction of a women's dormitory named for his father. His aim in setting up the foundation was to attract to DePauw many of the best and brightest graduates of Indiana high schools by awarding scholarship grants covering all college fees to 100 young men of high academic standing and character each year. Women were originally excluded from the program on the grounds that their rising numbers at the university were overtaxing housing and other facilities. Later this ban was lifted and eligibility also extended to graduates of any commissioned high school in the

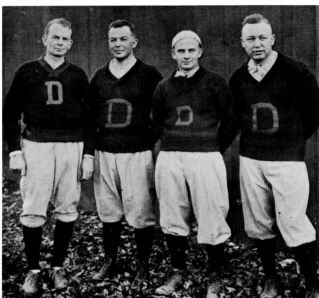

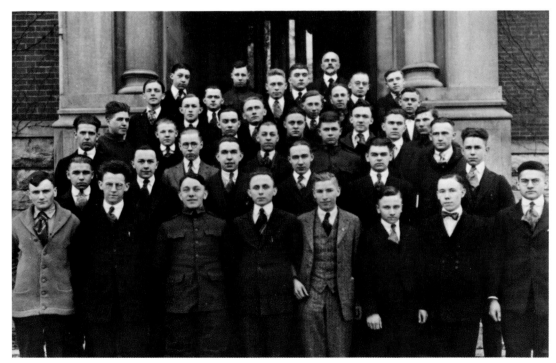

The first class of Rector Scholars in 1919-1920, which included many who went on to distinguished careers in many fields. Dr. Longden is standing in the last row.

In 1922 President Grose was on leave of absence in China to write a biography of Bishop Bashford. The Mirage of 1922 provided this cartoon.

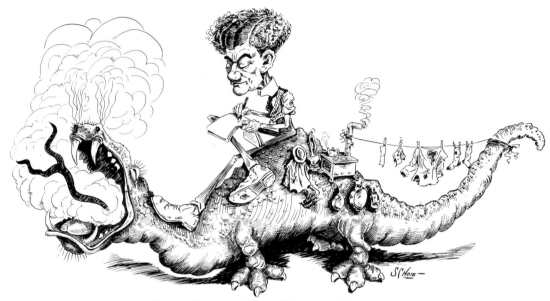

PREXY RIDES IN STATE THROUGH CHINA

The 1923 DePauw Debate Team. Top row, from left: Jerome Mikesell, Erwin Keller. Second row: Glenn Funk, Robert Conder, William McFadden, Robert Cushman. Bottom row: Professor Harry Gough, Eleanor Theek, Lawrence Cloe, Professor Robert Williams.

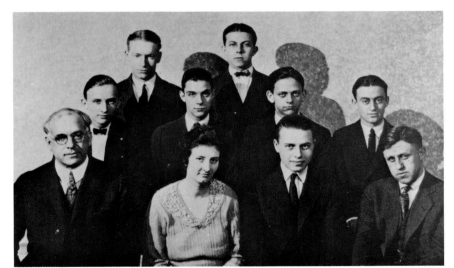

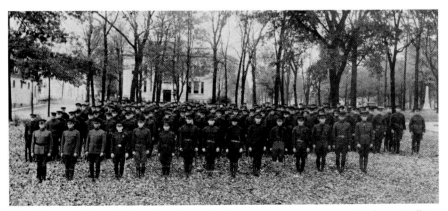

The Reserve Officers' Training Corps lined up on the present site of Asbury Hall in 1921. In the background is the Carnegie Library and in the right rear, the Roberts Grave.

country, not only those in Indiana.

Rector named Professor Henry B. Longden the first secretary of the foundation, which eventually reached a total funding of nearly $2.5 million, a considerable addition to the university's resources. Moreover this farsighted program contributed immensely to the intellectual life of the university by helping to subsidize the DePauw education of thousands of highly qualified students, many of whom would be otherwise unable to attend college.

President Grose spent the 1921-22 academic year in China on a special leave granted him for the purpose of gathering materials for a biography of James Bashford, the well-known Methodist bishop in that country. He published his findings in book form in 1922. Upon Grose's return to campus he devoted most of his remaining tenure as president to the successful prosecution of a million-dollar endowment campaign. Finally, in 1924 he was himself elected a bishop of the Methodist Episcopal Church and left Greencastle to take up his new post in China. He later returned to the United States to become the editor of a religious periodical in California. A final contribution to DePauw University was a short biographical sketch of Edward Rector published in 1928. Grose died in 1953.

To replace Grose the trustees sought an experienced college administrator, preferably a DePauw alumnus, who could attend to the internal affairs of the university at a time when enrollments were burgeoning and student unrest was rising. They turned to Lemuel H. Murlin, who had earned both a B.A. and S.T.B. from DePauw and had served as president of Baker and Boston Universities. At 63, Murlin was far older than any other president of the university at the time of election to that office and admittedly in poor health.

He accepted the post on the condition that he not be called upon to undertake a financial campaign and undoubtedly looked upon it as less taxing than the presidency of Boston University, which he had just led through a period of major growth. His wife, the former Ermina Falass, was also familiar with DePauw, having earned one of the first Ph.D.s awarded by the institution and taught in the preparatory department. The Murlins did not arrive on campus until February 1925, when they moved into rented accommodations until the new presidential home—a large Georgian Revival structure on Wood Street purchased by the university—was ready for occupancy.

President Murlin set the tone for his administration by canvassing students, faculty, alumni, and others to obtain suggestions concerning the university's needs. In an attempt to strengthen the academic program he established faculty committees dealing with educational policy and the curriculum. A new statement of purpose that stood unchanged for decades was adopted. In it the university's intellectual aim was described as "to encourage the search for truth, to develop the ability to think clearly, accurately, constructively, and fearlessly on all subjects, and to express (one's) thoughts effectively." On Murlin's recommendation the faculty also voted to restrict admission to the university to those graduating in the upper two-thirds of their high school class.

One of Murlin's first steps was to deal with the athletic situation at DePauw. Dissatisfaction had been mounting with the alumni-controlled Athletic Board, which managed all intercollegiate sports, hiring and firing coaches, recruiting athletes, and handling financing. Persuading the trustees to eliminate the Athletic Board, he restored control of intercollegiate sports to a committee composed of members of the faculty and administration and named William L. Hughes to the dual position of professor of physical

Left: Lemuel H. Murlin was president of DePauw from 1925 to 1928. A graduate of DePauw in 1891, he came to preside over the university after 13 years as president of Boston University.

Right: Ermina Fallass was one of three who earned a Ph.D. degree from DePauw (1888). She then taught history and mathematics in the preparatory department from 1888 to 1891. She became the wife of President Lemuel H. Murlin (1925-1928) and left a bequest to endow the President's office.

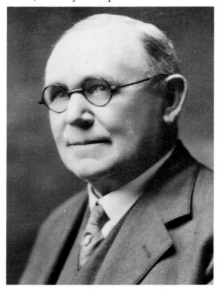 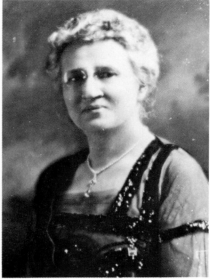

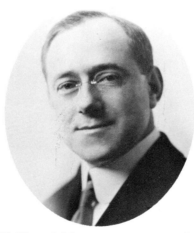

W. Henry McLean was assistant to the president for seven years from 1923 to 1929. He was designated Alumni Secretary in 1923 and was editor of the Alumni Bulletin. He was also instructor in a class in College Essentials.

education and director of athletics. For the first time all athletic activities, both intercollegiate and intramural, as well as the required physical education work, came under the authority of a regular department of the university. Besides Hughes the physical education department gained the services of William E. Search, Donavan C. Moffett, and Catherine Riggs, who joined Leroy C. Buchheit, Rachel J. Benton, and Lucy T. Bowen.

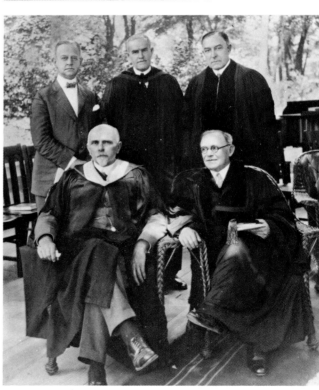

The Lemuel H. Murlin inauguration in 1925 brought together top row, left to right: benefactor Edward Rector, Bishop Frederick Leete of the Indiana Methodist Episcopal Church, Roy O. West, president of the Board of Trustees. Seated: Vice-President Henry B. Longden, and new president Lemuel H. Murlin (1925-1928).

Robert Guy McCutchan came to DePauw in 1911 as Dean of the School of Music and Professor of the History of Music. A graduate of Simpson College, he had a Doctorate in Sacred Music from Southern Methodist University. Director of the University Choir, McCutchan created a truly professional Music School. He retired in 1937 after 26 years on the faculty.

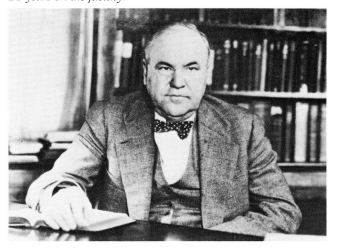

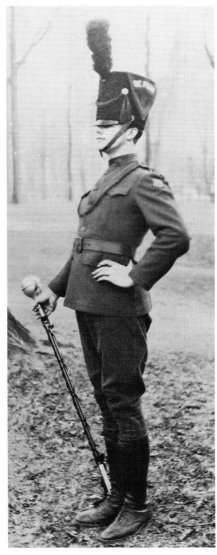

Drum Major Earl Morton of the class of 1924.

DEAN ALVORD: DEPAUW'S UNCROWNED QUEEN

For 21 years from 1915 to 1936, Dean Katherine Alvord ruled over the personal and social life of DePauw coeds with a kindly but firm hand. She was the first member of the faculty with primary responsibility for such a task, though she also taught a course in American colonial history each semester. Holding a B.A. from Michigan and M.A. from Columbia, she came to DePauw at the age of 44, having taught both high school and college classes and supervised a women's dormitory at the University of Wisconsin. She also was strongly recommended by the author of a recent book on the then new profession of dean of women.

She proved more than adequate to the difficult task of guiding the university's policies and practices for female students. Her tenure lasted from the prewar period through the social rebellion of the 1920s and 1930s and the accompanying changes in dress, behavior, and the social, economic, and political roles of women. Balancing pressures from the Methodist Church, the faculty and trustees, and traditional parents, she maintained discipline while gradually liberalizing regulations and expanding the horizons of her charges. Dean Alvord knew the name of every coed and was held in awe and admiration by most.

Ahead of her time, she advocated university sponsorship of social dancing and remedial gymnastic exercises for women. She extended the permission for men to visit women in the parlors of their living units from two evenings to any evening in the week. "Any night but not every night," was her prescription for dating. She also helped to organize the Women's Self-government Association, the Association of Women Students and the Women's Sports Association, as well as the DePauw chapter of the women's honorary society, Mortar Board. Though she would not have called herself a feminist, Dean Alvord encouraged DePauw coeds to be independent-minded, widen their vocational opportunities, and strive to attain self-fulfillment.

She retired in 1936 to her home in Gaylordsville, CT, with the final statement, "I've thoroughly enjoyed my work, almost every bit of it." She died in 1960 at the age of 88. There is a plaque in her honor in Rector Hall. Perhaps even more appropriate to her memory are the anonymous lines found on a mimeographed sheet in her correspondence in the DePauw archives under the title, "Dean Alvord: The Uncrowned Queen."

"We will march, march on down the field
Shouting for a real DePauw.
Break through Dean Alvord's line her strength to defy.
We'll give a loud cheer for DePauw's men,
We're here to win again.
FIGHT, FIGHT DEAN ALVORD TO THE BITTER END."

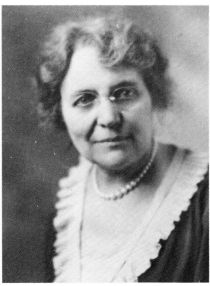

Katherine S. Alvord was Dean of Women and Professor of History from 1915 to 1936, a period of great change at DePauw in the status of coeds.

ATHLETICS

The Naiad women's swim team shown in the old Bowman swimming pool - steam pipes, wooden benches, and all. After 1932 Naiad was most active in syncronized swimming meets and prepared elaborate water pageants.

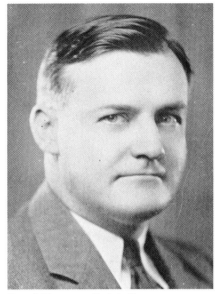

Coach Donovan C. Moffett.

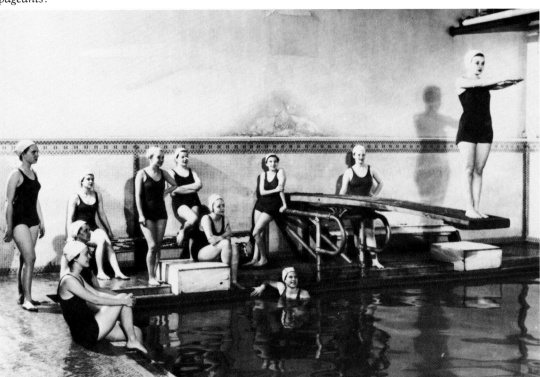

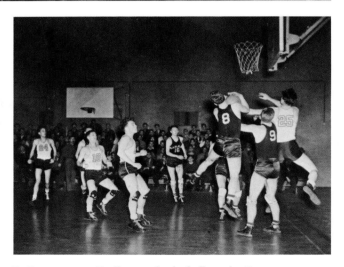

DePauw versus Earlham in basketball on the Bowman Gymnasium floor in 1938-39.

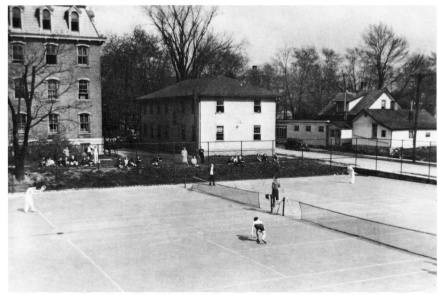

The university tennis courts behind Bowman Gymnasium. In the rear, from left to right, are part of the Music School, the Music School Annex, and across Chestnut Street the back of the Double Decker campus "hangout."

Pep talk for the football team in the locker room of Blackstock Stadium by Coach Raymond "Gaumey" Neal who led the 1933 undefeated, untied, unscored upon team. Neal's record at DePauw for 14 years was 80-34-6.

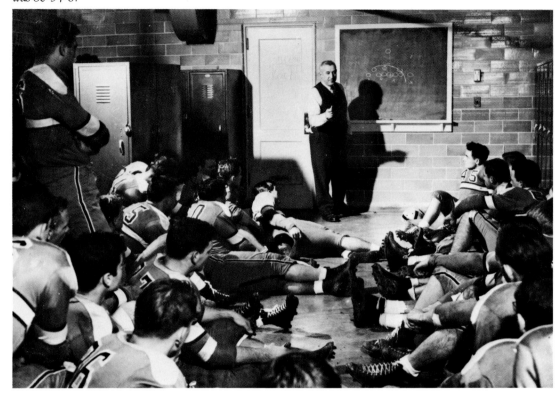

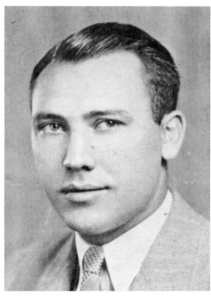

Coach Lloyd Messersmith

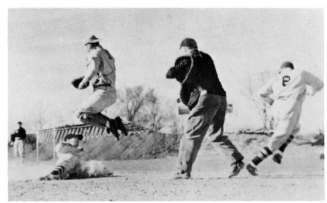

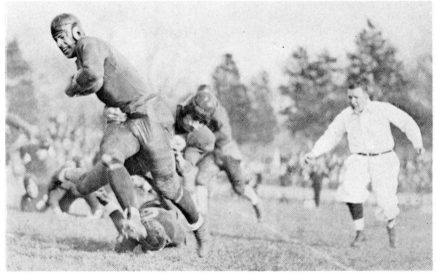

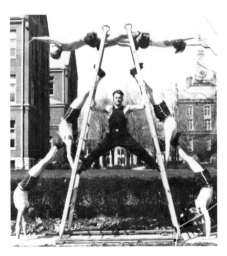

Above left: *The baseball team in action in back of Blackstock Stadium in 1941.*

Above: *Robert Fribley, member of the all-State team, is being tackled in the Wabash game of 1935, which DePauw dropped to Wabash 7-6.*

Left: *Work on the Roman Ladders in gymnastics shows an early emphasis in the DePauw athletic program.*

Under the new system interest in athletics rose to greater heights. Hundreds of students, both men and women, participated actively in intramural sports, while varsity teams chalked up winning seasons in baseball, football, basketball, and track. A disproportionately large number of the first persons named to DePauw's Athletic Hall of Fame came from this period, including John W. Ward '27, Andrew J. Ramsey '30, Marion L. Crawley '30, and Mary Washburn (Conklin) '28. The last went on to become the only DePauw athlete to win a medal in the Olympic Games, when she competed in the women's 400 meter relay race in Amsterdam in the year of her graduation.

To strengthen the administration, Dean Edwin Post was joined in 1926 by an associate dean who was placed in charge of academic affairs. The first incumbent of this office, Professor William W. Sweet of the history department, resigned the next year to accept a position at the University of Chicago. He was succeeded by Professor William M. Blanchard of the chemistry department, who was to have a long tenure in the deanship. Moreover, two decades after the naming of a dean of women, the post of dean of men was created in 1926. Named to that position was Louis H. Dirks, an experienced school administrator from Indianapolis,

who was also appointed professor of secondary education. It is noteworthy, however, that all these administrators, as well as the dean of women and the dean of freshman men, remained part-time members of the teaching faculty.

The growing student body, which neared 2,000 by the mid-1920s, created a demand for an expansion of the faculty. Among those added to the teaching staff in the Murlin administration were Coen G. Pierson and William A. Russ in history; Mary G. Hamilton and Jarvis C. Davis in English; Ermina M. Mills in comparative literature; Harold Zink and Harry W. Voltmer in political science; Orrin H. Smith in physics; Grace Barkley in botany; Lester M. Jones in sociology; Carroll D. W. Hildebrand, another Boston Personalist, in philosophy; W. Vernon Lytle and Warren C. Middleton in the newly independent department of psychology; Waldo F. Mitchell in economics; Herold T. Ross in speech; Earl C. Bowman in education; Benjamin H. Grave in zoology; and William S. Martin in Romance languages. The School of Music added Kenneth P. Umfleet, Edna T. Bowles, Rowland Leach, and Marjorie Lower.

Murlin was also able to raise faculty compensation slightly, though the average full professor's salary remained below $3,500 a year. To meet the increasing

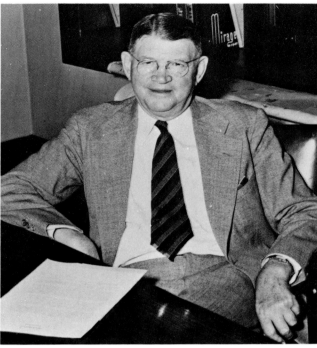

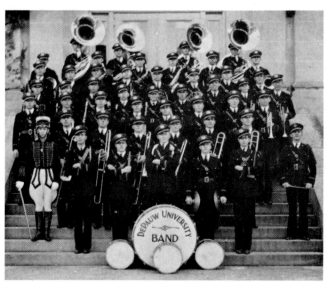

The DePauw University Band on the steps of Bowman Gymnasium in 1935.

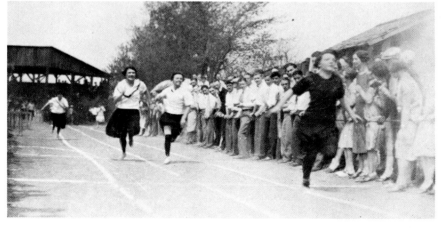

Mary Washburn, later Olympics runner and member of the DePauw Athletic Hall of Fame, leading the women's track race in 1927.

This group picture of faculty on the East College steps appeared in the 1924 Mirage.

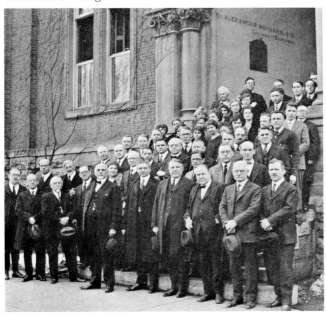

C. Howard Taylor, minister of the College Church and later Gobin Memorial Methodist Episcopal Church, was the father-in-law of later Professor Percival Allen and grandfather of DePauw astronaut Joseph Allen. In the main photo, students enter the College Church (old College Avenue Methodist) for Sunday service in 1927.

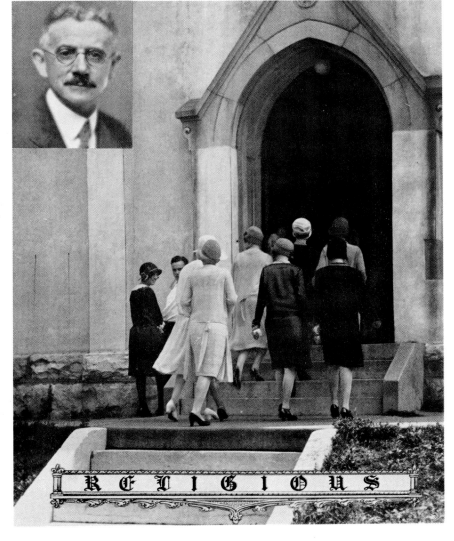

financial needs of the university he attempted to raise student fees but ran into the opposition of those who argued that DePauw would become a rich man's school. The board of trustees originally complied with his request by increasing the so-called incidental fee from a modest $85 to $125 per semester but rescinded it a year later.

As an experienced administrator, Murlin refused to be intimidated by outside attacks on the academic freedom of the faculty. When members of the North Indiana Methodist Conference circulated reports about the alleged lack of orthodoxy in the teaching of the English Bible at DePauw, he stood firmly by the professor involved. While urging the teacher to adopt a "better pedagogical method," he asked for "the broad, tolerant spirit and open mindedness of Gamaliel and of John Wesley" in his annual report to the Methodist Annual Conferences.

Perhaps the most significant accomplishments of the short Murlin presidency lay in the administration of student affairs. DePauw students had long chafed against the university's ban on social dancing (born of the traditional Methodist view that it was immoral, along with card-playing, theatre-going and the like). Increasing numbers of students were coming from homes where dancing was permitted, and it was becoming more and more difficult to enforce the unpopular prohibition.

When President Murlin arrived at DePauw in the fall of 1925 he found overwhelming student sentiment in favor of lifting the ban but a divided faculty on this issue. Seizing upon the fact that the General Conference of the Methodist Episcopal Church had slightly relaxed its stand on the question in 1924, Murlin initiated an experimental program. Social organizations would be permitted upon special request to include dancing as part of the entertainment at one formal party each year. Official chaperones were required, as well as written permission from parents of those who participated in such dancing.

This new policy was incorporated in the 1926 *Student Handbook*, along with an excerpt from the *Methodist Discipline* warning against the evils of dancing and similar amusements. The die was cast, and, despite vehement opposition from some church quarters, social dancing soon became a recognized part of DePauw's campus activities. It has been suggested that the venerable president was able to defy conservative Methodist opinion in this matter because at his age he had no ambition for a bishopric.

Murlin also attempted to regulate such matters as fraternity rush and hazing. The introduction of house mothers — required in sorority houses since 1919 — into fraternity houses in 1926 undoubtedly served to ameliorate the sometimes rowdy behavior of their residents. A most important innovation was the creation of Freshman Week at the beginning of the fall semester as a period of orientation for new students conducted by members of the teaching faculty.

The mid-1920s was a period of intense activity in the remodeling of old and the construction of new chapter houses for the social fraternities. Nine fraternities erected rather large houses and five sororities somewhat smaller ones. Other organizations were content with the refurbishing of existing structures: Delta Upsilon in The Towers after it ceased to be used as the presidential home, and Kappa Alpha Theta in Beechcroft, the former home of Professor James Riley Weaver on South College Avenue. Some of the new residences, described by President Murlin as "large and expensive houses (covered with large, elegant, and gilt-edged mortgages)," would become a financial burden to later generations of students.

The desire to provide residential facilities for non-affiliated men and women at least equal in comfort to the best chapter houses was brought to fruition by the final gifts of Edward and Lucy Rector. At his death in 1925 Edward Rector bequeathed $500,000 to the university for the construction of two dormitories. Longden Hall, erected in 1927 and named for Professor Henry B. Longden, secretary of the Rector Scholarship Fund, offered male residents the same modern features as Rector Hall had furnished women 10 years before.

The next year Lucy Rowland Hall, named for Rector's widow, was constructed on the site of Music Hall, which was moved catty-corner to a new location next to Bowman

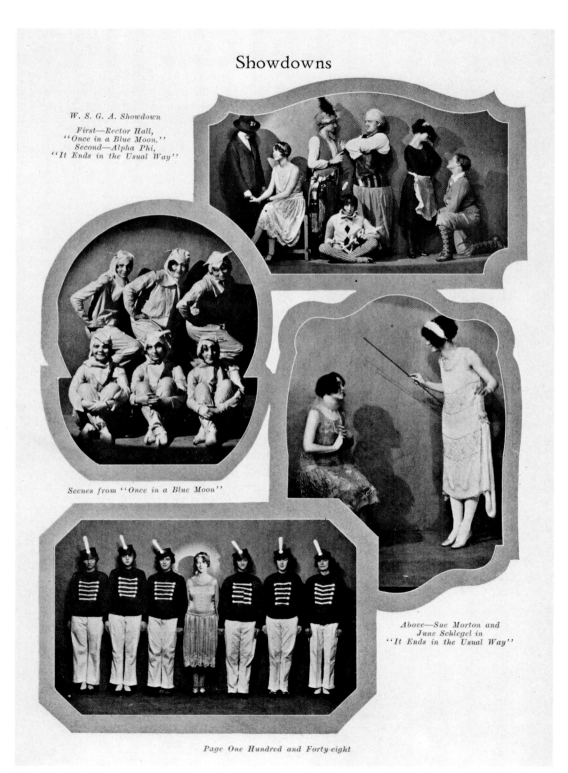

Showdowns

W. S. G. A. Showdown

*First—Rector Hall,
"Once in a Blue Moon."
Second—Alpha Phi,
"It Ends in the Usual Way"*

Scenes from "Once in a Blue Moon"

*Above—Sue Morton and
June Schlegel in
"It Ends in the Usual Way"*

Showdown first began in 1925 with a series of skits by women's groups under the auspices of the Women's Self-Government Association. Sometimes men's groups joined. Some Showdowns were so popular that they played before sell-out crowds at the Voncastle movie theater. President Murlin called his first one "a pale reflection of cheap vaudeville" whose jazz would split his head open. This picture is from the 1926 Showdown.

HUMOR AND
LITERARY MAGAZINES

In December 1914 there appeared on the DePauw campus the first issue of the *Yellow Crab*, a humor magazine sponsored by the journalism fraternity, Sigma Delta Chi. Its editors announced that the journal would accept no advertising and contain "nothing literary, nothing serious, nothing sensible." Subsequent issues, published irregularly over the next several years, became increasingly brash and risqué, often provoking the same kind of official displeasure as the boguses of an earlier era. In 1919 the faculty decreed that no further numbers could be issued without approval by university authorities. Despite this form of censorship the *Yellow Crab* continued to be a lively student publication, excerpts from it appearing occasionally in the national journal *College Humor* in the 1920s.

With its penchant for caricature and coarse humor, the magazine was unable to avoid conflict with the university administration. A former business manager, George Smock, has related how it successfully met one such challenge in 1927. Called into the Dean's office to receive a stern lecture on the offensive character of the current issue, he contritely promised to halt further sales of the issue and destroy all unsold copies. During his extended conference in the administration building, however, his energetic business staff had managed to distribute the entire printing run!

Finally, in the fall of 1932 the administration reacted to the ever racier and more audacious contents of the *Yellow Crab* by suspending its editors from the university. The national office of Sigma Delta Chi went so far as to revoke its parent chapter's charter for a time. Though the students involved were eventually reinstated and the journalistic fraternity's charter restored, *Yellow Crab* never resumed publication.

Less controversial was the *DePauw Magazine*, founded in the fall of 1919 by Professor Raymond W. Pence as a means of encouraging student literary expression. This quarterly journal contained a variety of articles, short stories, poetry, and book reviews as well as a few local advertisements to help pay printing costs. In the early 1920s Doubleday, Page, & Company collaborated with the editorial staff in the award of an annual O. Henry prize to the student submitting the best short story. The prize consisted of a complete leather-bound set of the collected works of William Sydney Porter, who wrote under the pen name O. Henry. From 1935 to 1937 the *DePauw Magazine* was issued in a larger and more attractive format, with a colorful cover and black and white illustrations. Financial constraints, however, brought about its demise in the latter year. It was not to be revived for nearly two decades.

Its successor, the *Boulder*, began publication in 1936, combining the character of both a literary and a humor magazine. Somewhat livelier than the *DePauw Magazine*, it boasted a handsome cover and filled its pages with photographs, wood-block illustrations by student art directors such as Don Booty, and short stories, poetry, a humor column, and feature articles, often controversial in content. In 1941 the *Boulder* created a minor literary sensation by publishing verses allegedly written by a former DePauw professor who had hidden them in the belfry of East College before his mysterious death in 1889. The journal also included a fictitious biography and blurred portrait of the poet. Editor Robert Hair and Professor Wisner Kinne of the English department eventually confessed to the hoax, but not before area newspapers had picked up the story and publicized it far and wide. The *Boulder* survived the war years and lingered on until 1952. While tending to become more of a general magazine dealing with campus life during its later years, it retained a solid literary section, where the early fiction of DePauw authors Jack Kennedy and John Jakes appeared.

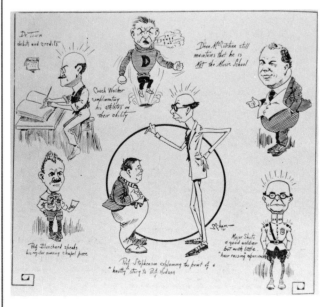

Cover of the Yellow Crab *in 1930. Controversial, clever and collegiate might be appropriate terms for this "notorious" campus humor magazine, particularly prominent in the "roaring twenties."*

Typical of Yellow Crab *humor was this cartoon depicting faculty in the December, 1930 issue of the humor magazine.*

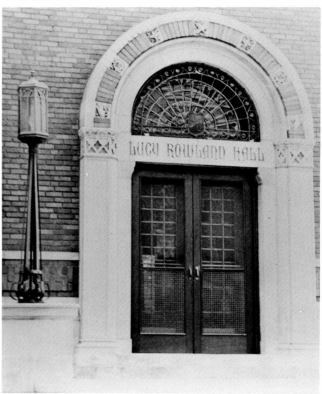

The elaborate entrance to Lucy Rowland women's dormitory erected in 1928.

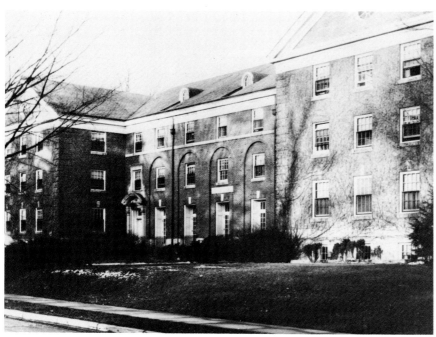

Longden Hall was completed on South College Avenue in 1927 to accommodate 117 men with its own dining room and kitchen. For the first time dormitory accommodations for men equal to those of women were provided. It was named after Professor Henry B. Longden.

Gymnasium on Hanna Street. (There, provided with a basement and a frame annex in the rear, the relocated building continued to house the School of Music for nearly a half century longer.) The construction of the new dormitory adjacent to Mansfield and Rector Halls created a residential quadrangle which housed freshman women as well as upperclass non-affiliated women. Both Lucy Rowland and Longden Halls were designed in his usual Beaux Arts eclectic style by architect Robert F. Daggett. In 1927 Katherine M. Mills became responsible for the oversight of these facilities as director of residence halls.

Longden Hall became the center of the activities of Men's Hall Association, an organization of independent men founded a few years before by a group of Florence Hall residents. M.H.A. soon became a significant force on campus, hitherto dominated by the Greek-letter social fraternities. For several

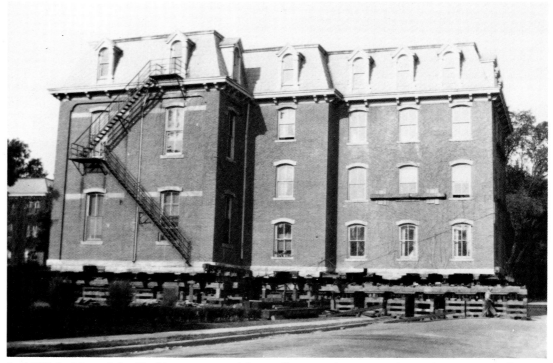

In 1927 the Music School building was moved diagonally across the street to the southwest corner of Locust and Hanna Streets to make way for the new Lucy Rowland Hall.

Meharry Hall in the 1920s with the Bowman Memorial Organ given in 1913 by President Bowman's daughter Sallie Bowman Caldwell. At that time the entire faculty would sit on the stage for each university convocation. Also the tradition had the freshman men compelled by their fraternities to sit in the balcony.

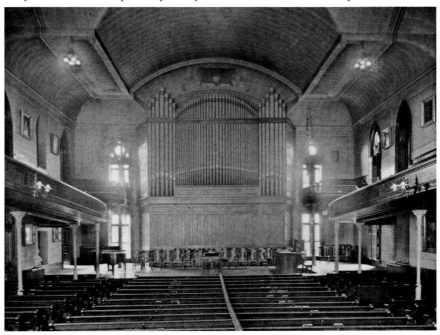

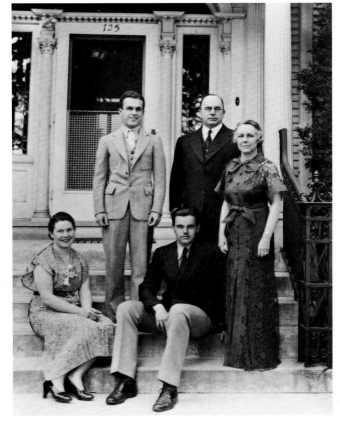

President G. Bromley Oxnam, his wife Ruth Fisher Oxnam, and their three children, Ruth, Robert, and Philip are on the steps of the President's home at the foot of East Seminary Street.

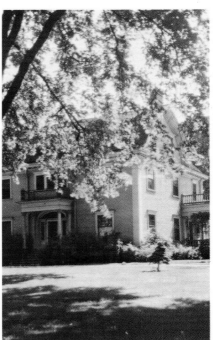

In 1926 the university purchased for its presidents the Van Arsdel home built at the foot of East Seminary Street in 1908. First occupied by the Murlins, remodelled extensively by the Oxnams, it served as the presidential home until the late 1970s when the Rossers purchased their own home closer to campus, the former St. John's Episcopal Church on East Seminary Street.

decades the independent organization competed actively in intramural athletics, student politics, and social activities. No such alternative to sorority affiliation seems to have existed at this time.

The Murlin presidency, brief as it was, covered an eventful, transitional period in DePauw's history. In 1928 the quiet but effective administrator, after experiencing repeated bouts of illness and encountering some opposition to his policies, reluctantly submitted his resignation to the board of trustees. He later served for a time as pastor of the American Church in Berlin and died in 1935. His widow bequeathed his library to the university, together with a small endowment to support the presidential office.

G. Bromley Oxnam, whom the trustees chose as Murlin's successor, was a quite different sort of college president than any of his predecessors. A graduate of the University of Southern California and the Boston University School of Theology, he had served as pastor of a large Los Angeles church before becoming professor of social ethics at Boston University. A vigorous, charismatic person, with strong convictions and a forceful speaking style, Oxnam was to achieve a high level of national and international recognition and bring DePauw an unprecedented amount of public attention during his presidential term. After taking up residence in Greencastle he not only continued his ardent advocacy of world peace and social reform but also proved to be an activist administrator bent on remolding the university in accordance with his own views.

The financial crash of 1929 and the ensuing depression created major problems for the university. Endowment income was reduced severely together with revenue from student fees as enrollment rapidly

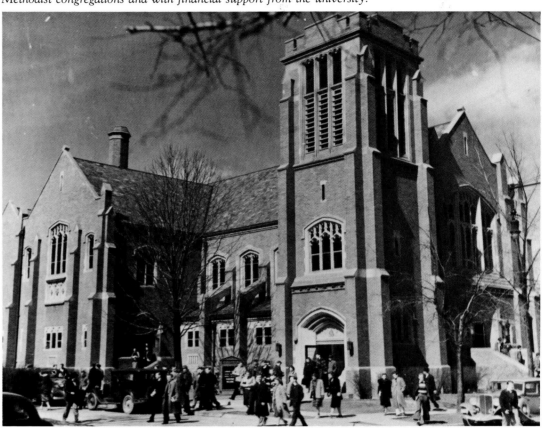

declined. The student population fell to 1600 by 1932 and dropped to the 1200 level during the mid-1930s. Despite draconian measures undertaken to balance the budget, including raising tuition fees and trimming salaries, the university books once more recorded annual deficits. Under the leadership of its president, Roy O. West, the board of trustees restructured the university's investments in an attempt to increase revenue. Real estate holdings that were producing poor returns were liquidated in favor of high-grade bonds and similar securities promising higher current income. By means of such measures DePauw managed to weather the economic storms of the period.

Part of the university's financial difficulties stemmed from the large indebtedness incurred in acquiring the two buildings formerly occupied by the Locust Street and College Avenue Churches and in constructing a new classroom building to replace the badly deteriorated West College. In 1929 the two Methodist

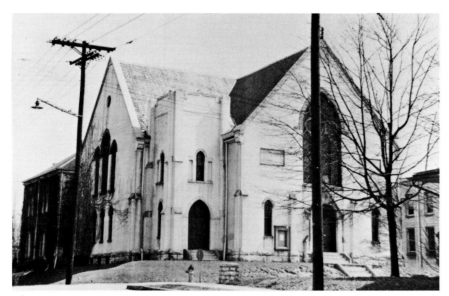

Minus its steeple the College Avenue Methodist Episcopal Church in 1929 was remodelled into Speech Hall. It housed the Speech and Education Departments (1943-1965) and its sanctuary was converted into the Little Theatre. It was torn down the summer of 1978.

congregations, having agreed to merge when the Conference boundaries separating them were redrawn, erected a large new edifice in late Gothic Revival style on university-owned land at the corner of Locust and Simpson Streets. Meanwhile the Locust Street church, its steeple removed, was utilized briefly for university theatrical performances before being refitted as an armory for the use of the R.O.T.C.

The College Avenue church, also minus its steeple, was stuccoed and remodeled into Speech Hall, which survived for five decades as the home of the Little Theatre and the speech and education departments. The university had originally planned to erect a building in conjunction with the new church which would house both the latter's educational facilities and DePauw's departments of English Bible, philosophy, and religious education and bear the name of its late

After 1927 the Locust Street Methodist Church was used by the department of public speaking to 1929 and then became the armory for the ROTC until it was disbanded in 1934. It was torn down that year.

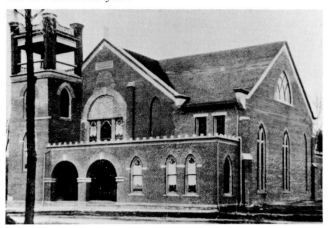

president, Hillary A. Gobin. When this project proved financially unfeasible, the newly merged congregation agreed to name its new edifice the Gobin Memorial Methodist Church in consideration of DePauw's help in paying off the building debt. In turn DePauw was permitted use of the sanctuary for chapel and similar services. While Gobin Church's architectural style and yellow-brick exterior did not harmonize closely with most of the academic buildings, the cathedral-like structure was conveniently located and came to be regarded as virtually an integral part of the campus.

In the meantime West College, the oldest building on campus, had been condemned as unsuitable for classroom use. Many alumni hoped that "Old Asbury," as the former Edifice was sometimes known, might be restored. But the trustees decided to replace the once-rebuilt structure with a new classroom facility perpetuating the memory of the pioneer Methodist bishop after whom the university had originally been named. In 1930 Asbury Hall was erected on West Campus, across from Middle College. Its construction was made possible in a time of economic depression by borrowing from the university's endowment fund as well as by special gifts. Housing the social

EDWARD AND LUCY ROWLAND RECTOR

Among the most generous benefactors of DePauw University were Edward and Lucy Rowland Rector. The wealthy, refined, childless couple virtually adopted the university—faculty, students, administration—as part of the family and lavished upon it the gifts which made possible a financial resurgence in the 1920s.

Born in Bedford, Ind. in 1863, Edward Rector worked at odd jobs after leaving school in his teens when his father suffered financial reverses. In 1882 he moved to Cincinnati, where he clerked in a law office while attending law classes. He graduated from the University of Cincinnati Law School in 1885 and began a career as a patent attorney, first in Cincinnati and then in Chicago. Through his friendship with another Chicago lawyer, DePauw alumnus and trustee Roy O. West, Rector became acquainted with DePauw President George R. Grose and took an immediate interest in the affairs of the Greencastle institution. He was named to the board of trustees in 1916 and played a large part in the capital fund campaign initiated that year.

While dining with President Grose in New York at the time of the General Conference of the Methodist Episcopal Church in the summer of 1916, Rector, a devout Methodist layman, is reported to have asked his companion what facilities DePauw University most needed. When Grose replied immediately, "a women's dormitory," the Chicago attorney pledged his personal gift of $100,000 to construct one. Rector Hall was completed in 1917 and was named for the donor's father, Isaac Rector, who had served as a trustee of the university in the late 1860s when coeducation was introduced. Two years later came the creation of the Rector Scholarship Foundation to provide scholarships at DePauw for 100 of the brightest male graduates of Indiana high schools each year. Until his death in 1925 Edward Rector visited the campus frequently and kept in touch by correspondence with many of the Rector Scholars, whose hometowns he marked on a large map of Indiana in his Chicago law office. His gifts to the university, as he explained to his fellow trustees, were "investments in humanity, in the men and women who are to carry out the work of our country and of the world when you and I are gone."

In his will Rector left a considerable part of his fortune to DePauw, the bulk of it to finance the scholarship program. He also provided $500,000 to construct two additional dormitories, one for men and one for women. The first, Longden Hall, named for Professor Henry B. Longden, was constructed in 1927. The second, Lucy Rowland Hall, was completed in 1928 and named in honor of Rector's widow, who carried on her husband's interest in DePauw for many years until her own death in 1949. Altogether, by lifetime gifts and bequests, Edward and Lucy Rector contributed a total of more than $3.8 million to DePauw.

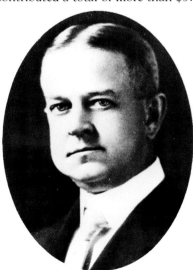

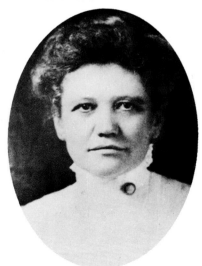

Edward Rector, trustee from 1916 to his death in 1924, founded the Rector Scholarship Foundation and was the donor of Rector Hall, Lucy Rowland Hall, and Longden Hall. He was a prominent Chicago patent lawyer.

Lucy Rowland Rector, after whom Lucy Rowland Hall was named, was the wife of donor Edward Rector. She continued a strong interest in DePauw into the 1930s and added about $143,000 in her own bequest to the Rector Scholarship Foundation.

FACULTY

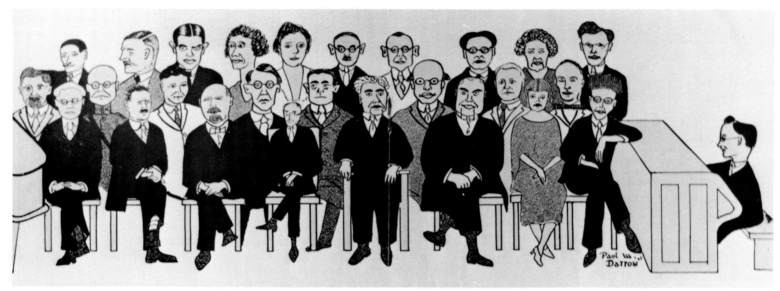

This faculty caricature appeared in the Yellow Crab in 1923. How many can you identify? We think we see Gough, Blanchard, Longden, Post, Grose, McCutchan, Alvord, Beyle, Shute, Bundy, Carson, Pence, Stephenson, Tilden, Eckardt, Hudson, Shearer, Manhart, "Rock" Smith, Thompson.

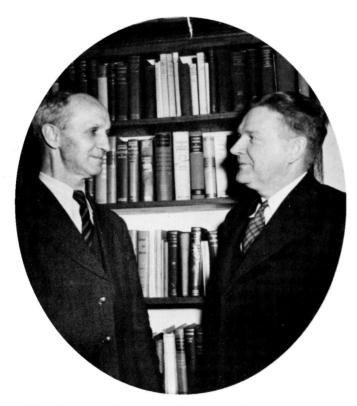

Two favorite professors were Lisgar R. Eckardt and Hiram L. Jome. Eckardt had studied at Toronto and Boston universities and taught at Iliff School of Theology before coming to teach philosophy at DePauw from 1913-45. Jome was head of the economics department from 1931-58.

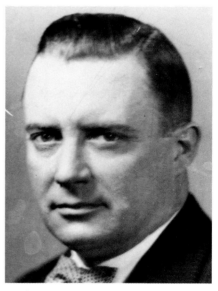

Walter E. Bundy of the class of 1912 studied theology at Boston University and Basel, where he served as vice consul during World War I. He began his 36 years of teaching and writing in Bible, particularly the synoptic gospels, in 1919.

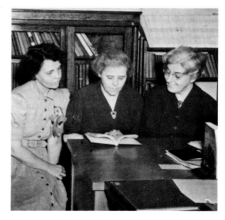

Marguerite Andrade, Anna Olmstead Raphael, Mildred Dimmick, Romance languages.

The DePauw Faculty in 1937 on the steps in front of the entrance to Lucy Rowland Hall. Left to right:
Row 1: Dirks, Ritchie, O. H. Smith, Carson, Ross, Fay, Hickman. Row 2: McCutchan, Pence, Nichols,
, , Dudgeon, Crandall, Evans, Jome, Bowman, Shearer, Taylor. Row 3: Studebaker, Riggs, Tilden,
Calvert, Yuncker, Cade, Welch, Giddings, Mueller, Rutledge, Ramsay, Mills, Thompson. Row 4:
Mintle, Huggard, , , ,Bowles, Wickersham. Row 5: Riebsomer, Arnold, Williams, Pierson,
Greenleaf, Manhart, A. A. Smith, Fulmer, Shadbolt. Row 6: Bundy, Moffett, Harlow, Stout, Siewart,
Dimmick, Voltmer, Salzer, Brooks, Messersmith, Davis, Umbreit, , Winsey, Turk, E. R. Smith, Baerg.

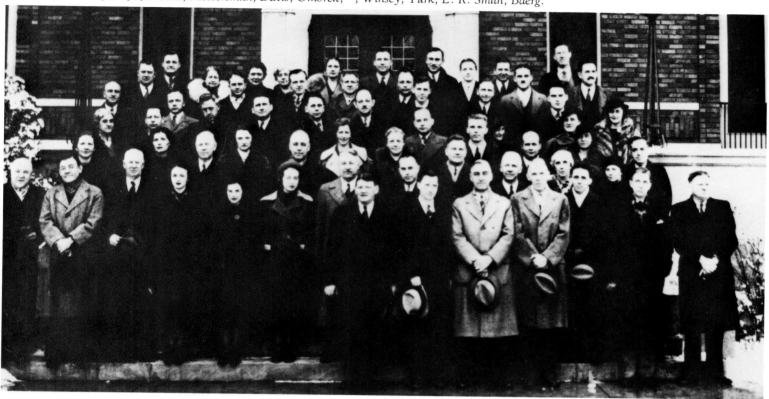

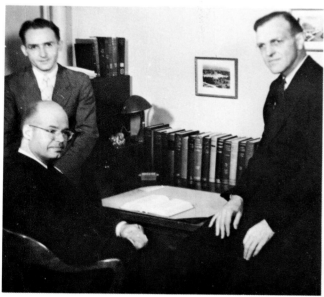

Above: Vernon Van Dyke, Harold Zink, and Harry Voltmer,
all of the political science department.

At right: William Eddington, Herrick Greenleaf, and
Clarke Arnold, of the mathematics department.

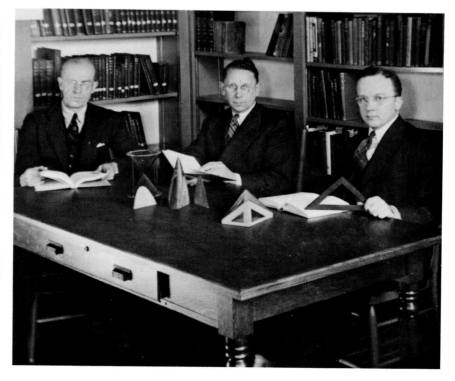

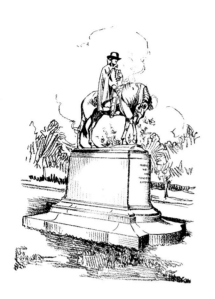

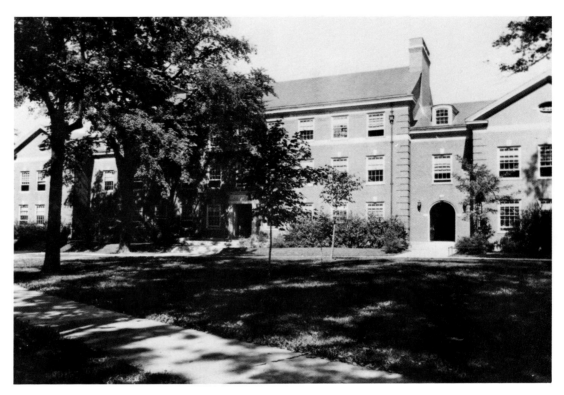

science and humanities departments, Asbury soon became one of the most frequented places on campus. A few years later West College was razed, but President Oxnam's plan for an equestrian statue of Francis Asbury on its site was never realized.

Asbury Hall also represented a new type of architecture on campus. It was designed by the indefatigable Robert F. Daggett in the Georgian or Colonial Revival mode which the board of trustees had adopted in 1929 as the official architectural style for future DePauw buildings. Its wide chimneys at either end of the central section, dormer windows and reverse-gable roof on the outer sections, and red-brick walls were typical features of the Colonial Williamsburg style that was becoming popular on many university campuses at the time and was to dominate DePauw architecture over the next few decades. In 1935 the Publications Building, financed largely by means of revenues from the student newspaper and yearbook, was constructed next to Asbury Hall in the same style. Some living units built in this period were also designed in Colonial Revival style, such as the Sigma Nu house on the corner of Seminary Street and

College Avenue. Other additions to the campus in the Oxnam administration were a new maintenance building erected behind Middle College in 1930 and a small fieldhouse at Blackstock Field, paid for from student athletic fees, in 1933. In the summer of 1931 four concrete tennis courts were built behind Bowman Gymnasium.

In the early morning hours of Sunday, October 12, 1933, fire broke out in Mansfield Hall, causing damage estimated at $100,000 to the oldest women's dormitory on campus. An intrepid coed carried Mildred Dimmick, the housemother, who had sprained her ankle, out of the burning building, but the only casualty was the president's son, Robert Oxnam, who was struck but not seriously injured by a piece of plaster while taking part in the rescue of residents' belongings. Most of the displaced women were assigned to Johnson House, a frame building on Walnut Street donated

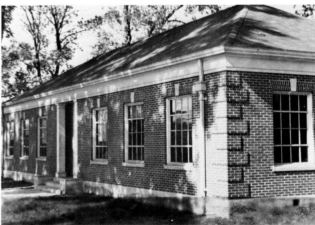

Above left: President Oxnam suggested in 1931 this type of statue honoring Bishop Asbury to be placed where the present Roy O. West Library now stands. The project never moved beyond this concept stage. Above right: Asbury Hall was dedicated in 1930. Largely housing classrooms and offices for the humanities and social science departments it has probably been the busiest building in the second half of the 20th century on the DePauw campus. Bottom photo: The Publications Building immediately west of Asbury Hall was built in 1936 entirely from funds generated by student publications.

The morning fire of October 15, 1933 gutted Mansfield Hall.

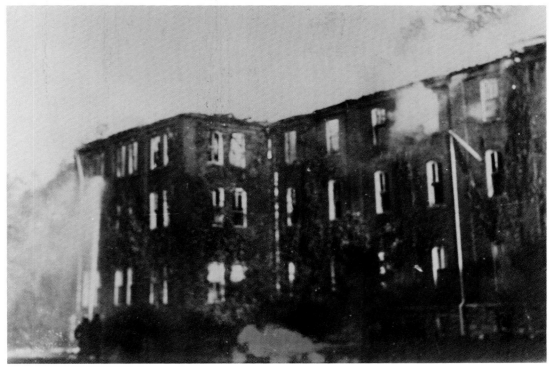

to the university some years before by Greencastle resident D. B. Johnson and used up to this time for housing male students. A few freshman sorority pledges were allowed to take up residence in their chapter houses.

After an appraisal of the partly-destroyed building that indicated the unfeasibility of restoring it, Mansfield Hall was razed and the site landscaped. The threat of fire to another building of the same vintage and type of construction brought about the evacuation of Middle College not long afterwards. The botanical and zoological laboratories were moved from the building's upper stories to a frame structure first erected as an annex to Florence Hall. Other departments were relocated in Asbury Hall, and in 1934 the old college building that had been originally designed as a men's residence hall was finally demolished, the third such campus landmark to disappear in this period. Financial constraints postponed the planned construction of a new women's dormitory, a

science classroom building, and more capacious facilities to replace the outdated Carnegie Library.

President Oxnam, concerned about reports of falling church attendance, inaugurated a special interdenominational vespers service on Sunday evenings that proved popular with students. Daily morning chapel was continued on a voluntary basis, but with religious services only on Wednesday. By 1933 this worship chapel and the Sunday evening vespers were conducted in the sanctuary of Gobin Memorial Church, its ecclesiastical setting and the robed university choir adding much to the dignity and solemnity of the occasion. On other weekdays chapel was held in Meharry Hall, featuring talks by the president, professors, or visiting speakers, with usually a musical program on Friday. President Oxnam himself was a frequent chapel speaker, sometimes choosing controversial topics dealing with

contemporary social issues or discussing his summer travels in Europe or the Orient. Through his wide contacts with pacifist and social reform circles he was able to bring to campus leading figures in those movements, including Norman Thomas, Kirby Page, and Sherwood Eddy. One program in 1935 was devoted to a student demonstration for world peace.

Shortly after his arrival on campus President Oxnam gave evidence of his own antimilitarist views by issuing an administrative order making participation in R.O.T.C. voluntary rather than compulsory. Both the faculty and the student body had discussed this idea before but without any decision being made. Despite outcries from the American Legion and similar organizations, Oxnam went even farther in 1934, calling upon the trustees to abolish the entire R.O.T.C. program at DePauw. The board quickly complied with his wishes, ending the university's second experience with student military training in peace time. On the whole, both the university and church constituency came to the support of the president in this matter against his many detractors in other quarters.

Oxnam was also eager to continue the work of his predecessor, President Murlin, in reorganizing and strengthening the university's administration. When Post retired from the deanship in 1930, Murlin elevated William M. Blanchard to dean of the university. Blanchard had been assisting Dean Post since 1927. Blanchard also acted as director of admissions, though much of the work of reviewing transcripts and the like fell to an enlarged registrar's office, headed first by Vera Worth and, after her marriage to the widowed dean in 1933, by her assistant, Veneta J. Kunter. Also active in admissions decisions was the secretary of the Rector Scholarship Foundation, Henry B. Longden.

When Longden finally retired in 1935 at the age of 75, the office of Rector secretary fell to G. Herbert Smith, who also served as dean of freshman men. To assist the admissions process, recent DePauw graduate Robert J. Farber became the first field representative, visiting Indiana high schools to interview students interested in attending the university. The dual post of director of publicity and alumni secretary was created in 1931, with F. Russell Alexander named to that office. Five years later Alexander issued the first number of the *DePauw Alumnus*, the glossy-page successor to the earlier *Alumni News*.

When the long-time treasurer, Salem B. Town, stepped down in 1929, his assistant, Harold E. Robbins took his place. Fund raising came under the jurisdiction of Byron H. Wilson, executive secretary of endowments and promotion. In 1930 Ralph E. Schenck, a civil engineer who had supervised the building of much of the physical plant in recent years while in the employ of an Indianapolis construction firm, was appointed superintendent of engineering, construction, and maintenance.

It was not until near the end of his administration, however, that President Oxnam was able to persuade the trustees to authorize the centralization of all business affairs in the new post of comptroller. Named to this office in 1935 was Superintendent Schenck, who proceeded to concentrate in it all matters relating to finances, purchasing, real estate, and the physical plant. Ernest H. Smith became the first chief accountant.

A major concern of the Oxnam administration was to strengthen the operations of the library, which did not come up to the standards of institutions with which DePauw liked to compare itself. Until 1931 the titular librarian was Professor Francis J. Tilden of the comparative literature department, who left most

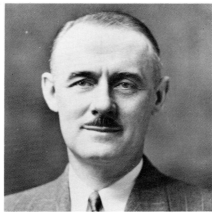

Ralph E. Schenck, representing the Colvin Construction Company, supervised the building of Longden, Lucy Rowland, and Asbury Halls, the Gobin Memorial Methodist Church and the move of the Music School. After 1930 he was superintendent of engineering, construction, and maintenance. In 1935 he became controller until faculty dissatisfaction forced his resignation in 1941.

of the work of supervising the library in the hands of an assistant, Margaret Gilmore. In that year Vera Southwick Cooper became the first professionally trained librarian to serve the university. She was soon able to increase the book budget and engage additional library staff, though the limitations of physical space in the Carnegie building prevented the enlargement of resources needed to meet the desired standards fully.

In 1932 the School of Music was completely restructured and integrated into the university. It had previously been operated more or less autonomously under the direction of Dean Robert McCutcheon. He rented facilities from DePauw and managed the school's affairs personally — collecting student fees, employing faculty, and even providing musical instruments and equipment. Now the instructional staff became regular salaried members of the faculty for the first time. Moreover, a music major and minor were accepted as part of the liberal arts degree

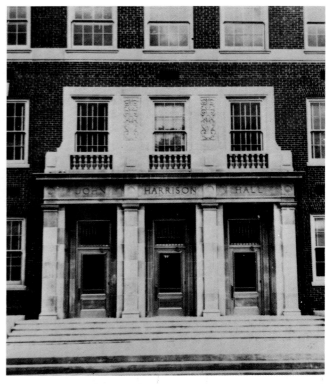

program, while the bachelor of music program was continued in force.

The residential graduate program that had existed in name since 1884 was expanded and reorganized. Several departments offered graduate work leading to a master of arts degree, and in 1931 the School of Music announced the establishment of a master of music degree. In 1934 the president appointed a graduate council to oversee the graduate program, headed by Professor William E. Edington of the mathematics department. Graduate enrollments at DePauw grew slightly but remained only a small fraction of the total and never threatened the university's basic commitment to undergraduate education.

In an endeavor to encourage high scholarship, the university in 1931 revived an honors program that had flourished in the last decades of the 19th century. Various departments

Harrison Hall, built for the departments of botany, zoology, geology and psychology, was first occupied in 1940.

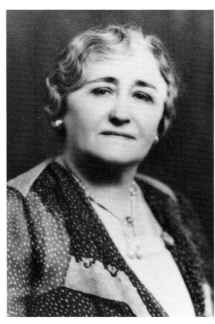

Margaret Gilmore presided behind the desk at the University Library from 1910 to 1934. Officially titled Assistant Librarian, she was in charge of routing library affairs until the arrival of a trained professional librarian in 1931.

HENRY B. LONGDEN

Henry Boyer Longden was born in Vevay, Ind., in 1860, the son of a Methodist minister. Attending both the preparatory and college departments of Indiana Asbury University, he graduated in 1881 with the intention of becoming a physician or surgeon. After trying briefly to raise money for this purpose by selling books door to door, he returned home one day to find a letter from President Alexander Martin inviting him to teach Greek and science in the preparatory department. Later he taught Latin in the College of Liberal Arts and in 1892 was named professor of German language and literature, a post he held until his retirement in 1935.

Though he had no formal graduate training, Longden was able to study at Goettingen and Leipzig during a leave in 1888-1890 and again in 1898 at Munich. A later sabbatical leave was spent at Amherst College and the University of Chicago. DePauw awarded him the A.M. degree in 1884 and an LL.D. in 1925. A sympathetic interpreter of German civilization, he was often referred to by his students with affection as "Kaiser" Longden.

Besides teaching, which was his main love, Longden held many administrative posts, including registrar and librarian early in his career. In 1919 he was named secretary of the Rector Scholarship Foundation and in 1922 vice president of the university, a largely honorary position, though it placed him in charge of the university affairs during presidential absences in 1921-22 and 1924-25. Longden Hall, constructed in 1927 through the generosity of Edward and Lucy Rowland Rector, was named for the veteran German professor.

Professor Longden became a veritable institution at DePauw during his 73 years as student and teacher-administrator. For many years he was called upon to give the welcoming address on the opening day of college. He once wired an entering student this recipe for a successful college career: "Choose men, not subjects; attend chapel daily."

Longden was married to DePauw graduate Mary Louisa Johnson, who preceded him in death in 1935. Their descendants are active participants in DePauw activities to this day, and his daughter-in-law, Hazel Day Longden of the class of 1916, remains a continuing link with the institution's past. Professor Longden lived on in Greencastle after retirement, dying in 1948 in his 88th year.

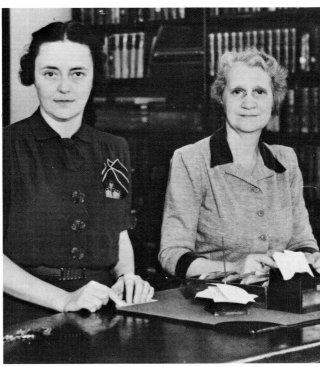

Alumna Vera S. Cooper (on the right) became the first professional university librarian in 1931 and remained for 25 years, retiring in 1956. Lucille Wickersham was assistant librarian from 1937-47.

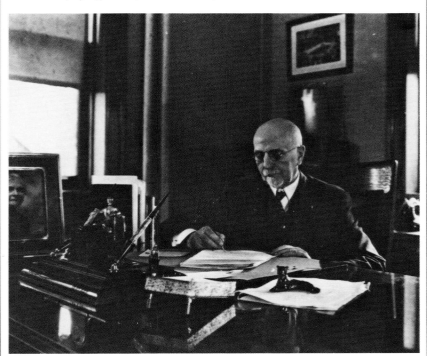

Henry B. Longden graduated from Indiana Asbury in 1881. He immediately joined the faculty of the preparatory department and soon the college, teaching Greek, Science, Latin, and German as well as serving as sometime Registrar, Librarian, Acting President, and Director of the Edward Rector Foundation. He is shown here in his administrative office in Studebaker Hall. The picture on his desk is that of Mrs. Longden.

One of the traditions at DePauw was inviting the student mothers to campus on May Day and the fathers on Dads' Day. Usually they formed living unit clubs of particular financial importance in enhancing the living conditions. Here are the charter members of the Phi Kappa Psi Mothers Club in 1929. In the center of the first row is Mrs. H. A. Gobin, widow of a former president.

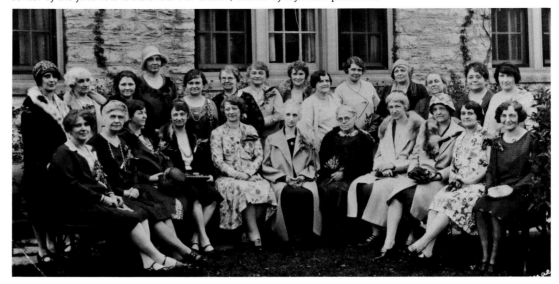

offered honors work in this period, eventually including history, economics, sociology, political science, psychology, and education. Students accepted for this program spent much of their junior and senior year in independent study under the direction of one or more members of the faculty in their major field. A preliminary examination was given at the end of the junior year, followed by both oral and written comprehensive examinations in the senior year. Each successful candidate for honors also submitted an extensive research paper in some field of specialization.

President Oxnam's recommendation to the faculty in 1932 that all students be required to pass a comprehensive examination was not acted upon at this time. The only major change in graduation requirements adopted by the faculty was to add six hours in philosophy or religion, a partial reversion to the role of those subjects in the former prescribed curriculum that dated back to the founding of the university.

A few significant changes took place in the organization of the liberal arts curriculum. In 1928 botany and zoology, which had been merged from time to time into a department of biology, regained independent departmental status. The department of public speaking was renamed the speech department in 1929. Taking up new quarters in Speech Hall (the former College Avenue Methodist Church), the department was able to expand its work in both forensics and Little Theatre.

An interesting development was the formation of a separate women's debating team which took part in intercollegiate competition along with the men's team. Upon the death of Professor Adelbert F. Caldwell in 1931, his department of English literature was merged into the department of English—formerly

called English composition and rhetoric—under the headship of Raymond W. Pence. In 1934 an art department was created. It absorbed the courses in art history taught by Professor of Greek Rufus Stephenson, and expanded the studio work carried on by the School of Music since the demise of the art school in 1913.

In seeking increased administrative centralization of the university President Oxnam undertook a complete reorganization of the faculty and departmental structure. As early as January 1930 he began grouping all departments into six divisions under chairmen appointed by him. The latter were to preside over fortnightly meetings of the faculty within each division. Together with the president, vice president, and the dean of the university, they constituted an educational policy committee.

General faculty meetings, held once a month under President Murlin, were to be convened only upon call. The six divisions with their first chairmen were as follows: Classical and Modern Languages (Edwin Post); English, Speech, and Fine Arts (Raymond W. Pence); Sciences (Orrin H. Smith); Social Sciences (W. Wallace Carson);

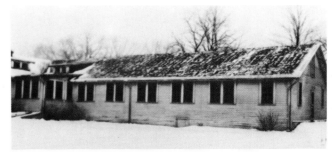

This "temporary" frame building of 1921 was used as the Florence Hall Annex, then for the botany and zoology departments after Middle College was razed, and finally known as "Termite Terrace" for the art department until it was torn down in 1951.

Education, Philosophy, and Religion (Walter E. Bundy); and Physical Education (William L. Hughes).

In the fall of 1930 a committee from the Commission on Survey of Educational Institutions of the Methodist Church visited the campus and submitted an elaborate report that endorsed the notion that divisions rather than departments be made the administrative units of the university. Thus encouraged in his vision of a more efficient and centralized system of operations, the president in May 1933 announced the abolition of the departmental structure altogether. Department heads were also eliminated, their functions being assumed by the division chairmen.

This view from the East College Bell Tower is a favorite, showing the Boulder and a few hangers-on. The bulletin board was also a longtime campus landmark.

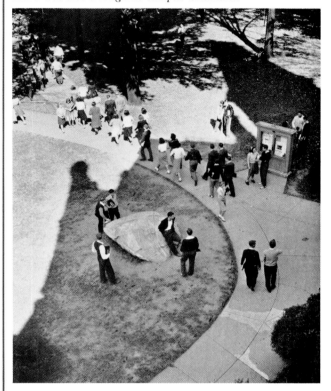

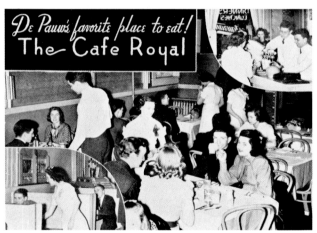

Above: For students in the 1930s and 1940s the major dining place was the Cafe Royale on East Washington Street next to the Voncastle theater managed by the Gerneth sisters. It was a favorite for weekends with parents, but particularly for a Sunday night supper with a date.

At right: A favorite student haunt in the 1930s was the U Shop across College Avenue from the Library. For most of its history this building served as a confectionary, ice cream parlor, bookstore, the Barn and eventually Faculty Office Building.

STUDENT LIFE BETWEEN THE WARS

In the aftermath of World War I there began a gradual relaxation of the older and stricter standards of student behavior that generally prevailed at DePauw up to the 1920s. University authorities, constrained by a relatively conservative faculty and board of trustees, to say nothing of still-potent ties to the Methodist Church, adjusted its policies and practices in this regard only slowly. Though the absolute ban on social dancing was lifted in 1926, coeds who wished to attend campus dances were required as late as 1935 to secure written parental permission, according to the official "Blue Book" defining student rules and regulations. Closing hour at all women's living units was 10 p.m., extended eventually to 11 p.m. on weekends and occasionally to midnight for special events such as the Junior Prom. After May Day senior women were permitted to stay out until 11 o'clock on any night of the week.

Male students could call upon women in the front parlor of their residence halls and also invite coeds to the public rooms of the fraternity houses on Friday and Saturday evenings. Housemothers and chaperones were a constant presence. No party which both men and women were expected to attend could be held without a hostess approved by the dean of women.

More informal dating took place on weekdays without university supervision, including "meeting at the Boulder" to attend chapel together and sharing a coke at the U-Shop or the Double Decker. Couples could also find a measure of intimacy in one of the three movie theaters in town—the Granada, the Chateau, and the Voncastle—or on a long walk out to Forest Hill Cemetery or the glens behind Blackstock Stadium. With sufficient funds in hand a young man might invite a coed to a dinner date in one of the local restaurants, such as the Cafe Royale, the Crawford Hotel, or the Elms, or even escort her via the Interurban to the English Theatre in Indianapolis.

The coming of the automobile brought few changes in dating patterns because the university maintained a strict policy regarding its use. Except for the first and last days of the academic year, students were prohibited from having cars on campus without special permission. Such permission was granted only to those needing transportation to jobs or student teaching assignments and to commuters from nearby communities. Later upperclassmen with outstanding academic records were also allowed the use of cars upon application to the dean of men. The rule forbidding women to ride in automobiles after seven o'clock in the evening effectively limited their usefulness in dating.

Card-playing, formerly banned along with social dancing, became a popular activity among both men and women. Bridge games, and an occasional bridge tourney, occupied a great deal of many students' free time. Most fraternities and sorority houses and some residence halls had their own card rooms as well as "bum rooms" for informal indoor recreation.

The university continued to enforce its prohibition of alcoholic beverages. Information gathered from student polls in the Oxnam administration seems to indicate the vast majority of undergraduates observed this rule, at least while on campus. Those who were apprehended in any infraction of the drinking code were punished summarily by expulsion from the university. Smoking, also officially banned on campus, proved more difficult to control. While a fair number of men apparently took up the habit after the war, it was still considered rather shocking for a coed to light up a cigarette at DePauw, according to the recollections of alumni from the 1920s and 1930s.

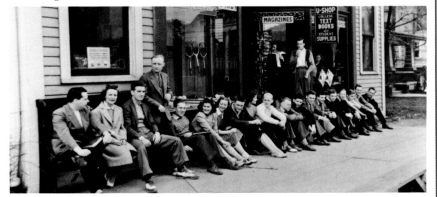

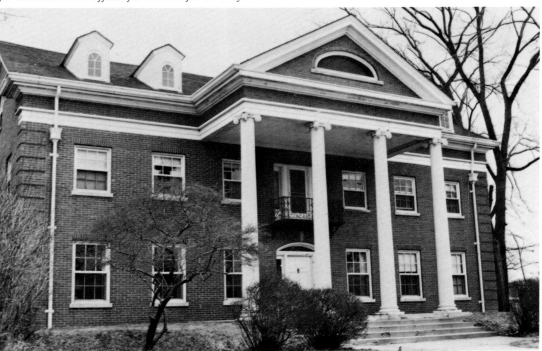

In place of the faculty as the supreme authority in educational matters was a new body, the senate, composed of the division chairmen and the administrators who were formerly designated as the educational policy committee. Pence and Carson retained their chairmanships, while the retired Post was replaced by Gerhard Baerg, Hughes by Donavan Moffett, Bundy by Fowler D. Brooks, and Smith by Truman Yuncker. It was argued that the new divisional organization would free faculty members from administrative detail and permit them to devote more time and energy to teaching, as well as help create a sense of the interrelatedness of knowledge.

The new scheme of university governance, imposed in such an arbitrary manner, proved decidedly unpopular with a large part of the faculty. Many thought, and some said openly, that the president's actions were inconsistent with his well known advocacy of democratic social ideas. After an overwhelming majority of the faculty voted to restore the former organization, the president relented and in January 1935 asked the trustees to reinstate the powers of the faculty. The departments once again became the chief instructional units, though the divisions were retained without any administrative authority as a gesture in the direction of interdisciplinary cooperation. The faculty proceeded to reorganize itself according to a plan produced by an informal committee, with regular monthly meetings and five standing committees. To four of these committees the faculty elected representatives nominated by the divisions.

Although a number of younger professors were dismissed during the early years of the depression for financial reasons, the Oxnam administration added many new names to the faculty roster. Included among them were Hiram M. Stout in political science; Franklin V. Thomas, Laurel H. Turk, and

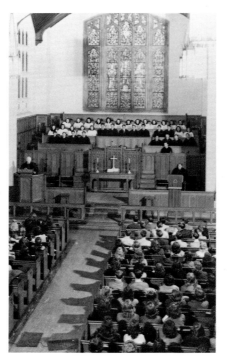

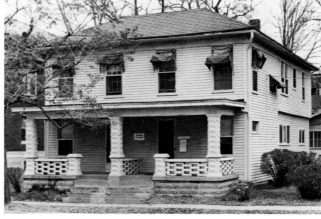

At left: A college chapel in Gobin Memorial Methodist Church. This view shows the university choir, President Wildman at the pulpit, Dean Bartlett behind the lectern, and organist Van Denman Thompson's head appearing slightly above the organ console.

Above: In 1927 this house on South Locust Street immediately south of the Administration Building was adapted for use as the Home Management House of the home economics department.

Alumnus G. Herbert Smith became dean of freshmen in 1932, director of the Rector Scholarship Foundation in 1935, and dean of administration from 1935 to 1942 when he left to become president of Wilamette University. A strong supporter of Beta Theta Pi he served as national president when the local chapter celebrated its centennial in 1945.*

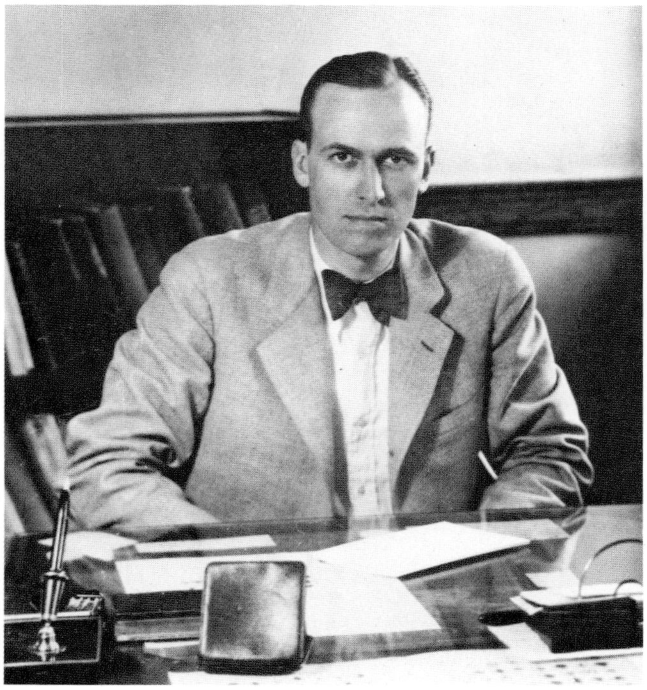

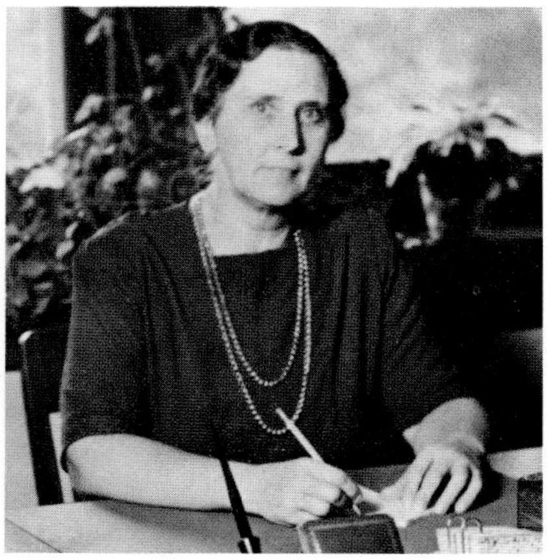

Helen Salzer came in 1931 to assist Dean Alvord and become DePauw's second Dean of Women from 1936 to 1943. She left to marry the Rev. Frederick H. Blair, much to the surprise of students who assumed that women deans could never have romance in their hearts by the nature of their position.

Marguerite Andrade in Romance languages; Elsie F. Waldo, George L. Bird, George E. Smock, and T. Carter Harrison in English; Lucile Calvert in speech; Marion H. Griffitts, G. Hans Grueninger, Gerhard Baerg, and Edward M.G. Mueller in German; William A. Neiswanger, Hiram Jome, and Fred Ritchie in economics; Francis M. Vreeland in sociology; Fowler D. Brooks and Paul J. Fay in psychology; William Edington in mathematics; Glenn W. Giddings in physics; Albert E. Reynolds in zoology; Winona H. Welch in botany; Jervis M. Fulmer, Jesse L. Riebsomer, and Percy L. Julian in chemistry (the last appointed to a position as research assistant in lieu of a professorship which the trustees were not yet ready to grant to a black candidate, no matter how highly qualified); A. Reid Winsey in art; Vera L. Mintle in home economics; and Raymond R. Neal, Lloyd L. Messersmith, Willard E. Umbreit, Martha Taylor (Inglis), and Harold Hickman in physical education.

New members of the Music School faculty included Kenneth R. Umfleet, Vernon R. Sheffield, Dorothy L. Fleetwood, Henry B. Kolling, Louise P. Walker, Franklin P. Inglis, Bjornar Bergethon, Margaret Dennis, Herman C. Berg, Carmen E. Siewert, Leah Curnutt, Mary E. Herr, Edward G. Shadbolt, and Edris King (Loveless).

President Oxnam involved the university in a serious controversy over the issue of academic freedom and faculty tenure by refusing in 1933 to renew the contract of Professor Ralph W. Hufferd, a member of the chemistry department since 1920. Hufferd was a highly respected, though admittedly rather tactless, chemistry teacher, as well as an officer in the U.S. Army Reserve, who may have been uncomfortable with Oxnam's pacifist pronouncements. At any rate he incurred the president's displeasure by his outspoken criticism of administration policies and his participation in an interdepartmental quarrel with a division chairman. At his request the American Association of University Professors dispatched a committee to Greencastle to investigate the case. Finding the president uncooperative and the methods of faculty appointment, promotion, and dismissal vague and uncertain, the committee decided to look into the whole system of tenure at the university. Its final report to the executive board of the A.A.U.P. not only condemned Hufferd's dismissal on the grounds of unsubstantiated charges and the lack of any hearing process but also severely criticized President Oxnam's wide, unchecked authority in tenure matters.

At its annual meeting in November 1934 the A.A.U.P. voted to remove DePauw University from the "eligible list" of institutions of higher education, a measure amounting to a general censure of the administration. One constructive result of this unfortunate controversy was the adoption by the board of trustees in 1935 of a "Statement of Academic Freedom and Tenure," which belatedly brought the university into compliance with the accepted professional standards of the A.A.U.P. and similar bodies.

Whatever his differences with the faculty, President Oxnam was generally popular with the student body. Many former students have attested to his magnetic personality and interesting chapel addresses, to the air of excitement he brought to the quiet and rather isolated campus. His socially prominent wife and active young family also may have contributed to a more sophisticated image of the contemporary Methodist university presidency.

It is not altogether clear how much Oxnam's progressive ideas on politics and society may have influenced undergraduates. In the fall of 1932 a straw poll revealed that a large majority of students favored the re-election of Herbert Hoover, a result consistent with the prevailing Republican predilection of the DePauw constituency. More suprisingly, 245 students cast their ballots for Norman Thomas, the Socialist candidate who had spoken on campus at the president's invitation. After the election of Franklin Roosevelt and the enactment of his New Deal reform measures, the Oxnam administration worked closely with the federal government to help students find employment opportunities on campus. Hundreds of students took advantage of jobs provided through the National Youth Administration and similar agencies to augment their resources in working their way through college.

Despite the economic hard times undergraduates found ways to enjoy the good times associated with the college experience. With the ban on dancing at campus parties lifted by the previous administration, social life flowered in the Oxnam years. DePauw's first Junior Prom took place on May 19, 1930 in Bowman Gymnasium. Formally dressed couples danced to the music of Don Bestor's Victor Recording Orchestra from Pittsburgh in a setting designed to resemble a Japanese garden. Two years later coeds sponsored a Leap Year Ball, which in turn inspired the subsequent annual Gold-Diggers' Ball. In a reversal of roles, women invited men to these dances, furnishing them with ingenious, and sometimes outrageous, corsages and calling for them at their living units. Besides such all-campus affairs, the fraternities and sororities each included one formal and one informal dance in the campus social calendar. Interestingly enough, the handful of black males at DePauw held their own annual prom in these years at The Elms, a popular off-campus restaurant, inviting women from Indianapolis and elsewhere as their dancing partners.

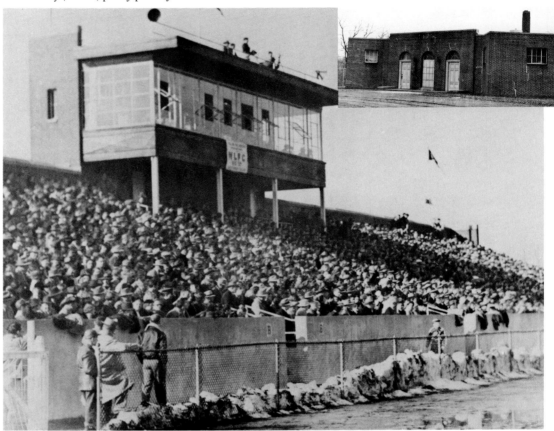

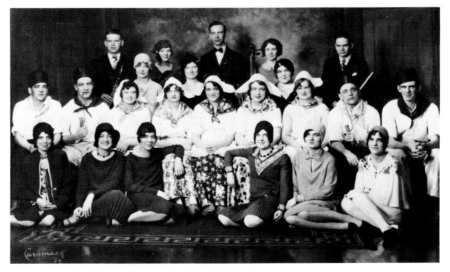

The February 1929 Phi Mu Alpha and Mu Phi Epsilon presented Hulda of Holland *with villagers, milkmaids, and farmhands from the two honoraries and the operetta class. Edna Tyne Bowles, voice instructor, directed.*

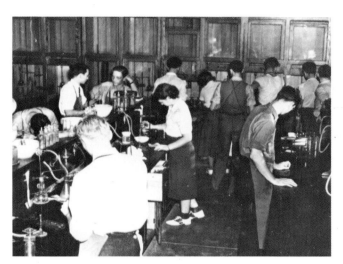

Chemistry laboratory in Minshall Hall

Senior Week became a DePauw institution in the late 1920s and early 1930s. It consisted of a series of chapel programs, the first of which was "coming out" day for seniors, who wore caps and gowns for the first time, after securing them against theft by underclassmen. The president or a favorite professor addressed the assembled student body in Meharry Hall, the juniors and sophomores occupying their assigned places behind the black-garbed seniors on the main floor. Men and women were still separated on either side of the room, and freshmen sat in the balcony, the normal practice in daily chapel.

One or two days were given to recognition chapel, when awards for athletic and scholastic excellence were presented and elections to senior honoraries announced. The Old Gold Gown was passed down from the senior woman holding it to the junior woman chosen for that honor. Senior men of Blue Key—later Gold Key—solemnly tapped new initiates from the junior class with the cane that served as their badge of office. The climax came with the presentation of the Walker Cup, given to the university in 1926 by alumnus Guy Morrison Walker and originally awarded at Commencement time, to the senior deemed to have contributed the most to DePauw. This high honor, the

WILLIAM MARTIN BLANCHARD

William Martin Blanchard left Rose Polytechnic Institute in Terre Haute in 1901 to begin a 40-year career as professor of chemistry at DePauw. A 28-year old North Carolinian with a Ph.D. from Johns Hopkins, he was to have a profound influence on the university. He chaired the enlarged chemistry department, and later became academic dean, helping to guide the institution through the difficult years of the Great Depression.

In January 1903 Blanchard was able to move the department of chemistry from its far-from-adequate quarters in the basement of East College into the north wing of the newly erected Minshall Laboratory. He presided over the installation there of modern laboratory equipment and a special chemistry library named for his predecessor, Philip S. Baker. He began attracting a corps of excellent students who went on to become leading chemists and physicians. The Chemistry Club, which he founded in 1908, often met in his Greencastle home. Despite a heavy teaching load he found time to publish research articles as well as a chemistry textbook and laboratory manual.

In 1927 President Lemuel Murlin persuaded Blanchard to take on administrative responsibilities as an associate of aging Dean Edwin Post. Upon the latter's retirement in 1930 Blanchard assumed the full duties of the deanship in addition to heading the chemistry department. He was also the longtime chairman of both the admissions and the athletic committee. A heart attack in 1938 slowed down the hard-working Blanchard, who took a leave of absence to recover his health. Unable to continue his scientific research during his convalescence, the versatile professor turned to writing poetry. He gave up the chemistry headship in 1939 and retired from the university fully two years later.

At alumni chapel in June 1941 former students lavished praise upon Blanchard as a teacher, scientist, humanitarian, administrator, and poet. He suffered a stroke and died in 1942, survived by his second wife, Vera Worth Blanchard, who had been registrar of the university at the time of her marriage. One of his most distinguished students, Percy L. Julian, whom Blanchard had brought back to DePauw as a research fellow in the mid-1930s, penned a poetic tribute to him that began:

From him I learned that Truth and Grace
Do not belong to but one race.

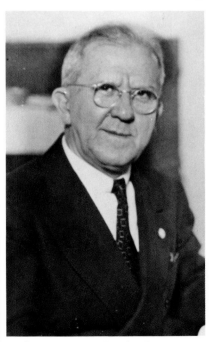

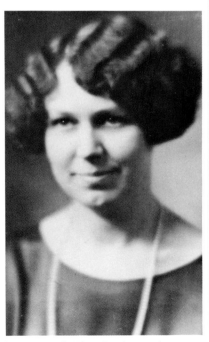

William Martin Blanchard came to DePauw in 1901 as professor of chemistry and remained until his retirement in 1941. Appointed associate academic dean in 1927 and dean in 1931, he served both the Oxnam and Wildman administrations.

Vera Worth Blanchard was the second wife of Dean William M. Blanchard. She was university registrar from 1923 to 1933 and before her retirement served as secretary to the Student Union.

STUDENTS

YWCA fete in the late 1930s with an impromptu band and bottled Coca-Cola.

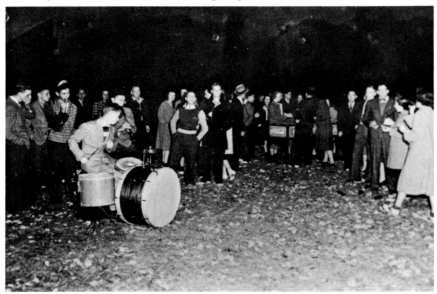

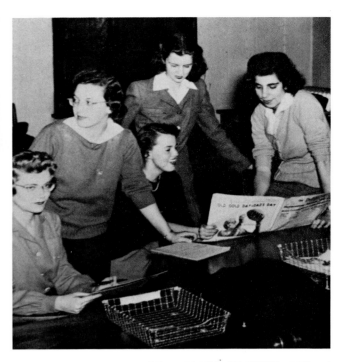

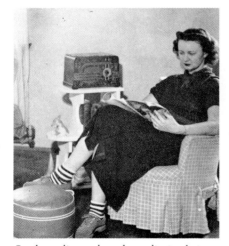

Students listened to the radio in their rooms in 1937.

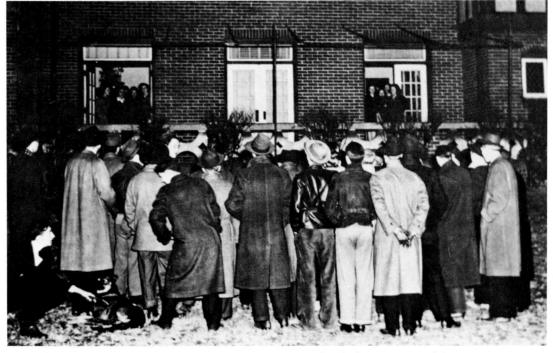

Top right: Representatives from the chapter of Theta Sigma Phi which was instituted for women journalists in 1919. The coeds published the May Day and Old Gold Day issues of the DePauw. Bottom: The boys serenading the Alpha Chi Omega sorority in 1939. Notice the student, probably a freshman monotone, making sure a dog does not enter into this sentimental moment.

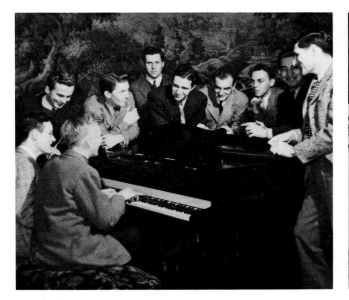

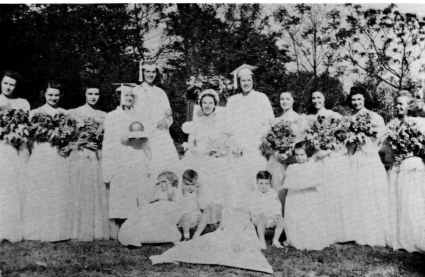

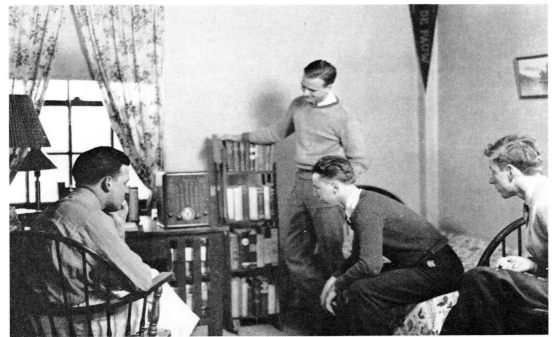

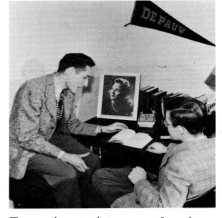

Two students in their room at Longden Hall. On the desk beside the edition of Plato is an enlarged picture of the student's mother.

Above left: An informal gathering of students around the piano in Longden Hall. Styles have changed by 1987.

Above right: The May Day Court with the queen and her escorts in 1941. Pages were usually borrowed from faculty families.

Bottom: A group of boys in their room listen to the radio, a common form of entertainment in the era.

After being caricatured frequently in Mock Chapel the faculty retaliated by their own parody of May Day. Seated: President Oxnam and Dean McCutchan. Among the flower girls may be found Jarvis Davis, Lloyd Messersmith, Gerhard Baerg, A. W. Crandall, Fowler Brooks, Van Denman Thompson, Rufus Stephenson, Carter Harrison, Willard Umbreit, P. G. Evans, Donovan Moffett, Raymond Pence, Robert Williams.

recipients of which were chosen jointly by vote of the senior class and the faculty, went only to males until 1941.

But for many the high point of Senior Week was the mock chapel which took place on Friday morning. With the entire faculty occupying the front rows of Meharry Hall, members of the senior class appeared on stage performing skits intended to caricature certain prominent administrators and professors. The more successful performances evoked howls of appreciative laughter from the students and a few smiles and an occasional frown from the subjects of the skits. On one occasion President Oxnam and some of the most often-caricatured members of the faculty retaliated by staging their own parody of the annual May Day festivities. Decked out in flowing gowns and garlanded with flowers, they marched into chapel impersonating the May Queen and her court before the astonished but delighted student body.

Group singing had a large part in campus life. Each fraternity and sorority had its own songs, sung almost nightly at the dinner hour and on special occasions. Many of these were collected in a volume published by two alumni, Raymond E. Smith and Wade Hollinghead, under the title *University, Fraternity and Sorority Songs of "Old DePauw."* This collection also contained alumna Vivien Bard's "A Toast to Old DePauw," which soon became the official university anthem, sung at Commencement, Old Gold Day, and Alumni Day and on other ceremonial occasions. Each spring the Greek letter organizations competed for prizes in the interfraternity and intersorority sings. A frequent campus happening was the fraternity serenade, when men from one chapter house would gather in front of a women's residence after closing hours to entertain the occupants with song,

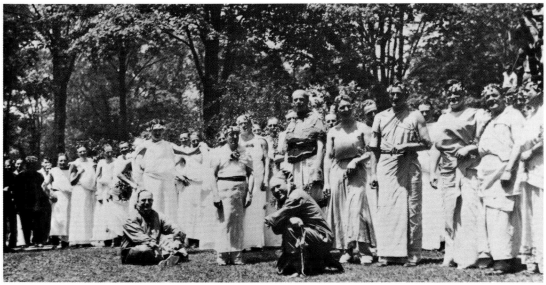

sometimes arriving with a piano installed in the bed of a truck for accompaniment. A chief excuse for such an event was one of the brothers bestowing his fraternity pin upon a coed as a token of his affection, an action that often led to eventual marriage. Professor Oliver W. Robinson, himself a graduate of DePauw in 1933, has described the custom in one of the stories of fictionalized fraternity life published in his nostalgic collection, *The Pillared Porch Stands Tall:*

Even the pin serenade was a flop.... All of us Alpha Yoops stood under the dormitory windows in the snow and the moonlight singing our fraternity sweetheart song. Then Peter crooned I Love You Truly for Harry. Elaine sang her own reply, and the dormitory girls stationed at various strategic windows tittered throughout. It was almost more than the dignity of Alpha Sigma Upsilon could endure.

The newly remodeled Speech Hall furnished spacious facilities for all kinds of theatrical productions. It was dedicated on Old Gold Day in 1929 with a performance of "The Goose Hangs High" by Lewis Beach. The

following February, the Association of Women Students sponsored the first Monon Revue, called the "Moan-on Revue." This musical entertainment, written and directed by students, was performed annually for several years. Other student-organized events that flourished in this period were the annual Gridiron Dinner, put on by the journalistic fraternity Sigma Delta Chi, and Matrix Table, sponsored by its counterpart for women, Theta Sigma Phi. These were chiefly occasions for "roasting" or "razzing" prominent members of the student body. Gridiron also awarded a serious honor, the *leather medal,* for the person making the greatest contribution to the university. Theta Sigma Chi usually invited a leading woman journalist to address Matrix Table and receive recognition for her achievements.

Interest in intercollegiate sports remained high. DePauw joined the Buckeye Conference in 1930 and, before dropping out two years later,

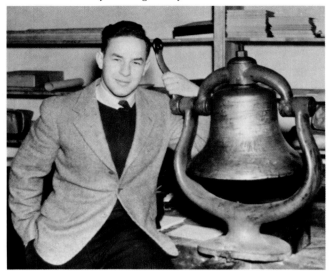

Joe Barr, captain of the 1938 football team and later Congressman and U.S. Secretary of the Treasury, is shown with the Monon Bell always held by the victor of the DePauw-Wabash football game after 1932.

competed actively with such Ohio colleges as Denison, Ohio Wesleyan, Wittenberg, Cincinnati, and Miami University of Ohio. In 1932 the Chicago, Indianapolis and Louisville Railroad Company (the "Monon") donated one of its locomotive bells to be held by the winner of the annual football game between DePauw and Wabash, an ancient rivalry. Since the game played in the fall of 1932 ended in a 0-0 tie, neither institution could claim the prize. It remained for the near-legendary undefeated, untied, and unscored-upon team of 1933 coached by Raymond "Gaumey" Neal to bring the Monon Bell home to Greencastle with its final victory of the season in Crawfordsville.

DePauw's "apostolic succession" was renewed when Oxnam was elected a bishop of the Methodist Episcopal Church in 1936, making him the last of six presidents to attain that office. His subsequent long career as a major ecclesiastical leader brought him national and international acclaim. At times he remained a controversial figure, as

PROFESSOR'S SYSTEM UNDONE

One of the ploys students used to further their education with the least effort was the fraternity file system. As students completed tests these results were placed in the house file for use by future students. To thwart such a system and make learning an individual effort, one enterprising and demanding professor refused to return test papers to students, choosing rather to hand each one a bit of paper with his score written on it. There would be no discussion of the test unless, of course, the student wanted to go over it privately with the professor.

As in wrestling, there is a counterhold for each hold; so with students, there is a countermeasure for anything that thwarts their path to a chosen goal. Students in one fraternity decided to manage the test storage plan without the tests. Several students in that class would simply divide the test questions among them, each one being responsible for a certain set of questions. At the close of the testing session they reassembled and wrote the questions they were responsible for, thus reconstructing the test. These questions were then researched and the correct answers with the test were then placed in the file.

In every class this professor's tests were assembled for the files. Believing he had thwarted storage of his tests, the professor seldom changed the test questions, and several generations of students coasted through his tests without the requisite study he thought necessary to master his material. No one ever knew whether he was aware of the fact that his method had been breached and that his tests were available to all. At any rate, he continued to use the same questions over and over again.

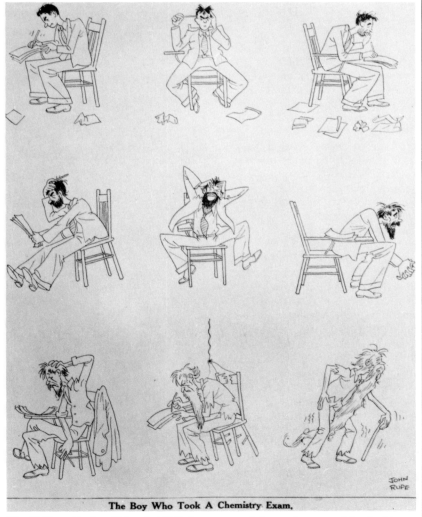

The Boy Who Took A Chemistry Exam,

The Yellow Crab of March 1930 demonstrated the student anguish of taking an examination and how it presumably ages students.

during his spirited defence of civil liberties in the 1950s. He died in 1963. Among his and his wife's generous contributions to the university was a valuable collection of Bret Harte first editions presented to the library in 1958. Oxnam himself published a total of 16 books in his lifetime, six of them while president of DePauw. In later years he apparently had second thoughts about his administration of the university. According to Jerome Hixson's memoir, *Past Perfect*, Oxnam stated on his return to campus three decades after leaving the presidency: "Oh, how I wish I could come back and do it all over again! There are so many things I would have done differently."

In the aftermath of the controversies of the Oxnam erea, the trustees decided to seek the participation of the faculty in choosing a new president. A search committee was formed which included Professor Walter Bundy of the English Bible department as the elected representative of the teaching faculty. Bundy distributed a questionnaire to his colleagues in an effort to obtain their views in regard to presidential qualifications. He found a fair degree of consensus in their replies, which described the ideal candidate for president as a man of high Christian principles and solid educational experience; an articulate but uncontroversial, fair and impartial leader. Many also indicated a preference for a layman in place of the long series of ordained ministers occupying the presidency.

The person ultimately selected to become the next president of DePauw was Clyde E. Wildman, who appeared to fit these criteria very well, except for the fact the he had been ordained to the Methodist ministry. Both Wildman and his wife, Forest Kyle Wildman, were

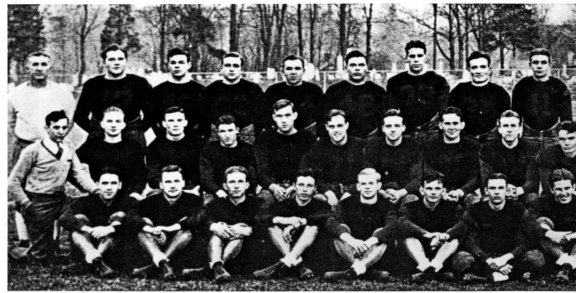

The 1933 football team, coached by Gaumey Neal, was undefeated, untied, unscored upon.

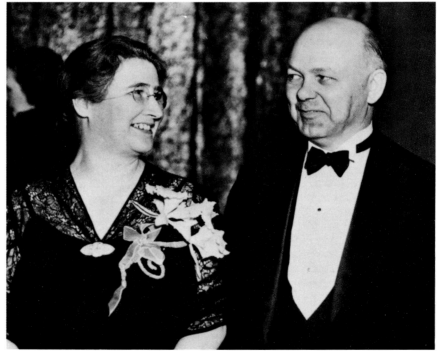

President Clyde Wildman (1936-1951) and Mrs. Forest Kyle Wildman.

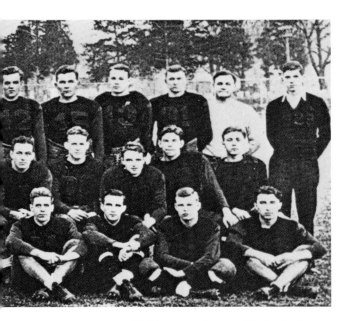

DePauw graduates. He had also earned an S.T.B. and Ph.D. from Boston University, making him the first president of this institution to hold an earned doctorate. Currently a professor of Old Testament at the Boston University School of Theology, Wildman had spent most of his career as a college or seminary teacher, with a brief stint as an administrator. Moreover he had served a term as president of the Boston University chapter of the A.A.U.P., not an insignificant item in light of recent events at DePauw. Clearly the new president brought with him an intimate knowledge not only of the university itself but also of faculty governance and Methodist educational institutions.

The Wildman administration began auspiciously with the A.A.U.P. voting to restore DePauw University to the eligible list at its annual meeting in December 1936. This action, taken in recognition of the change in administrations, has never been reversed, perhaps because the DePauw chapter of the A.A.U.P. has exercised a watchful eye over questions relating to academic freedom.

The 1936-37 academic year also marked the 100th anniversary of the founding of the university. In honor

FRANCIS CALVIN TILDEN, ONE OF DEPAUW'S "GRAND OLD MEN"

One of the most popular professors ever to teach at DePauw was Francis Calvin Tilden. The Illinois native entered the DePauw Preparatory School in 1890 and graduated from the university seven years later with Phi Beta Kappa honors. While in college he played on both the varsity football and baseball teams and edited the *Mirage* in his junior year and the *DePauw* in his senior year. After earning his A.M. degree at Harvard and studying briefly at Oxford and in the British Museum, he joined the DePauw faculty in 1900 as an instructor in English literature, only the third person to teach that subject here.

Leaving DePauw in 1904, he edited the *Greencastle Herald,* a forerunner of the *Banner,* and served for two years in the Indiana General Assembly as a Democratic senator from the district comprising Putnam, Marion, Morgan, and Owen counties. Near the end of his term he was invited to deliver a series of lectures at his alma mater on the relationship between literature and life.

In 1911 he returned to DePauw as professor of comparative literature. For the next 29 years Tilden introduced students to the works of such writers as Tolstoy and Dostoievski and placed them in their social and intellectual context in his popular courses, Great Modern Writers, Social Ideals, and Religious Ideals. Much in demand on the lyceum circuit, he often delivered 15-25 public lectures each winter. During 1917-18 he traveled around Indiana lecturing on behalf of the State Council for Defense.

It has been estimated that Professor Tilden had in his classes nearly three-quarters of all the students attending DePauw during his 33 years on the faculty. In his last year of teaching alone he had 555 students enrolled in his classes. The popular and much-admired professor retired in June 1940. He died in 1958 at the age of 85 and was buried in Forest Hill Cemetery. His wife, Ethel Arnold Tilden, who preceded him in death in 1950, was a widely recognized poet as well as housewife and mother. A Greencastle native and graduate of DePauw, she was perhaps best known for writing the words to an oratorio composed for the 150th anniversary of Methodism by Van Denman Thompson, "The Evangel of the Western World."

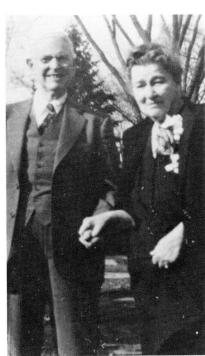

Professor Francis C. Tilden and his wife, the poet Ethel Arnold Tilden, taken in 1948.

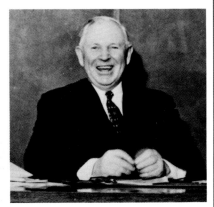

Professor Francis C. Tilden graduated from DePauw in 1897. He joined the faculty as instructor in English Literature in 1900. Except for a brief period as editor of the Greencastle Herald (1904-1911) he taught 33 years on the faculty until 1940. He was one of the university's most popular professors with large classes in comparative literature.

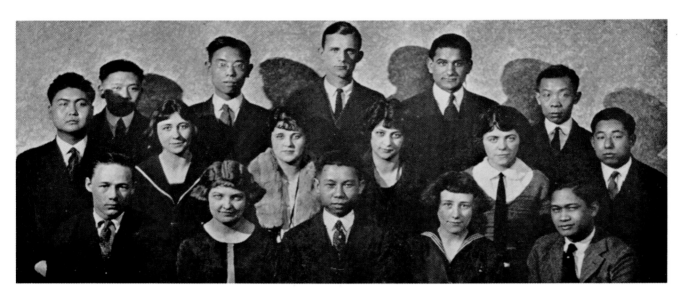

In 1923 the Cosmopolitan Club promoted friendship among foreign students at DePauw. There was one American student for each foreign student.

of the centennial the university sponsored a series of four conferences entitled "Life Looks at the College." Attending the first three were representatives of the churches, the business community, and the legal, medical, and teaching professions. The last conference was devoted to the role of women, a highly relevant topic in view of the 70 years of coeducation at DePauw. In 1937 William W. Sweet, a former head of the history department, published the first full-length history of the institution under the title *Indiana Asbury-DePauw University, 1837-1937.* Poet Max Ehrmann from the class of 1894 composed a "Centennial Ode" prophesying a "glorious rebirth" of Alma Mater.

DePauw's financial situation brightened as the nation gradually began to recover from the worst effects of the Great Depression. By the late 1930s the university was operating in the black once more. But new dormitory, classroom, and library facilities were still needed. In January 1937 President Wildman inaugurated the Centennial Fund campaign with a goal of $500,000, later raised to $1 million. By 1941 the campaign had raised slightly less than half that figure, but other gifts and bequests brought the total amount received during that period to nearly $950,000. Chief among

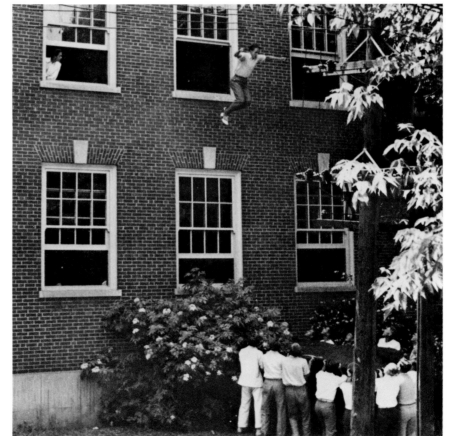

these was a bequest for $422,000 from Augustus L. Mason, an alumnus, trustee, and onetime dean of the Law School. Finally after long litigation the estate of former student John H. Harrison, a wealthy

In 1938 Alex Vraciu opened the window of his psychology class in Asbury Hall and, to the amazement of Professor Paul Fay and his classmates, jumped out. This picture is a publicity replay showing how his fraternity "saved his life."

Dedication ceremonies for John H. Harrison Hall on June 10, 1938 included Board President Roy West, Chairman of the Building Committee Charles Barnaby, Mrs. John H. Harrison, Professor Emeritus Henry B. Longden, President Clyde Wildman, and editor and publisher of the Danville, Illinois Commercial-News, Edwin C. Hewes.

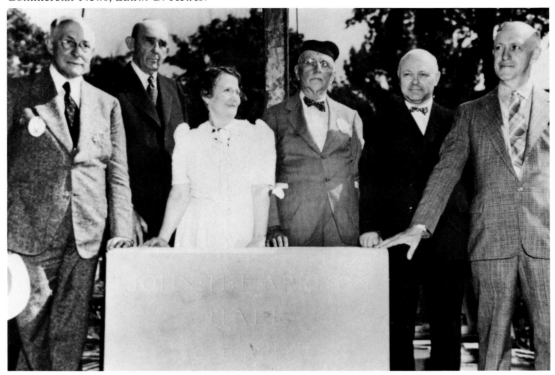

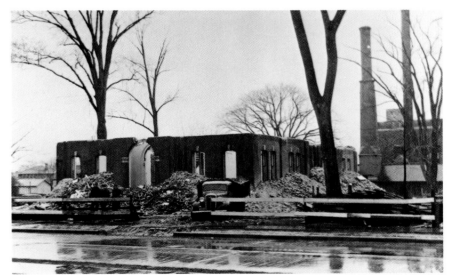

The razing of Middle College in 1939. In the rear is the enlarged heating plant with its high smoke stacks. Virtually all campus buildings, including Gobin Church, were heated through underground campus tunnels from the central heating plant which students were reminded of by the little steam geysers dotting the campus.

newspaper publisher in Danville, Ill. produced $600,000 for the university.

At last plans could be finalized to replace the razed Mansfield Hall and deteriorating Middle College. Part of the Mason bequest was used in the construction of a women's dormitory bearing his name on the site of the hall destroyed by fire seven years before. Half of the Harrison funds went into the building of a biological sciences facility, also named for the donor. Both Mason and Harrison Halls were completed by September 1940. Although Robert F. Daggett had submitted preliminary plans for Harrison Hall some years before, the university elected to save on the fees of an architect and general contractor by having the buildings designed and constructed in-house under the supervision of Comptroller Schenck and the department of engineering, construction, and maintenance. The blueprints were drawn up by M.G. Thompson of that department in conformity with the Colonial Revival mode decreed by the trustees and followed by Daggett in designing Asbury Hall.

Harrison Hall, located on the site of the former Middle College, was a handsome counterpart to Asbury Hall, standing directly across from it on the West Campus. The three-story red-brick structure, with its wide chimneys and dormer windows, echoed the design of the earlier hall with one major exception: the roof gables at either end were not reversed but ran in the same direction as the center section. An ornate central entrance made up for the lack of side doors found in Asbury. Inside, its long halls gave access to up-to-date classrooms and laboratories for the departments of botany, zoology, geology and psychology. Harrison Hall also contained the first elevator installed in any of the university's buildings. Plans for the construction of a new Colonial Revival-style library on the site of the razed West College to complete the academic quadrangle were put off for lack of funding.

The exterior of Mason Hall followed a very similar pattern, but with the front entrance on Anderson Street made conspicuous by tall classical columns on a semicircular portico looking out over a broad expanse of lawn. In the rear it abutted the quadrangle formed with Rector and Lucy Rowland Halls, with arched windows and entryways designed to harmonize with those of the latter building standing opposite it. The general effect inside the residential quadrangle was of a blending, rather than a clashing, of the Colonial Revival lines of Mason Hall with the more eclectic design of the older halls. Besides rooms for more than 100 women, Mason contained a spacious dining hall and an elegant lobby from the ceiling of which hung an elaborate glass chandelier imported from Czechoslovakia. Historian George Manhart has testified that it was long considered the "show place of the campus."

In 1938 the heirs of Robert L. and Eva H. O'Hair of Greencastle donated the large family residence on Seminary Street to the university. For a time this handsome red-brick structure was under consideration as

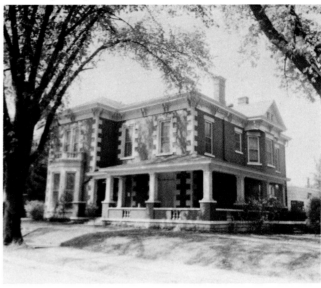

In 1938 the heirs of Robert L. and Eva H. O'Hair gave their family home to DePauw and it became the university health service until the 1980s when assigned to the office of the University Chaplain.

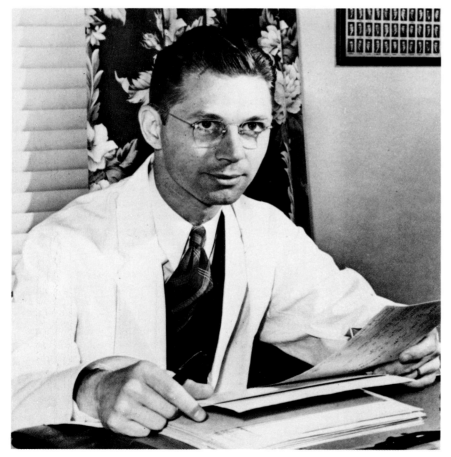

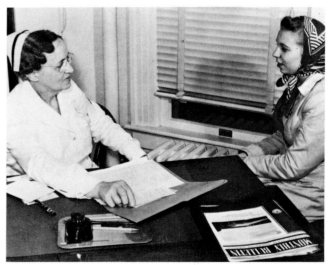

At left: George F. Parker, graduate of the University of Iowa, became the first University Physician and Director of the Health Service from 1941-1948. Like all university physicians his competency was questioned by students who yelled "Quack, Quack" and "Keep him away" when he walked onto the football field to take care of an injured player.

Above: A graduate of City Hospital in Indianapolis, Kathryn Davenport, a native of England, had the title of University Nurse from 1932 to 1950 and initiated the first formal health services. She is shown here with student Frances Tracy.

THE POSITION OF WOMEN STUDENTS AT DEPAUW

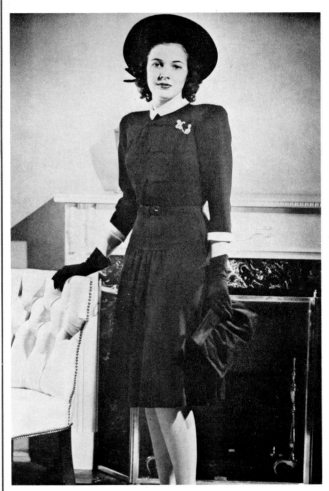

After 50 years of coeducation at DePauw, women students by and large still found themselves in separate—some might say subordinate—campus roles at the close of World War I. Excluded from membership, for example, in the all-male journalism honorary Sigma Delta Chi, coeds interested and active in journalism organized their own similar society, Theta Sigma Phi, in 1919. Sigma Delta Chi's arch-rival, the advertising honorary, Alpha Delta Sigma, also did not admit women. Though women were playing a larger part in staffing student publications, men continued for a long time to monopolize most of the chief editorial positions. In partial recompense, the members of Theta Sigma Phi published a special edition of the *DePauw* with an all-female staff on Old Gold Day and May Day. Not until 1939 did a coed become editor-in-chief of the *DePauw*, with the election of Betty Parker to that post for the second semester of the academic year.

Women were making progress in reaching top posts in other student publications. Mary Niblack won the position of chief editor of the *Mirage* as early as 1930, and Elizabeth Yout headed the editorial staff of the *DePauw Magazine* in the spring of 1937 and Virginia Bridge that of the *Boulder* in the fall of 1942.

But separate campus organizations for women persisted throughout this period. Ineligible for participation in the R.O.T.C. and its honorary society, Scabbard and Blade, a group of coeds formed a military auxiliary, Alpha Mu Phi in 1924. There were also a women's rifle club and even a women's debate team which took part in intercollegiate competition separately from the men. DePauw actually boasted a chapter of the women's scholastic and leadership honorary, Mortar Board, a decade before the formation of the all-male Blue Key in 1929.

With Old Gold Day in its early years chiefly oriented toward male participation in class scraps and interclass football games, May Day became the premier campus event for women. Held in early May the festivities usually began with a lantern parade on Friday evening—sometimes complemented by an unofficial "pajama parade" of male students to the women's dormitories after hours. The next day the Y.W.C.A. served an early morning breakfast on the East College lawn, which was followed by a women's tennis tournament or field day and a student-written and directed pageant. (In 1920 Margaret Mead, later the distinguished anthropologist, wrote the day's pageant, entitled "The Choice of American Girlhood.") The climactic events took place in the Dells behind Longden Hall, where gaily dressed coeds danced and sang, the seniors winding the May-pole, juniors forming a daisy chain, and the Queen of the May accepting her crown in the midst of her court. A play performed first in Meharry Hall and later in the theatre in Speech Hall concluded the day's events. Sometime in the 1930s May Day was combined with Mothers' Day and survived in that form down to recent times.

As at other coeducational colleges of the era where campus romances often led to the altar after graduation, DePauw women were judged in part by their femininity and desirability as marriage partners. Beginning in 1923 the college yearbook, the *Mirage*, annually featured a special section on "campus beauties," consisting of a half dozen photographs of glamorously posed coeds selected by vote of the male student body or by a well-known artist or other supposed expert on female beauty and charm. In 1931 the celebrated Broadway producer Florenz Ziegfield was called upon to make the final selection.

Coeds themselves collaborated by nominating candidates from their respective living units to participate in this competition. Despite attempts from time to time by reform-minded editors to modify this custom by instead presenting photographs of both men and women chosen as "representative students," the emphasis on feminine beauty and glamor continued to be a regular feature of the yearbooks as late as the mid-1960s.

The practice of naming selected coeds to reign over campus festivities proliferated in the 1930s and beyond. Besides the May Day Queen, there were soon the Old Gold Day Queen, crowned at halftime during the homecoming football game, the Dads' Day Queen in November, and the various Prom Queens chosen to lead the grand march with their male escorts.

A sign of coming changes in the perception of women's role on the DePauw campus could perhaps be seen in the awarding of the coveted Walker Cup in May 1941 to Rosa Neil Reynolds, the first coed to achieve that honor.

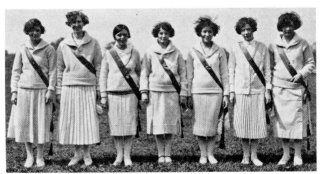

Top: May Day in the Dells. Middle: Another example of a Mirage beauty in 1941 was Aileen Perkins.
Bottom: A group of coeds in 1926 who formed a military auxiliary.

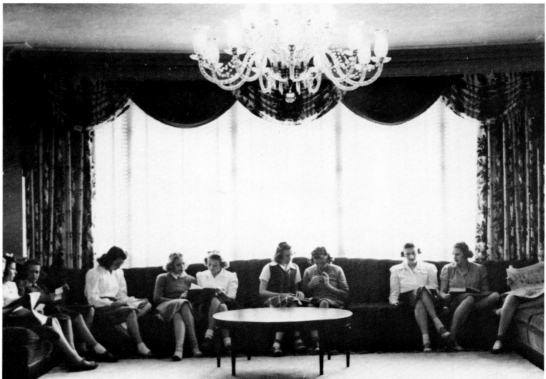

the site of a possible faculty club but instead was turned over to the university health services to provide much-needed enlargement of its facilities. By 1940 O'Hair House was remodeled into an infirmary, with a physician's office, X-ray room, laboratory, diet kitchen, and a few beds for student patients. At the same time the university engaged the services of its first full-time physician, Dr. George F. Parker, who operated the infirmary with the assistance of long-time staff member Kathryn Davenport and other nurses.

Another important addition to the physical plant was the construction of a permanent stadium in 1941 to replace the wooden bleachers at Blackstock Athletic Field. The gift of Mary H. Blackstock, who continued to show an active interest in her husband's alma mater long after his death, the stadium was built to seat approximately 4,000 persons and contained an enclosed press box as well as commodious dressing rooms for both home and visiting teams. Mrs. Blackstock later became the first woman elected to the DePauw board of trustees.

The early years of the Wildman administration brought some shifts in administrative personnel. In 1936 the formidable dean of women, Katherine Alvord, retired and was replaced by her assistant, Helen C. Salzer, who served until 1943. Wildman strengthened and expanded the office of academic dean, assigning to it some of the duties formerly handled by the president himself. The incumbent, William Blanchard, was encouraged to give up his teaching responsibilities in the department of chemistry in order to devote himself fully to the supervision of the entire academic program as well as the work of the registrar's office, the library, and the recently integrated Music School. Upon Blanchard's resignation in 1941 after suffering a severe heart attack, the president named to that post a

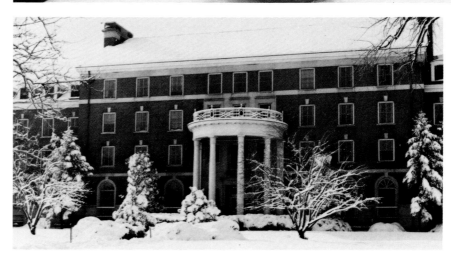

Mason Hall facing Anderson Street and site of the old Locust Street Methodist Church was first occupied in 1940 as a dormitory for women, particularly upperclass independent women.

fellow Boston University alumnus, Edward R. Bartlett, who had organized and led the department of religious education since 1923.

President Wildman faced a difficult personnel question in the case of Comptroller Ralph Schenck, whose handling of university business affairs had come under severe criticism from the faculty. In early 1941, a special faculty committee investigated the charges

against him and brought its findings, largely unfavorable, to the attention of the president and the trustees. Schenck submitted his resignation as comptroller along with a bill for his services in connection with the design and construction of Mason and Harrison Halls. The board of trustees eventually settled with him for half the amount of money he had requested. In his place the president

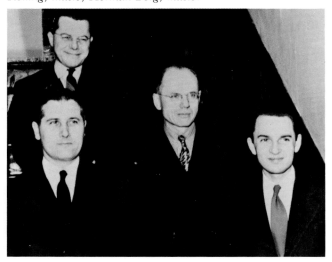

Franklin Inglis, music; Karl T. Schlicher, art; Henry Kolling, music; Herman Berg, music.

appointed Howell H. Brooks comptroller and M. Arthur Perry superintendent of buildings and grounds.

New appointments were made to the teaching faculty, helping to fill out to some degree the ranks depleted by the reduction of the early years of the depression. They included Wisner Kinne, Paul J. Carter, William H. Strain, and Frederick L. Bergmann in English, the last of whom also served for a time as director of publicity for the university; Gerald E. Warren and Carl W. McGuire in economics; Harriet M. Hazinski in art; Lester B. Sands in education; Vernon Van Dyke in political science; Harry J. Skornia and George F. Totten in speech; Joseph C. Heston in psychology; D. Keith Andrews in English Bible; Howard R. Youse in botany; Walter E. Martin in zoology; Jonathan S. Lee in physics; Milton C. Kloetzel in chemistry; Mary E. Smith in mathematics; James Y. Causey and Julia Crawley (Shumaker) in Romance languages; and Helen J. Cade in home economics. In 1937 Van Denman Thompson, professor of piano and organ as well as university organist, succeeded Dean Robert McCutcheon as director of the School of Music, a new title selected as more in accord with the new status of that institution. Added to the

VAN DENMAN THOMPSON: ORGANIST AND COMPOSER

Van Denman Thompson served in the School of Music under six presidents for a period of 45 years. University organist and a teacher of organ, piano, and composition since 1911, he also directed the School of Music from 1937 until his retirement in 1956. He was a graduate of the New England Conservatory of Music and earned the degree of B.Mus. from Lincoln-Jefferson University in 1919 and was elected a fellow of the American Guild of Organists in the same year. DePauw awarded him an honorary doctorate in music in 1935.

Outside of his work in the Music School and as organist and choir director at Gobin Methodist Church, Thompson was best known for his brilliant organ recitals and witty chapel entertainments. Diminutive in stature and painfully shy, he revealed a remarkable sense of humor in his public appearances. His colleague Jerome Hixson has described him as a "lesson in the gentle art of not taking himself too seriously." Seated at the console of the Bowman organ in Meharry Hall he would improvise in the style of Bach, "My girl's a hullabaloo; she goes to D.P.U.," exhibit his mastery of Boogie Woogie to the delight of the assembled students, or hunt for the "Lost Chord," finally finding it at the end of the performance. One morning word spread that a second daughter had been born to his wife, and students shouted, "Thompson, speech!" Slipping from behind the organ bench and drawing himself up to his full height of about five feet, he confirmed the report with the explanation that "we had rather hoped for a boy, but we decided to name her Patience." (Patience Thompson Berg grew up to become a concert performer and teacher of violin and viola at the university.)

Van Denman Thompson was a prolific composer of hymns, anthems, cantatas, and oratorios, and a principal contributor to the 1935 edition of the *Methodist Hymnal* edited by Dean Robert McCutcheon of the Music School. Commissioned in 1934 to compose an oratorio in the honor of the 150th anniversary of American Methodism, he wrote the music for "The Evangel of the New World" (with words by a faculty colleague's wife, Ethel Arnold Tilden). Its premier performance was given on the DePauw campus by the university choir under Thompson's direction.

A devoted family man, vegetable gardener, and reader of encyclopedias, the versatile organist was also a gourmet cook, specializing in pastries. When he purchased a bright red convertible in his later years, he justified its acquisition by the typical Thompsonism, "We can only be young twice." He retired to his home in Greencastle, where he died in 1969 at the age of 78. His wife, Eulamai Bogle Thompson, who was blind and herself a musician and composer, as well as a celebrated seamstress and mother of six, died in 1954. Van Denman Thompson's portrait, painted by Harold McDonald, hangs today in the Recital Hall named for him in the Performing Arts Center on the DePauw campus.

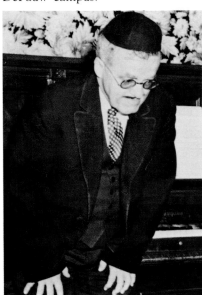

A demure and mild mannered musician, Professor Van Denman Thompson could also be a cut-up as shown in this picture taken about 1948.

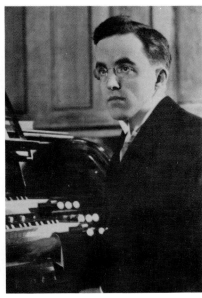

Van Denman Thompson taught organ and served as University Organist at DePauw from 1911 to 1956. He was Director of the School of Music from 1937 until his retirement.

FRATERNITIES/SORORITIES

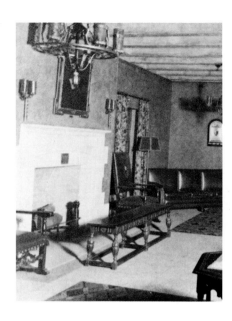

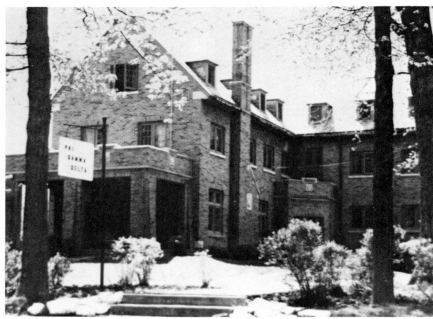

Top left: Living room interior of the Delta Tau Delta fraternity house.

Top right: The old Phi Gamma Delta fraternity house on South College Avenue.

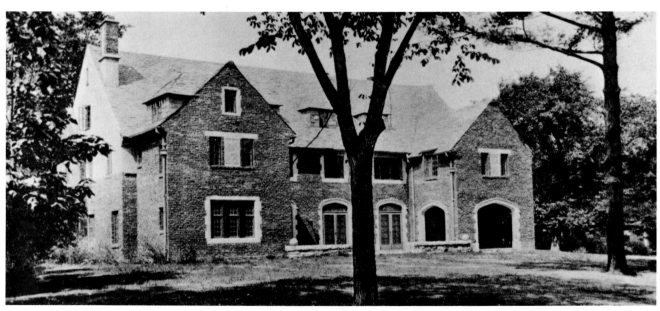

The original Lambda Chi Alpha fraternity house on Bloomington Street.

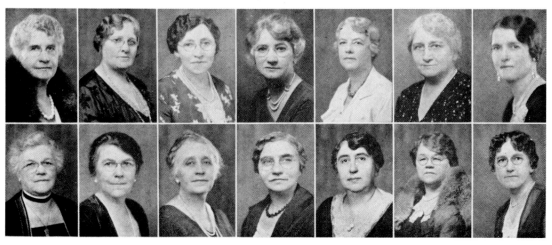

Fraternity housemothers

Old Gold Day decorations in front of the Phi Delta Theta fraternity house show the damage to be done to the University of Evansville Purple Aces.

Sorority housemothers

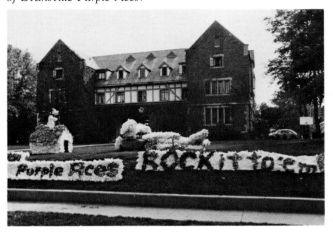

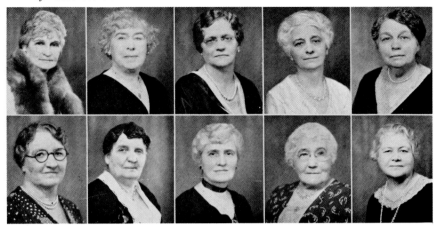

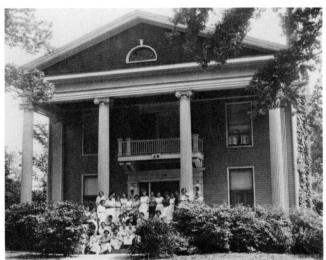

Above: The Alpha Phi sorority house on East Seminary Street with a group of sisters in the 1930s.

The old Alpha Omicron Pi sorority house on the northeast corner of Bloomington and Anderson Streets.

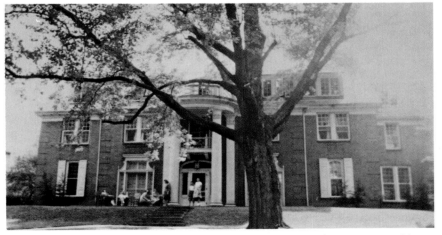

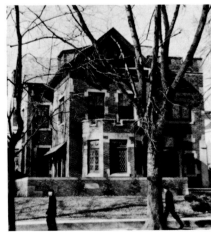

The Delta Zeta sorority house on East Washington Street was the reconstructed home of two prominent Greencastle historians, John Clark Ridpath and Jesse Weik.

The old Alpha Gamma Delta sorority house on South Locust Street.

corps of music instructors were C. Edmond Jarvis in voice and Howard B. Waltz and Helen Harrod (Perry) in piano.

Minor changes were effected in the organization of the College of Liberal Arts. Speech, which had been merged briefly with English, regained departmental independence. History and political science, which had been under a single head in the Oxnam years, were granted separate leadership. A similar development took place in the psychology and education departments. The latter greatly expanded its academic mandate in 1936 by initiating a program of training elementary school teachers in addition to its traditional role in the preparation of secondary school teachers and administrators. This return to the practice of the former DePauw Normal School resulted in large increases in enrollment, chiefly young women looking for careers in elementary school teaching. When Professor Francis Tilden retired in 1940, his department of comparative literature was discontinued and some of its subject matter taught in the English department.

A short-lived but very significant innovation was the creation of a department of anthropology in the fall of 1936. Eli Lilly, grandson of the founder and chairman of the board of the Indianapolis pharmaceutical firm bearing the family name, who was himself an enthusiastic amateur archaeologist, agreed to underwrite the expenses of such a department on a trial basis for five years. Named to conduct the work of the department was Charles F. Voegelin, a young anthropologist educated at Stanford and the University of California. He instituted courses in native American language and culture. With his wife, Erminie Wheeler-Voegelin, a trained ethnologist, he carried on various research projects on the same subjects. At the expiration of the Lilly grant in 1941, however, the

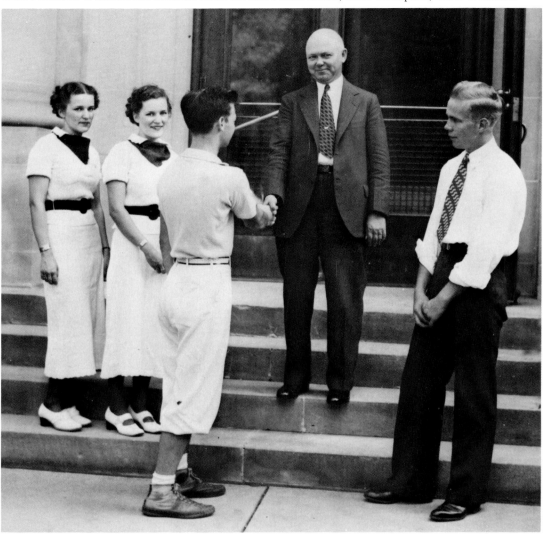

department was discontinued for lack of funds, and the Voegelins transferred their activities to Indiana University.

DePauw University also pioneered in the development of a systematic student foreign exchange program. Drawing in part upon educational contacts in his native Germany, Professor Hans Grueninger of the German department inaugurated a series of annual exchanges of students between DePauw and various European universities in 1935-36.

Over the next several years a few DePauw students spent their junior year in Berlin, Cologne, or Freiburg, while students from those institutions enrolled at DePauw. Some Greek-letter living units cooperated with the program by providing board and room to foreign exchange students, and the Rector Scholarship Fund made scholarship funds available. Eventually the program was expanded to include universities in France, Switzerland, Austria, the Scandinavian countries, and South America, though the

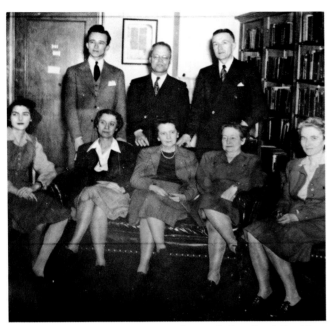

Some members of the English faculty, including (top) Fred L. Bergmann, Jarvis Davis, Jerome Hixson; (bottom) Elizabeth Mullins, Ermina Mills, Edna Taylor, Virginia Harlow, and Mary Fraley.

outbreak of the Second World War brought about a temporary interruption of student exchanges in the years after 1939.

By the end of President Wildman's first five years in office—just one-third of his 15-year tenure—DePauw University was well on its way toward recovery from the economic crises and academic controversies of the preceeding era. Wildman's administrative skills, tact, and geniality had won over both faculty and students and created an atmosphere of confidence and optimism within the entire university constituency. But ahead lay a new disruption of normal college life brought about by four long years of U.S. involvement in an unprecedentedly destructive world war.

RAYMOND WOODBURY PENCE: TEACHER OF WRITING

DePauw's most revered teacher of writing, Raymond Woodbury Pence, came to the university in 1916 as professor of English composition, only the second person to hold that title at the institution. An Ohio native with both bachelor's and master's degrees from Ohio State University, he had taught at state normal schools in Washington and Oregon and at Denison University. At DePauw he headed the department of English composition and rhetoric until 1931, when a merger with the department of English literature created the English department, which he led until his retirement in 1952. The tireless Pence continued to teach freshman English and a seminar in the department for the next 15 years.

From the beginning of his career at DePauw, Pence emphasized the acquisition of superior writing skills and encouraged his students' literary aspirations. In 1919 he founded the *DePauw Magazine* as a vehicle for student literary expression and served as its managing editor until its demise in 1937. A demanding teacher, he was a perfectionist who reviewed the work of undergraduates rigorously and asked for repeated revisions of their manuscripts. "This is too good not to be better" was a comment he often wrote on student papers. Anthropologist Margaret Mead has claimed in her autobiography that she never found elsewhere instruction in English composition equal to that of Pence, under whom she had studied during a year's residence at DePauw. Other of his students who became successful authors and editors have been lavish in their praise of his teaching as an indispensable aid to their writing careers.

The engergetic Pence, who held office hours at 7 a.m., found time from his teaching and departmental administrative duties to publish a dozen or more textbooks. Among them were several anthologies of short stories, essays, and plays, as well as editions of Shakespeare's *Hamlet* and *Midsummer Night's Dream*. In addition he was the author of *College Composition*, (1929), *Style Book in English* (1944), and *The Craft of Writing* (1944), and the co-author of *A Grammar of Present-Day English* (1947) and *Writing Craftsmanship* (1956).

As the veteran English professor, who was both feared and loved by students, neared retirement age, the *Boulder*, successor to the *DePauw Magazine*, carried on its front cover a picture of him with a caption asking the question, "Will the Bulldog Go?" "Pop" Pence, or the "Bulldog," as he was variously known for his fierce paternal regard and tenacious spirit, reluctantly accepted emeritus status in 1952 with a promise by President Russell J. Humbert that he could continue teaching at the university for as long as he wished. Hundreds of former students, many of them "Pence majors," contributed to a fund to furnish a seminar room in the English department in his honor. Dedicated on Old Gold Day in 1959, the Raymond Woodbury Pence Seminar Room on the third floor of Asbury Hall, with its oak paneling, a large photomural of Stratford-on-Avon, and elegant furniture in Old English style, provided a gracious setting for English classes at DePauw.

Pence finally left teaching altogether in 1967. He died 10 years later at the home of his daughter in Wilmington, Delaware. His wife, Robin Purdy Pence, preceded him in death in 1970.

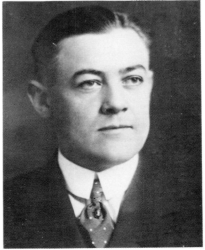
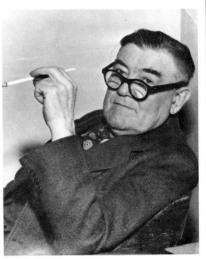

Raymond W. Pence early and late in his career as Professor of English. He came to DePauw from Denison University to teach in 1916.

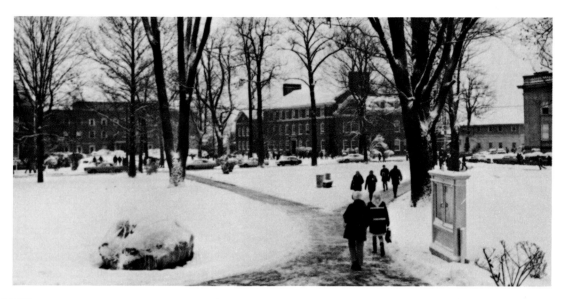

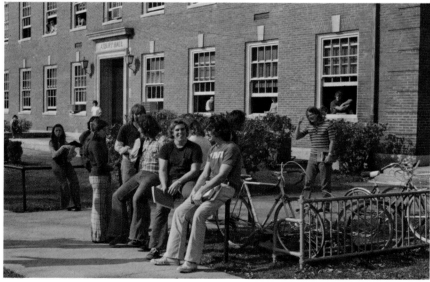

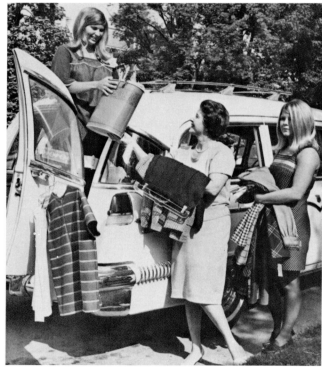

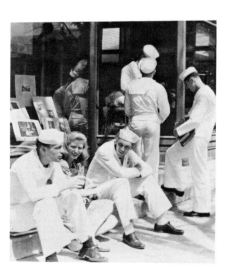

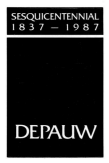
Chapter 4

DEPAUW SINCE 1941

The outbreak of the war in Europe in September 1939 had little impact at DePauw or other American colleges, where both academic and social life continued for the most part on its usual course. The intellectual climate on campus reflected the political isolationism then so prevalent in much of the nation, particularly in the Middle West. It is true that since the mid-1930s increasing attention was being paid to current events in Europe and Asia in chapel and convocation programs as well as in certain courses in the college curriculum. International affairs, however, probably seemed very remote from the interests of many undergraduates of that time, who were presumably more concerned with the immediate problems of economic recovery at home and jobs after graduation.

Under the Selective Service Act passed by Congress in September 1940, DePauw men 21 and over registered for the military draft, but few were called up because of the law's liberal provisions for deferment of college students. As the war went on, campus polls revealed a strong measure of sympathy for the Allied cause but little inclination toward either personal or national involvement. In 1940 a half dozen professors joined the Indiana Committee for Defense, a body affiliated with the ardently interventionist Committee to Defend America by Aiding England, while most remained on the sidelines. By November 1941 the *DePauw Alumnus* could report that 45 graduates of the university were already actively participating in the war and that 26 former students were residing in various parts of East Asia under threat of Japanese aggression.

Japan's surprise attack on the United States naval base at Pearl Harbor in Hawaii on December 7, 1941 and the subsequent declaration of war on the Axis Powers by Congress brought greater changes to the campus than any previous military crisis. The immediate response was an outburst of patriotic display along with jittery nerves and apprehension about the future, particularly among men eligible for military service. The 1942 *Mirage* reported this reaction: "The Stars and Stripes were uncovered and rolled out the windows; rifles were snatched from corners and platoons were maneuvered about East College...Everywhere students swapped rumors and prognostication; everywhere radios chanted communiques." By February 1942 a local national emergency committee was formed, later joined by a committee of defense, both consisting of representatives of the student body and the faculty and staff. The ordinary round of student activities and social life gradually gave way to community service, farm chores, paper and scrap-metal collection drives, first-aid classes, and accelerated study programs.

Before the end of the 1941-42 academic year 37 men had withdrawn from the university to enter military service and another 105 had been accepted, but were temporarily deferred under the provisions of the Selective Service Act. Six members of the faculty, the first of whom was Professor of History Andrew W. Crandall, a World War I veteran, also answered the call to the colors. By fall 1942 male enrollment dropped by nearly 100, and a year later only a handful of civilian men remained on campus, chiefly pre-theological students, conscientious objectors, and those exempted from military duty for health reasons. Faculty ranks also continued to thin as more professors joined various branches of the armed forces. Eventually 22 faculty members saw active military service, and seven others participated in some phase of war work. The possibility loomed of DePauw becoming almost an all-female institution for the war's duration.

In November 1942 President Clyde Wildman and Dean Edward Bartlett visited Washington, D.C. to offer the university's facilities for possible use in military training programs, consulting especially with DePauw alumnus Howard Peterson, then a special assistant in the War Department. The Navy showed an interest in the institution's offer and sent a team from the Great Lakes Naval Training Station to survey DePauw's facilities. As a result the university was selected as the site of one of 20 Naval Flight Preparatory

On opposite page, clockwise from top:

Campus snow scene looking from East College toward Asbury Hall.

Freshmen arrive at college in the 1960s

Men from the Navy V-12 unit in front of the old U Shop in 1944, soon to be transformed into the Barn.

Students take in sun and scholarship in front of Asbury Hall.

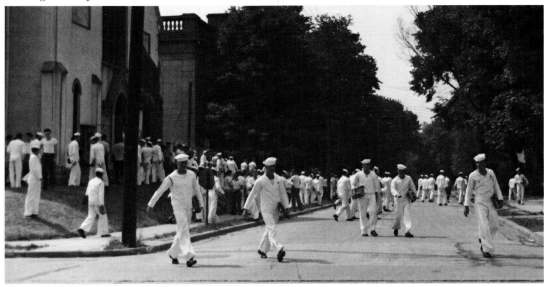

Apprentice seamen of DePauw's V-12 unit emerging from Speech Hall at the close of one of their regular morning assembly sessions.

Schools (V-5). The first V-5 unit of 200 men arrived in Greencastle in January 1943.

Headquartered in Asbury Hall — rechristened the "Good Ship Asbury" — the units were under the command of Naval officers but were taught largely by DePauw professors, four of whom were sent to William Jewel College for an intensive five-day course in navigation in order to prepare them to teach that subject. Altogether 31 members of the DePauw faculty took part in the program, along with 14 other instructors brought in for that purpose, mostly from high schools. Dean Bartlett acted as director, while Lester B. Sands of the education department, who had been a Naval Academy cadet, was named coordinator of the curriculum. Navy Lieutenant Edwin N. Dodge was the commanding officer.

Locust Manor became the Navy V-5 administrative center, and the Music School Annex was converted into a military hospital. The men were housed in Longden and Florence Halls and the Delta Chi fraternity house, and marched in formation to classes. By the end of the program in August 1944, 2,463 men had undergone the requisite three months of Navy training on the DePauw campus.

Later DePauw was host to another, quite different Naval training program. The Navy V-12, a college training program for qualified students preparing to be commissioned as Naval Reserve officers, arrived in July 1943 and remained until October 1945. Again the resident faculty was responsible for most of the curriculum, which consisted in large part of academic subjects studied in regular college classes with civilian students. Under the command of Lt. Commander William B. Dortch, the 400 apprentice seamen in the Navy V-12 program lived in Rector and Lucy Rowland Halls. Their number was later increased to 600 after the last V-5 unit departed. Eligible to participate in athletics, these Navy students made it possible for DePauw to continue in

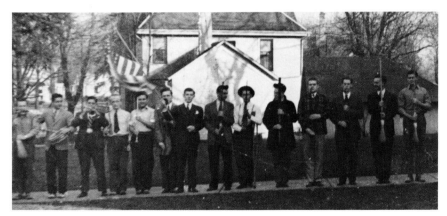

When the Japanese attacked Pearl Harbor on December 7, 1941, the men of Phi Delta Theta lined up in the front yard to protect their country. (Heath C. Steele '45)

intercollegiate sports competition during the course of the war. Altogether the two Navy training programs played a large role in helping the university survive at a time when there were few civilian male students available. "We have served the nation," President Wildman said in summing up DePauw's experience with the Naval units, "in helping to give training to its officer personnel and we have in turn been helped through some extremely difficult years by their presence on campus."

Life was far from normal at DePauw during wartime. Besides the Naval trainees, there were about 900

women and less than 100 men in the student body. Unaffiliated and freshman women were housed in Mason Hall and the empty fraternity houses. Near the end of the war women were also able to reside in Florence Hall, Locust Manor, and Johnson House. Beginning in 1943 the academic calendar was revised to add a summer term to the fall and spring semesters making it possible to attend classes all year, in accordance with the Navy V-12 schedule. New courses were added in meteorology, interpretation of maps, nautical astronomy and navigation, military German, Russian and German history and government,

The Barn for students in the 1940s did not survive the building of the Union. In time the location became the Faculty Office Building and was torn down by the early 1980s.

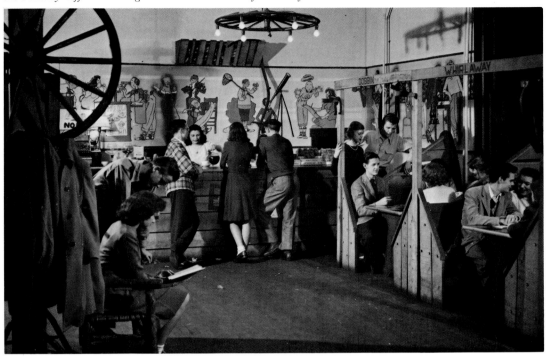

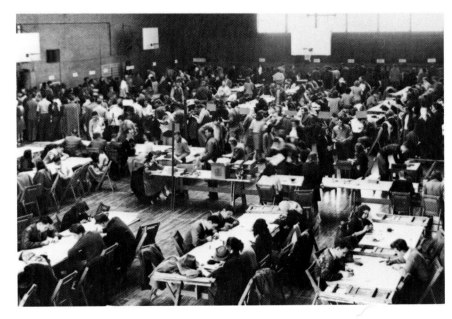

Registration in Bowman Gymnasium was always a major ordeal each semester, often lasting several days. This picture was taken in the late 1940s.

and "women in war." On the other hand a few advanced courses had to be dropped for lack of enrollment, the honors program curtailed, and a recently adopted plan for senior comprehensive examinations postponed.

Women students found new opportunities to demonstrate their abilities. For the first time coeds acted as cheerleaders at athletic events and joined the marching band. The varsity debate team became coeducational and was indeed composed chiefly of women during the war years. In 1943-44 a coed, Katharine Draper, served as president of the senior class. Women were particularly numerous on the staffs of and in leadership positions on the student newspaper, the literary magazine, and the yearbook. The Y.W.C.A. was unusually active in wartime, sponsoring a nursery school for underprivileged children and assisting in the services at the Maple Heights Church in addition to its regular programs.

The pace of social life moderated significantly as the academic schedule accelerated, but extracurricular activities did not come to a complete halt. The Association of Women Students established a social center for both Navy and civilian students in a two-story frame building located directly across from the Carnegie Library. Formerly known as the U Shop, it was dubbed The Barn. Dedicated by alumnus Ford Frick following a football game in the fall of 1943, The Barn served as a makeshift student union building into the early postwar years.

Food rationing and travel restrictions made necessary the curtailment of activities involving parents and alumni. Old Gold Day and Dad's Day were combined into a single holiday and Mothers' Day was omitted after 1943 for several years. Only the 50-year alumni reunions were celebrated at Commencement.

In May 1944 President Wildman appointed several committees in anticipation of postwar adjustments. On the recommendation of one such

Quonset huts from World War II provided efficiency apartments for veteran couples north of Florence Hall.

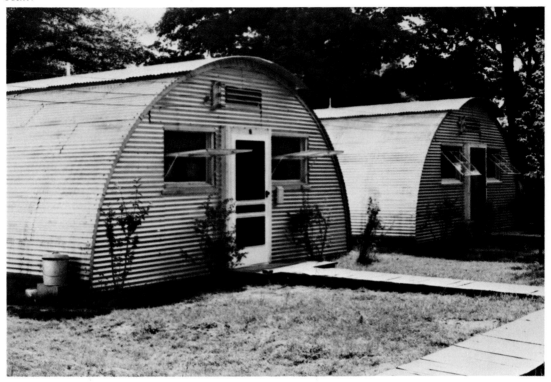

committee the Bureau of Testing and Research came into existence that fall. Directed by Joseph Heston of the psychology department, the bureau became responsible for freshman testing and conducted the first guidance clinic for prospective freshmen in the summer of 1945. Its functions were to increase greatly in the following years as a valuable adjunct to the whole instructional process.

Wartime additions to the faculty included Leota C. Colpitts, who succeeded Helen Salzer as dean of women in 1942; Edith Huggard, who introduced courses in typing and shorthand in what became known as the business education and later the secretarial science department; Mary Louise Miller and Mary Steele (Callaway) in physical education; Arthur W. Shumaker in English; Edward B. Stevens in classical languages; and Karl T. Schlichter in art.

Others were Audrey B. Beatty in home economics; Elizabeth J. Turnell in speech; Howard B. Burkett and Donald J. Cook in chemistry; and Paul A. Thomas in sociology. The Music School added Patience T. Berg, Franz Bodfors, and George W. Gove. New members of the library staff included Audrey Knowlton, Lois E. Goan, and Grace E. Mitchell. In 1943 Martha M. Cleavelin was named director of residence halls, and Elsie T. DePonte (Miller) began her long DePauw career, first as dietician and later as director of residence halls and university food service.

After successfully guiding the university through the war years the Wildman administration faced another crisis immediately after the termination of hostilities. An influx of veterans swelled enrollments, which rose from less than 1500 to just under 2300 in two years, straining university resources. Particularly affected was housing, which now had to be provided for wives and children in many cases. In 1946 six Quonset huts were erected just north of Florence Hall, each affording two small apartments. The university

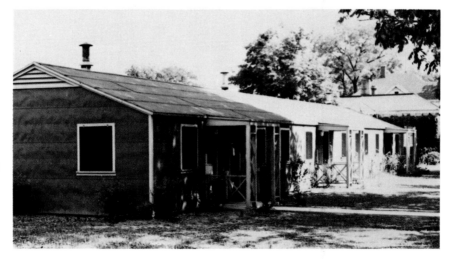

Former Army barracks were remodeled into modest veterans' apartments, later used for junior faculty housing.

also obtained 11 former Army barracks, which were placed on Locust Street, College Avenue, and in an area near McKim Observatory.

In addition 15 prefabricated cottages formerly occupied by the employees of a powder plant in Wilmington, IL were relocated to the south of the Observatory. Despite their somewhat insubstantial character, most of these buildings survived the postwar veteran influx

and found later uses. In 1950 the barracks on College Avenue was converted to a food laboratory for the home economics department and eventually furnished quarters for both the Air Force R.O.T.C. and the International Studies Program. The other structures continued to supply housing, sometimes barely adequate, for married students and junior instructors and their families for many years.

A PROFESSOR'S RECOLLECTIONS OF WARTIME DEPAUW

Professor Jerome C. Hixson retired from the English department in 1967 after 43 years of teaching a variety of subjects, including one of the most popular courses on campus called, "Living Language." He taught a few more years on a part-time basis before moving to Englewood, Florida, where he resides presently with his wife Margaret. In his memoir, *Past Perfect*, he describes his experiences teaching physics to the young men of the Navy Flight Preparatory School (V-5).

When the first classes started on January 1, 1943, the cadets did not have uniforms and other equipment. Many were marched into their classes by platoon leaders, all in civilian dress; but gradually military shoes, blouses, and other recognizable pieces of equipment appeared until the campus began to take on more of a military appearance. Of course for the remaining students, mostly women, regular classes went on as usual but not in Asbury Hall. They soon became familiar with the "one-two, one-two" as the cadets marched between Longden and Asbury, and to the athletic field. The cadets had no leisure time for social activities: they attended academic classes 48 hours a week, eight hours a day, six days in the week. The only way whereby Flight School could cover the required work was by strict attention to business. Christmas Day was a holiday only because the day's work was made up by extra classes on other days.

Inexorably, the examinations came under seal from Annapolis regularly each week. Inexorably, the weekly tests (4.0 was top) separated the fit from the unfit. On each crucial Saturday many cadets left offerings of pennies on the statue of Abraham Lincoln, then in the corridor of Asbury, in the hope of success so that they would not be "washed out" and lose all hope of becoming a flight officer...

Not only were uniforms and pieces of equipment lacking at the outset, but more seriously the rapidly assembled staff was obliged to plan and give courses before textbooks arrived. For example in the physics course which I was asked to give (on the basis of national emergency), we had to present the subjects of motion, heat, light, electricity, and sound with only a bare outline...

Early in the program a problem developed. Cadets became so appreciative of their instructors' work that some of them started presenting gifts such as hand-luggage. Of course, this had to be stopped. The instructors were only doing their duty. The sheer objectivity of the military regime completely obviated any dangers of favoritism. There was an inexorability in the impersonal questions which came in sealed envelopes from Annapolis and which were graded by machine...

Despite the necessary wartime regimentation in the V-5 school, there was some irrepressible fun. This happened in one of Reid Winsey's classes in flight. After the cadets had been marched into place by their platoon leader, the room was darkened for the showing of the film strips which were used in this and other branches of instruction. The warm, dark room provided an irresistable opportunity for needed rest. One cadet removed his military shoes and went to sleep on the back row. At the end of the hour, when the bell rang for the class to march out into the hall...this unfortunate cadet could not find his shoes. Some comrade with a dry sense of humor had thrown them out the window, and the luckless youth had to march as best he could without them, hoping not to be disciplined!

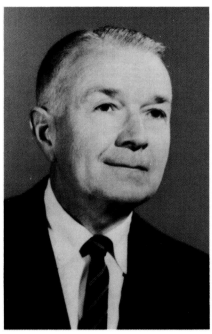

Professor Jerome Hixson, 1924-67.

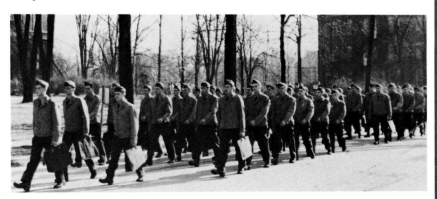

The V-5 unit of the Naval Flight Preparatory School marching down College Avenue to class in Asbury Hall. By its end in 1944, 2464 men had completed the three month training program at DePauw.

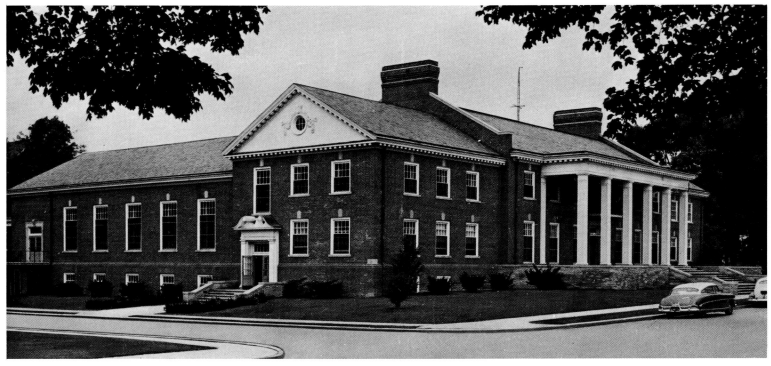

After making do with temporary quarters in the old Florence Hall Annex and one of the postwar Quonset huts, the art department in 1949 moved into the former Charles H. Barnaby home on East Washington Street, a handsome two-story structure that served its new purpose well as the University Art Center. In the same year a Quonset hut-type building was erected near Blackstock Field for use as a storeroom for the maintenance department.

As early as Old Gold Day 1945 students and alumni had begun a campaign to raise funds for a student activities building that could serve as an all-campus center for recreation and social life. The result was the construction of the Memorial Student Union Building, opened in 1951 and dedicated to the memory of the more than 100 DePauw students who had lost their lives in World War II. Designed by the Indianapolis architectural firm of McGuire and Shook in the prevailing Georgian Colonial style, the L-shaped building on the corner of Locust and Hanna Streets had at its main entry a broad portico supported by six columns facing the women's

dormitory quadrangle. Inside were a ballroom-auditorium, cafeteria and dining room, bowling alleys and billiard room, and a large central reception hall. Space was also found for the Alumni Office and a faculty lounge. A patio overlooked the East College lawn.

The new Union Building also contained specially designed studios for DePauw's 10-watt radio station, WGRE-FM. Radio broadcasts had begun on a regular basis from the DePauw campus as early as April 1941, when an arrangement was made with station WIRE in Indianapolis to carry two or three 15-minute educational programs a week from an improvised studio in the psychology department's experimental laboratory on the third floor of Harrison Hall.

In 1948 Herold Ross of the speech department, who had been named director of the radio program in 1945, applied to the Federal Communications Commission for a license permitting the university to operate a 10-watt F.M. station. The license was granted, and in April 1949 station WGRE-FM began broadcasting from studios in Rooms 318 and 319 of Harrison Hall, using a

transmitter donated by the General Electric Corporation. Named as program director to assist Ross, who became the station director, was a new member of the speech department who was to exert a major influence on the development of radio at DePauw, Elizabeth Turnell. In May 1951 WGRE turned back its studios in Harrison Hall to the psychology department and moved its operations to the new and improved facilities in the Memorial Student Union Building. Since then DePauw students have broadcast a wide variety of programs daily during the college year. In 1962 permission was obtained from the FCC to increase the station's power to 250 watts.

Some changes in departmental organization took place in the war and postwar years. In 1942 the Latin and Greek departments, which had suffered losses in enrollment with the growth and interest in modern languages, were consolidated as the department of classical languages. Four years later the departments of philosophy and religious education were also merged into a single department of philosophy and religion; Bible, however, remained a

The Memorial Student Union Building was completed in 1952 in memory of the DePauw students who died in World War II.

For many years students participated in local campus party campaigns and rallies for student offices. These students support the Union Party.

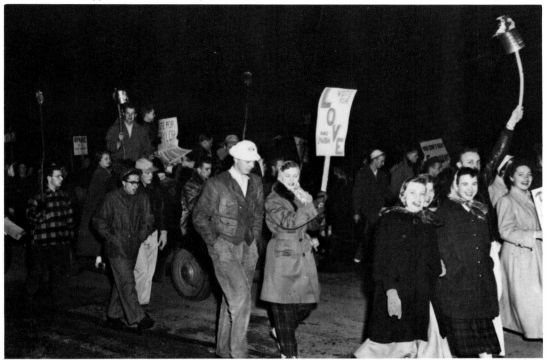

separate department until 1955. In the natural sciences the botany department added bacteriology to its title in 1947 to reflect an expansion of its course offerings in that area, and the geology department in 1948 added geography after having already listed courses in that subject in its curriculum for some years.

Shortly after the war's end Professor Hans Grueninger revived and enlarged the foreign study program begun in the mid-1930s. Student exchange programs with foreign universities in Europe and Latin America were revived and new ones instituted, notably with the Universities of Durham and Exeter in the United Kingdom. Selected DePauw undergraduates spent their junior year studying in Austria, Colombia, Denmark, Equador, France, Germany, Great Britain, Mexico, the Netherlands, Norway, Spain, Sweden, and Switzerland. A smaller number of foreign students attended classes at DePauw, living in dormitories and Greek-letter living units and participating to a large degree in the life of the campus.

Student life returned to normal after the austerities of wartime. Proms and other all-campus parties were held in the spacious ballroom of the new Student Union Building, while all the social fraternities reinstated an active social calendar. Greek-letter life was strengthened with the addition of a chapter of Sigma Alpha Epsilon for men and two new women's organizations: Pi Beta Phi and Delta Gamma.

Independent men and women also sought a larger voice in student affairs. In 1947 an Association of Independent Women was organized which lasted several years before disbanding. The well-established Men's Hall Association was especially active in promoting interracial housing at DePauw. As a result of their concern the administration assigned black males, who had formerly lived out in town, to rooms in Longden Hall in 1948. Black women, however, had to wait until 1955 to live in university residence halls.

The university re-emphasized its historical relationship with the Methodist Church while recognizing the growing religious diversity of its student body. In 1944 an interdenominational Council on Religious Life was formed, composed of representatives of the students, faculty, and administration. It took responsibility for the weekly vesper services on Sunday evenings and for Religious Emphasis Week, a series of special meetings held each spring dealing with the application of religion to personal and social life. Led by prominent preachers, these meetings provided a substitute for the evangelistic services once a regular feature of the Indiana Asbury-DePauw religious scene.

The daily chapel services were reduced, first to three or four mornings a week, and finally to one chapel service on Wednesday in Gobin Methodist Church and a Friday convocation in Meharry Hall devoted to a musical program or a lecture, often by an outside speaker.

In the early postwar years the faculty studied ways of strengthening the program of general education at DePauw. One result was the creation in 1948 of an area major, consisting of 48 semester hours in related fields, cutting across departmental lines. A special faculty committee devised an Experimental Curriculum during the 1947-48 academic year. Designed to introduce students to major areas of knowledge by integrating subjects normally taught separately, it included four-hour courses in physical science, biological science, the history of civilization, the social sciences, and basic communications. The last covered both oral and written composition. Fifty students enrolled for the first classes, but the number eventually declined. Originally approved for a five-year period, it was later extended to seven years.

In 1950 DePauw University completed arrangements for a binary pre-engineering program with Rose Polytechnical Institute, Case Institute of Technology and the Carnegie Institute of Technology. The plan called for three years on the DePauw campus and two years at one of the cooperating institutions, at

FACULTY *in the early 1960s*

Botany and bacteriology: P. Adams, T. Yuncker, W. Welch, F. Guernsey, H. Youse.

Romance languages: top row, left to right: P. G. Evans, W. Most, L. Turk, L. Tennis, H. Albro, A. Grundstrom. Bottom row: R. Carl, M. Andrade, E. Sublette, L. Kemp, R. Goetting, R. Grace, M. Wachs.

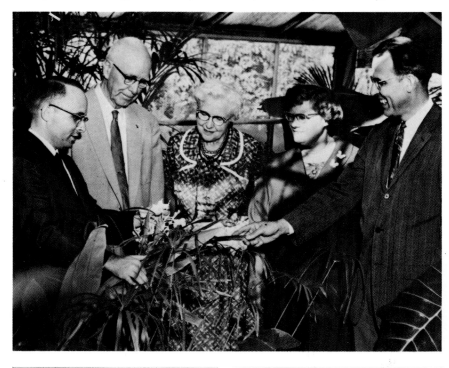

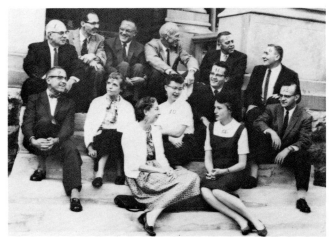

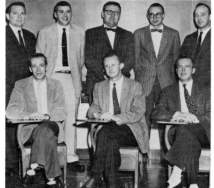

Psychology: Top: F. Goodson, J. Exner, P. Diem, C. Thomsen, F. McKenna. Bottom: R. Rector, K. Wagoner, H. Hawkins.

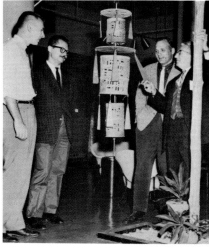

Art: G. Boone, R. French, R. Peeler, R. Winsey.

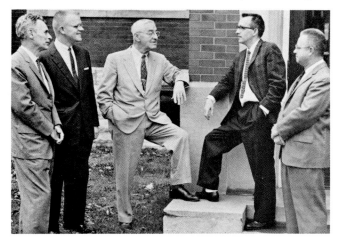

Sociology: J. Rhoads, P. Thomas, W. McIntyre, J. Reiling.

Physics, left to right: A. Sprague, W. Stoppenhagen, O. Smith, P. Kissinger, H. Henry.
(this is from mirage)

History: N. Risjord, C. Pierson, D. Ling, J. Wilson, C. Phillips, G. Manhart, A. Crandall, J. Baughman, J. Findlay.

Physical education: Top: E. McCall, R. Harvey. Second row: E. Snavely, T. Mont, T. Katula, C. Erdmann, J. Loveless. Bottom: C. Dumbrigue, M. Miller, N. Baldwin, J. Beckman, S. Watts.

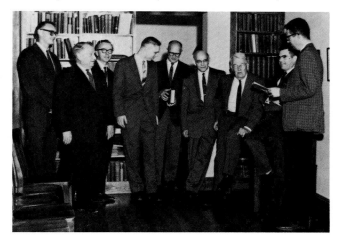

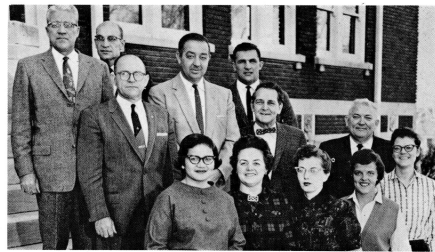

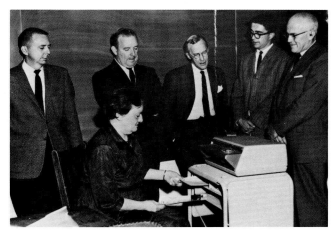

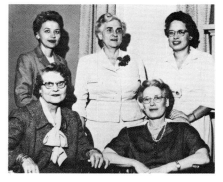

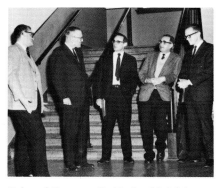

Economics: D. Maloney, E. Hadcock, F. Silander, J. Wyckoff, P. Frevert, J. Allen.

Home Economics: Top: B. Staggs, V. Mintle, B. Smith. Bottom: L. Barber, A. Beatty.

Political Science: S. Early, H. Voltmer, R. Sullivant, C. Norton, W. Morrow.

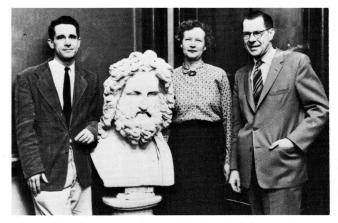

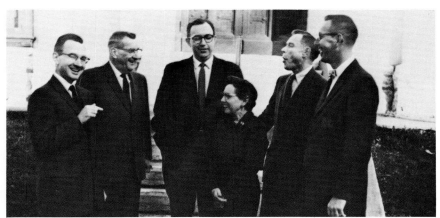

Classical Studies: B. Steele, M. Norton, E. Minar.

Speech: R. Weiss, D. Gooch, J. Foxen, E. Turnell, J. Elrod, J. Hammack.

FACULTY (continued)

Music: Top row: F. Bodfors, L. Curnutt, M. Strong. Second row: E. Jarvis, F. Peterson, C. Grubb, G. Sherman, G. Gove. Third row: A. Carkeek, H. Berg, R. Grocock, P. Lloyd. Fourth row: M. Trusler, D. Hanna, P. Lappan, S. Bielawski, H. Kolling.

Philosophy and Religion: W. Petrek, C. Hildebrand, R. Newton, J. Eigenbrodt, R. Eccles, E. Klemke, R. Compton, K. Thompson, R. Gustavsson.

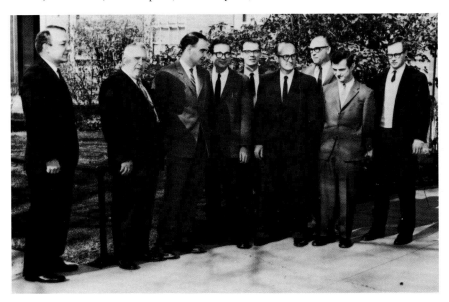

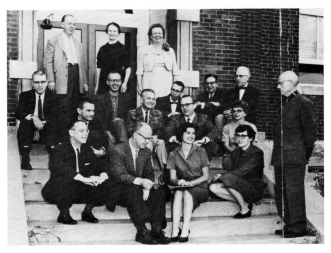

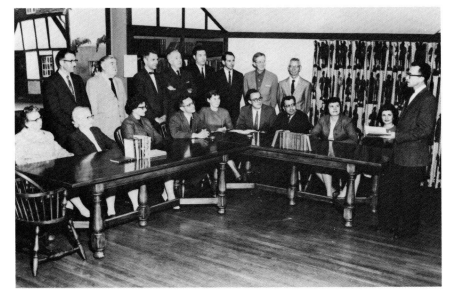

English: Top row: A. Shumaker, R. Pence, H. Spicer, J. Hixson, F. Nelson, D. McCall, O. Robinson, W. Huggard. Bottom row: E. Taylor, A. Harlow, H. Gilbert, R. Mizer, C. Lenhart, R. Cox, H. Garriott, E. Peebles, J. Morgan, F. Bergmann.

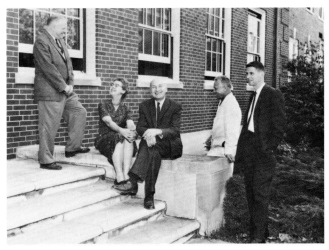

Zoology: C. Hickman, F. Hickman, A. Reynolds, F. Fuller, J. Gammon.

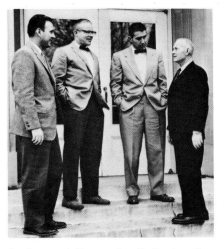

Geology and Geography: R. Loring, J. Madison, M. Schneider, C. Bieber.

Chemistry: J. Fulmer, H. Golding, H. Burkett, J. Ricketts, D. J. Cook.

German: H. Layh, G. Welliver, Z. Dabars, M. Baerg, H. Grueninger.

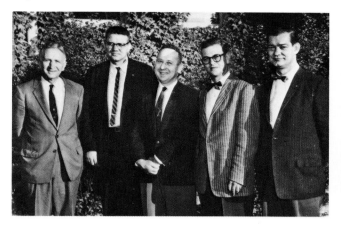

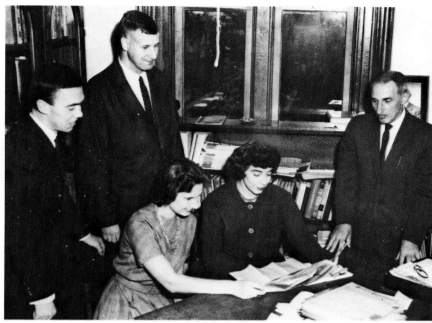

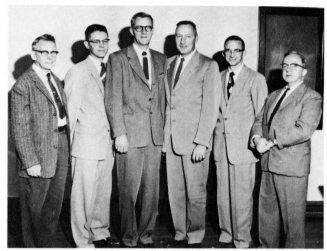

Mathematics and Astronomy: H. Greenleaf, R. Hultquist, C. Johnson, C. Gass, R. Thomas, C. Arnold.

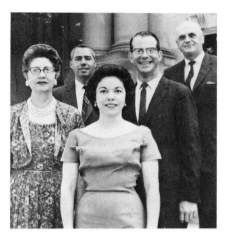

Education: F. Guild, D. Orlosky, M. Holland, N. McPhail, C. Green.

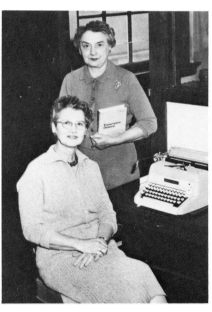

Secretarial Science: E. Huggard, A. Evans.

the conclusion of which students would receive a B.A. from DePauw and a B.S. from the engineering school. A somewhat similar program for forestry was arranged with Duke University and a cooperative system of nursing education with Methodist Hospital in Indianapolis.

A number of administrative changes took place in the last years of the Wildman administration. When Dean Edward Bartlett resigned in 1949 to become president of Iliff School of Theology, George B. Manhart was named acting dean for a year. Edgar C. Cumings came from the presidency of Canterbury College to assume that office until 1950, when Louis W. Norris of the philosophy and religion department was appointed to the position.

The student personnel offices were completely reorganized in 1948 following the retirement of Louis Dirks as dean of men and the resignation of Dean of Women Leota Colpitts. Named to the new post of dean of students was Lawrence A. Riggs, a graduate of the University of California with a doctorate from Columbia who had held a similar position at Willamette College. Working with him were three assistant deans: Lucille Scheuer, Ida Nelle Barnhart, and Robert H. Farber, the last having returned to university service after the war as secretary for veteran affairs. Trained counselors under the direction of Dean Barnhart were assigned to each of the four university residence halls for the first time. Dean Farber also acted as secretary of the Rector Scholarship Foundation and directed the Placement Bureau.

Willard E. Umbreit of the physical education department became the first full-time director of admissions. Upon the resignation of Comptroller Howell Brooks in 1950, his assistant, Deward W. Smythe, assumed that office. Longtime staffer Frank DeVaney became assistant comptroller. Wilbur J. Eckardt was appointed purchasing agent and Ralph Bee cashier. Frederick L. Bergmann acted as director of publicity in addition to his teaching duties in the English department, and

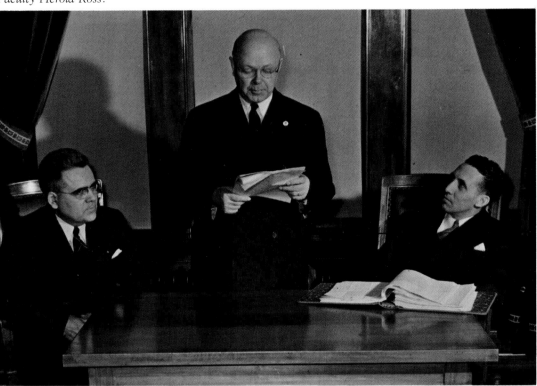

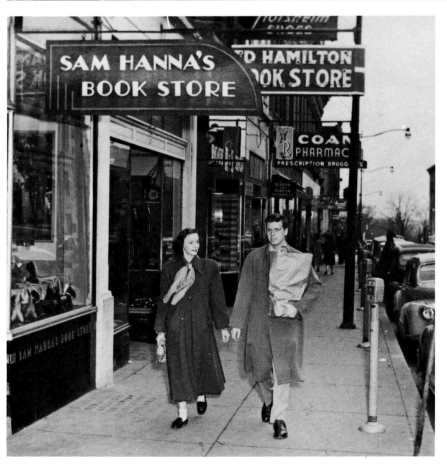

The downtown part of the campus on Washington Street in the late 1940s.

154

WOMEN TEACHERS OF ENGLISH AT DEPAUW

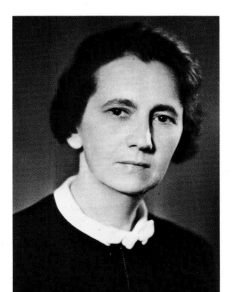

Edna Hayes Taylor, 1918-22, 1935-56.

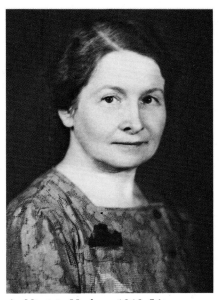

A. Virginia Harlow, 1919-56.

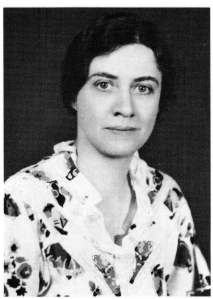

Ermina M. Mills, 1928-60.

The English department has enjoyed the services of more women teachers than any other department in the College of Liberal Arts. Three whose careers spanned several decades were Edna Hayes (Taylor), Agnes Virginia Harlow, and Ermina Murlin Mills.

The first to join the DePauw teaching staff was Edna Hayes, a graduate of Denison University with teaching experience there and at the high school level. She was appointed an instructor of English composition and rhetoric in 1918. Four years later she married James Taylor and left the university to raise a family. After her husband's death in 1935 she returned to DePauw to teach in the new English department, which combined both composition and literature. She earned an M.A. from Ohio State University in 1939. Known to generations of students as Mrs. Shakespeare for her devotion to the Bard of Avon, she was an inspirational and beloved teacher. Former students contributed to a fund to send her to England in the summer of 1952 for the coronation of Queen Elizabeth II. An ardent Anglophile, she wrote two prize-winning coronation poems while there. Professor Taylor retired in 1956 but continued to teach part-time for another decade and spent one year as a visiting instructor at the American Collegiate Institute in Turkey. She died in 1984.

Virginia Harlow came to DePauw in 1919 after two years of teaching at the State Normal School in Shippensburg, Pa. A graduate of Mount Holyoke in the same class as Anna Olmstead (Raphael), who joined the faculty in the same year as a member of the Romance languages department, she later earned an M.A. from the University of California and Ph.D. from Duke. Her doctoral dissertation, published by Duke University Press, was highly praised by literary historians. She was a demanding teacher, thorough in her scholarship and lucid in class presentation. In 1952 she was chosen to succeed veteran Raymond W. Pence as head of the English department, the first woman to hold that post. Reaching the mandatory age of retirement in 1956, Professor Harlow remained active in teaching both at DePauw and abroad for several years, including stints as a Fulbright-Hays lecturer at Hiroshima University in Japan and visiting professor of English at Seoul National University in Korea. She died in Greencastle in 1977.

The youngest of the three, Ermina Murlin Mills, was a graduate of Cornell College in Iowa who was brought to DePauw in 1928 as an assistant to Professor Francis Tilden in the department of comparative literature. The daughter of Henry A. Mills, former dean of the DePauw School of Art, she had earned an M.A. at Boston University and taught seven years at her alma mater, Cornell College. She was a prodigious reader who combined a knowledge of history and sociology in her interpretation of modern literature. Professor Mills remained a member of the comparative literature department until 1940, when upon Tilden's retirement it was combined with the English department. Transferring there she taught general European as well as English and American literature for two more decades. After her retirement in 1960 she continued to teach part-time for a few years before moving to Colorado, where she still makes her home.

Other women with shorter tenures at DePauw who made significant contributions to the teaching of English were: Lillian B. Brownfield, 1922-40; Judith K. Sollenberger, 1924-34; Mary Glenn Hamilton, 1928-34; Mary L. Fraley, 1938-48; Jean Butler Sanders, 1946-50, 1951-58; Marian Shalkhauser (Brock), 1955-57, 1961-65; and Elizabeth Ann Christman, 1969-76. Women are still well represented in the English department, which today includes Cynthia E. Cornell, Martha Rainbolt, Erin McGraw, and Jesse Lee Kercheval. The roster of part-time teachers who have served the department long and well contains the names of several others: Kathleen L. Steele, Julia D. Knuppel, Christina T. Biggs, and Ann L. Weiss.

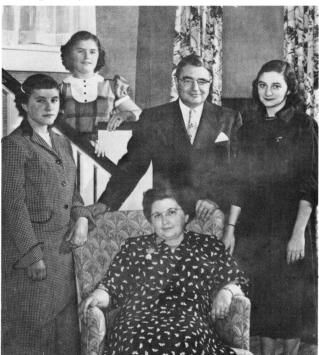

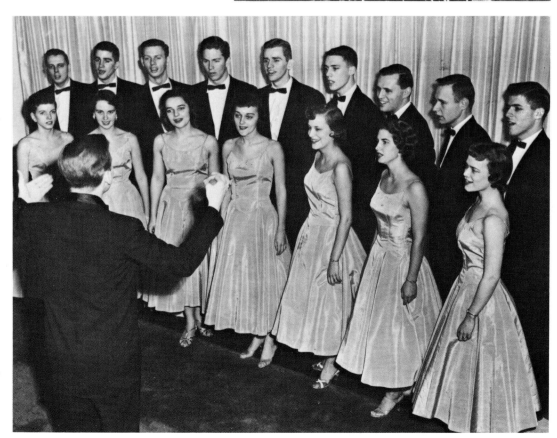

President Russell J. Humbert (1951-62) and his family in 1951. Seated is Margaret Lundy Humbert (Hixson) and standing Carolyn, Sarah, the President, and Martha.

Marga Bruning Voltmer was made editor of university publications. New by-laws approved by the board of trustees in 1947 expanded the membership of that body from 35 to 40 and authorized the appointment of a vice president to take charge of public relations and financial promotion. The person named to this position, William H. Butterfield, resigned after a few months, however, and the title was not to be used for another two decades.

Rising enrollments after the war prompted expansion of the teaching faculty. Among the new members of the faculty were Austin D. Sprague and Charles Ammerman in physics; Forst D. Fuller in zoology; Charles L. Bieber and Robert D. Loring in geology and geography; and Harry L. Hawkins and Kenneth S. Wagoner in psychology. Others were Jean Sanders, Harold M. Garriott, Oliver W. Robinson, Harold O. Spicer, and Edward L. Galligan in English; Woodrow L. Most, Ralph F. Carl, Ruth Grace, Edith Sublette, Ralph McWilliams, and LeGrand Tennis in Romance languages; Helen A. Leon and Raymond H. French in art; Forrest L. Seal in speech; Robert M. Montgomery in Bible; Louis W. Norris, Orville L. Davis, and Warren E. Steinkraus in philosophy and religion; Clinton C. Green and Herbert L. Heller in education; Clark F. Norton and Wallace B. Graves in political science; James M. Erdmann in history; and Edith A. Hadcock, Wallace O. Yoder, V. Judson Wyckoff, and H. David Maloney in economics.

Also added were Charles P. Erdmann, Edwin R. Snavely, Ethel A. Mitchell, and Martha F. Cornick in physical education; Lorna Barber in home economics; and Raymond A. Mulligan and Otto L. Sonder in sociology. The School of Music added May Agnes Strong, Donald H. White, Glen Sherman, Cassel W. Grubb, Arthur D. Carkeek, Evelyn Gibson, and Robert G. Grocock. New to the library staff was Marjory H. Royer.

President Wildman suffered a coronary occlusion in February 1950 and submitted his resignation to the board of trustees in June, asking that it take effect one year later. He recovered sufficiently to conduct the university's affairs during the 1950-51 academic year with the assistance of newly appointed Dean Norris.

One of Wildman's last official acts was to preside over the dedication ceremonies for the Memorial Student Union Building in May 1951. After his departure from Greencastle he taught Old Testament at the Perkins School of Theology of Southern Methodist University and later at Dickinson College, where he died suddenly in November 1955. His widow, Forest Kyle Wildman, survived him for over three decades, dying in 1987.

The board of trustees, given such early notice, was able to conduct a leisurely search for a new president, aided by a faculty committee appointed for that purpose. The choice finally fell upon Russell Jay

Joseph Flummerfelt directing the Collegians in 1957-58 as a student. He later returned to teach briefly at DePauw and then became director of the Westminster Choir.

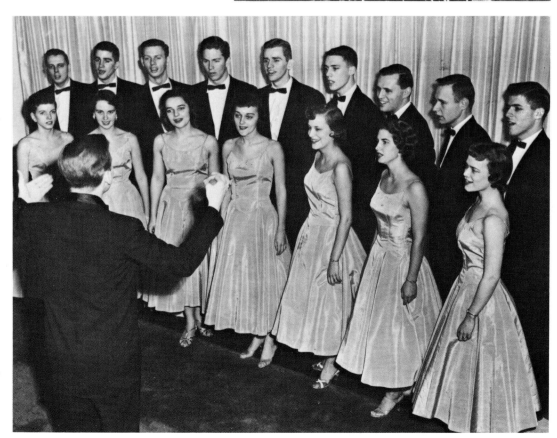

156

The Roy O. West Library was ready for occupancy in the fall of 1956.

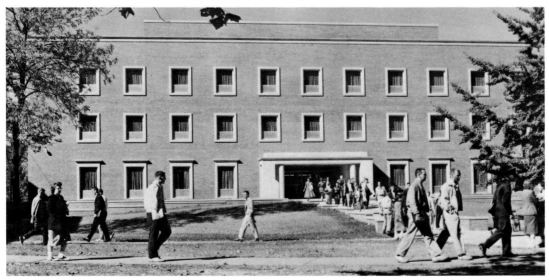

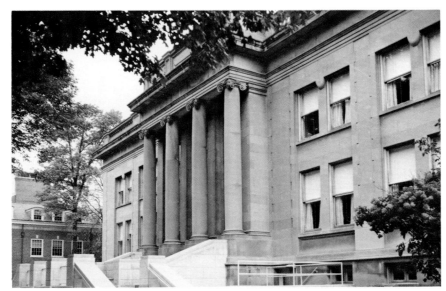

In 1958 the former Carnegie Library was converted to the Art Center. A new south entrance was created. In 1986 it was named the Emison Art Center after generous support from the Emison family.

Humbert, a graduate of the College of Wooster and the Boston University Theological School, who had served Methodist pastorates in Akron, Toledo, and Youngstown, Ohio. Less scholarly but a better speaker than his predecessor, the personable and gregarious Humbert proved to be a popular administrator and effective fund raiser. During the first year of his presidency alone he travelled over 50,000 miles, meeting with alumni clubs, attending 600 meetings, and making 322 addresses

– a striking contrast to Wildman, who is said to have spent a greater proportion of his time on campus than any other president in recent memory.

One of President Humbert's first major steps was to initiate the Greater DePauw Program, a 10-to-15 year plan to raise $10 million, about half for new buildings and half for endowment. Marts and Lundy, a consulting firm of which Humbert's father-in-law, George Lundy, was vice president, surveyed the needs of

the university and possible sources of financial support. Upon the firm's recommendation the first phase of the program was set in motion, a campaign to raise $1 million for a new library and $500,000 for other purposes, including faculty salaries. Willard Umbreit was transferred from the admissions office to direct the program. He was assisted by Orville Davis, who was named director of church relations, along with representatives of Marts and Lundy. By 1954 the campaign had collected $1,671,000 including a challenge grant of $150,000 from the Lilly Endowment. Approximately one-third of the alumni and former students solicited made contributions.

A building committee chaired by the librarian, Vera S. Cooper, began drawing up plans for the construction of a large modern library on the site of the former West College. Two specialists in library architecture, Joseph L. Wheeler and J. Russell Bailey, were called in to assist in planning a facility meeting both present and future needs of the university.

The resulting structure, designed principally by Bailey, a Virginia architect, departed radically from the Colonial lines of Asbury and Harrison Halls with which it formed an academic quadrangle. Cost considerations largely dictated its construction as a box-like, flat-roofed cube of reinforced concrete and brick. Named for distinguished alumnus and trustee Roy O. West and opened for use in 1956, the building provided sufficient space for the first time to house the university's library holdings and technical services.

The abandoned Carnegie Library was then made into the University Art Center, with considerable remodeling financed by contributions from alumni and friends of DePauw, and dedicated on Old Gold Day 1958. A new entrance with a large double stairway was added on the south side of the building, with its four great Ionic stone columns. Inside the former reading room of the library was converted into a spacious gallery for art exhibits, while the basement and upper floor furnished quarters for art studios, classrooms, a small theatre, and faculty offices. At the same time the university purchased the two-story frame building across College Avenue that had long served as a campus hang-out and remodeled it as an air-conditioned office building for members of the humanities and social sciences faculty.

The second phase of the Greater DePauw Program began in 1958 with another survey by Marts and Lundy. At the urging of President Humbert the goal was raised to $2 million. Led by Humbert himself, Norman Knights, the newly named director of public relations and financial promotion, and Robert Crouch, the secretary of alumni affairs, with Marts and Lundy, the campaign raised slightly more than the targeted amount by June 1961.

Just before it was completed the trustees authorized the construction of a new men's dormitory to replace antiquated Florence Hall. Constructed at a cost of $850,000 and designed by the same architectural firm, McGuire and Shook, that had drawn the plans for the Student Union, this was to be the last campus building to follow the Georgian Colonial pattern. It was named for the pioneer Indiana Methodist bishop, Robert E. Roberts, and opened for occupancy in the fall of 1961. Bishop Roberts Hall furnished living quarters for 150 men – later women – and dining facilities connected through a tunnel to the kitchen in nearby Longden Hall. The subsequent razing of Florence Hall left East College, Music Hall, and McKim Observatory as the only surviving 19th century structures on campus.

In academic matters President Humbert proceeded cautiously, perhaps in recognition of his inexperience in this area, and tended to rely heavily on the advice and guidance of senior faculty and

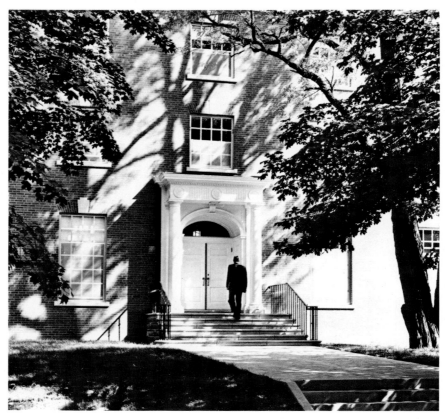

Front entrance to Bishop Roberts Hall which had accommodations for 150 men when built. It later became a freshmen women's dormitory.

administrative staff. To replace Dean Norris, who resigned in 1952 to accept the presidency of MacMurray College, he chose Robert Farber from the dean of student's office. Farber, who spent most of his adult life in various administrative posts at DePauw, was to serve as academic dean longer than anyone before or since. In 1952 DePauw alumnus John J. Wittich was named director of admissions and the Rector Scholarship Foundation, and another alumnus, Donald L. Tourtelot, was named the first full-time director of publicity and the news bureau.

The new position of dean of chapels was created to organize the weekly chapel and convocation programs, a task assumed by veteran Professor of English Jerome Hixson in addition to his teaching duties. In 1954, when a bookstore was added to the Student Union Building, Samuel T. Hanna was persuaded to become its first manager. The jovial "Sam" Hanna, a DePauw graduate who had operated his own bookstore

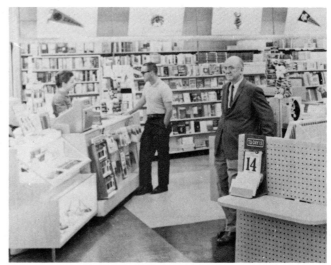

Interior view of the DePauw University Bookstore in 1962. Sam Hanna was manager from 1953 to 1970. Prior to that he had owned his own bookstore in downtown Greencastle. The Sam Hanna calendar he produced each fall has been a standard product for 40 years, still continued. A graduate of DePauw, Hanna was in the first class of Rector Scholars and a recipient of the Old Gold Goblet for an outstanding alumnus. His son Dan Hanna and later grandson Steve taught in the DePauw School of Music – a three-generation family working for DePauw.

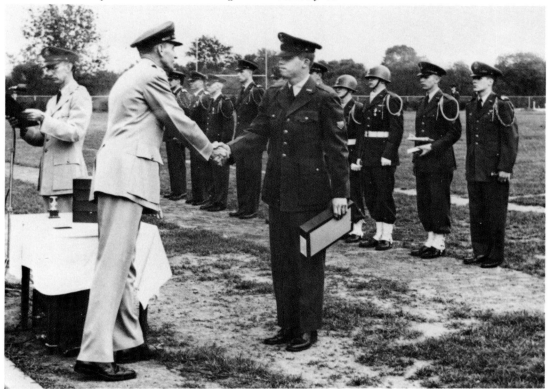

Air Force ROTC ceremony in 1955. Captain Joseph Campbell is at the microphone and Lt. Colonel Frederick Sanders presents the award to Eugene N. Holladay '57.

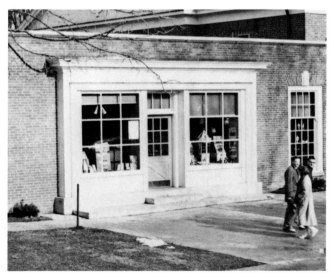

The University Bookstore was completed in 1954 as an addition to the Memorial Student Union. It was managed by Sam Hanna until his retirement in 1970, followed by 16 years with managers Donald Tunks to 1975 and Richard Conrad (1978-86). In 1986 the Bookstore became a franchise of Barnes and Noble with a separate notions store, The Annex, managed by Conrad and still a part of the university. It is located in the former Union Bowling Alley.

downtown for many years, made the university's entrance into the book business a success from the start.

Other administrative shifts included the appointment of David W. Robinson as assistant dean of students in 1952, followed by William McK. Wright in 1957. Ethel A. Mitchell moved from the physical education department in 1960 to take the place of Lucille Scheuer with the new title of associate dean of students. Upon the death of Veneta Kunter in 1952 her assistant, alumna Value Timmons Williams, became registrar. Successive directors of the Memorial Student Union Building were Glenn W. Timmons in 1952 and John Nanovsky in 1956. DePauw graduate James N. Cook was named editor of the *DePauw Alumnus* in 1954 and also acted as assistant secretary of alumni affairs. In 1961 Louis J. Fontaine succeeded fellow DePauw alumnus Wittich as director of admissions.

Worth M. Tippy, a retired Methodist minister who had graduated from DePauw in 1891, was responsible for establishing the Archives of DePauw University and Indiana Methodism in two small rooms in the basement of the Administration Building in 1951. Tippy, who was named the first archivist, had studied archival procedures in Washington, D.C. and began collecting the large quantity of documents which are now stored in specially equipped rooms in the Roy O. West Library. He also played an important role in the removal of Old Bethel Church from Charlestown, Indiana where it had been built in 1807, to the grounds of Gobin Memorial Methodist Church. The log structure, the first Methodist church building in Indiana, was dedicated on Founders' and Benefactors' Day in 1955. It stands there today as a tangible reminder of DePauw's Methodist origins.

The beginning of Humbert's presidency coincided with the establishment of a student military training program, the third such to be organized on the DePauw campus. United States military intervention in Korea under United Nations auspices in the summer of 1950 raised the specter of severely reduced enrollments as a result of male students being drafted into the Armed Forces. The administration, with strong faculty and student support, approached the federal government concerning the possibility of introducing some kind of military training program. In July 1951 the Defense Department responded by instituting a unit of the Air Force Reserve Officers' Training Corps at DePauw.

Under the command of Lt. Colonel Frederick A. Sanders, this unit, eventually known as the 235th Wing, enrolled nearly half of the male student body in its first years. Cadets were not only exempt from the military draft but also became eligible for commissions in the Air Force Reserve upon the completion

In the Commencement of 1958 British Prime Minister Harold MacMillan gave an address and received an honorary degree from President Humbert. His maternal grandfather, Joshua T. Belles, was a graduate of the Indiana Asbury Central Medical College in 1851.

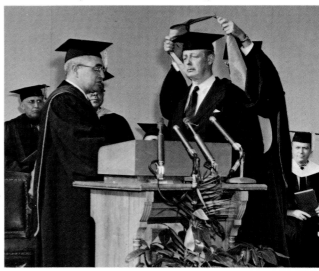

of two years of basic and two years of advanced training, plus summer camp. The bowling alleys in the gymnasium were converted into an indoor rifle range, and once more marching men in cadet uniforms became a common campus sight. A new honorary for advanced R.O.T.C. students was formed and called the Arnold Air Society, and interested coeds organized Angel Flight as a supporting group. Though enrollment in the unit declined in later years, the program survived by adapting to changing conditions.

A major accomplishment of the Humbert administration was the organization of the School of Nursing in 1955. The university entered into an agreement with Methodist Hospital in Indianapolis for a cooperative program in nursing education that included two years of pre-nursing classes at DePauw and two years of professional and clinical training at Methodist Hospital. Graduates would receive the degree of bachelor of science in nursing from DePauw University and become eligible to take the licensing

examination to qualify as registered nurses. Fredericka E. Koch of Methodist Hospital became the school's first director and was succeeded in 1957 by Catherine M. Friddle. Eight young women entered the program in the fall of 1955 and five graduated four years later. By 1961 enrollments had grown into double digits.

In 1955 a faculty self-study committee funded by the Ford Foundation for the Advancement of Education issued a report containing 56 specific recommendations for improving DePauw's academic program. Strongly supporting the university's commitment to the liberal arts, the committee endorsed the general studies courses that had emerged from the Experimental Program of a few years before and urged expansion of the honors program and comprehensive examinations for all graduating seniors. The report also suggested that the student body be expanded to 2000 and eventually 2500, and that faculty teaching loads be limited to 12 hours per week with a maximum

of 100 students. These ideas all helped shape the future direction of DePauw.

The committee recommended new graduation requirements, which were shortly afterwards adopted by the faculty. In all areas except physical education and foreign languages requirements were increased. Two hours of speech were added to the previously required six hours of freshman composition, with the proviso that any student could choose instead eight hours of combined oral and written work in the basic communications course offered under General Studies. In both the natural and the social sciences the minimum requirement for graduation was raised from six to nine hours. A new group requirement was added in the humanities, consisting of the former six-hour requirement in philosophy and religion plus six hours of work in art, music, or literature in either English or a foreign language. The latter six hours could also be fulfilled by the history of civilization course plus the senior colloquium in General Studies. The committee's recommendation that three hours of Bible be required of all students was not adopted.

Early capping ceremony of the nurses in Gobin Church. Frederika Koch, first Director of the School of Nursing (1955-57) presides and Opal Gilbert (1955-57), Assistant Director, assists.

PERCY L. JULIAN

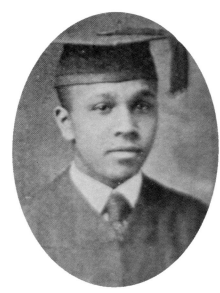

Percy L. Julian as a graduating senior in 1920.

Percy Lavon Julian was born in Montgomery, Alabama in 1899. He was the grandson of a slave and the oldest child of James Sumner Julian, a railway mail clerk, and Elizabeth Adams Julian, a schoolteacher. After graduating from a small normal school in his home town, he entered DePauw University as a "subfreshman" in the fall of 1916. At first he lived in the attic of a fraternity house, where he worked as a janitor and waiter in return for room and board. Later his parents moved to Greencastle to establish a home for Percy and his two brothers and three sisters, all of whom eventually graduated from DePauw.

Percy quickly made up his academic deficiencies and majored in chemistry under the guidance of Professor William M. Blanchard. The southern-born Blanchard recognized his protégé's scientific potential but recommended that he find a teaching position in a black college after graduation rather than undertake advanced training, because his skin color would limit his chances for success as a chemist.

Graduating from DePauw in 1920 at the top of his class, Percy accepted an instructorship in chemistry at Fiske University. Two years later he received a fellowship to study at Harvard, where he earned an M.A. in 1923. After two more years spent at Harvard on various research grants, he went to West Virginia State College for Negroes and later to Howard University to teach chemistry. Taking leave to study at the University of Vienna, where he received a Ph.D. in 1931, Julian found his career momentarily blocked at Howard and had to look elsewhere for a suitable position.

In 1932 his old mentor Professor Blanchard, now academic dean of DePauw University, invited Julian to return to his alma mater as a research associate in organic chemistry. For four years Julian carried on research in Minshall Laboratory that led to the successful synthesis of physostigmine, a drug used in the treatment of glaucoma. But DePauw lost the opportunity to retain the services of a brilliant scientist when the board of trustees proved unwilling to grant the black chemist a regular faculty position. Instead, in 1936 Julian became director of research for the Soya Products Division of the Glidden Company in Chicago.

During 17 years with that company he developed such products as fire-fighting foam and perfected methods for the mass production of hormones. In 1953 he formed his own company, Julian Laboratories, Inc. with headquarters in Franklin Park, Ill. and branches in Mexico and Guatemala. One of his major accomplishments was a process for the commercial production of the arthritis drug cortisone. Eventually selling the company to two large pharmaceutical firms, he organized Julian Associates and the Julian Research Institute in 1964, continuing his work as a research scientist and consultant until his death in 1975.

Throughout his life Julian maintained a deep interest in DePauw University, visiting the campus frequently as a guest lecturer, becoming a trustee in 1967, and even purchasing a farm near Greencastle as a country retreat. After his death his widow, Dr. Anna Johnson Julian, and their children, Faith and Percy Jr., established a trust fund to support research programs in the university's chemistry department and an annual Percy L. Julian Memorial Lecture. Also included was a scholarship fund to enable talented students to prepare themselves for careers in chemistry or related fields. Finally, in 1980 DePauw University rededicated the recently constructed building housing the mathematics and physical science departments as the Percy L. Julian Science and Mathematics Center.

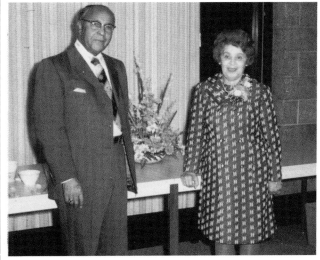

Percy L. and Anna Johnson Julian at the dedication of the Science and Mathematics Center in 1972. (Donald J. Cook)

In a special celebration for Business and Industry Day in front of the Roy O. West Library in 1957 Vice President Richard M. Nixon received an honorary degree from President Russell Humbert. In the rear are Professor Harry Voltmer (1926-66) of the political science department and longtime university marshal, Glenn W. Thompson, president of the board of trustees (1956-63) and Chief Executive Officer (1962-63) and Professor Herold T. Ross (1927-61), secretary of the faculty.

The language laboratory, a gift of Anne Hogate Hamlet in 1951, was first located in East College and later in the Roy O. West Library.

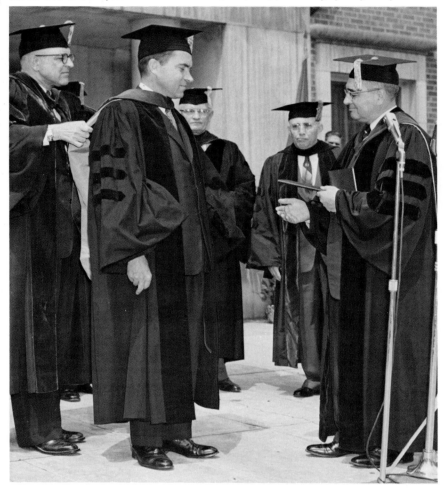

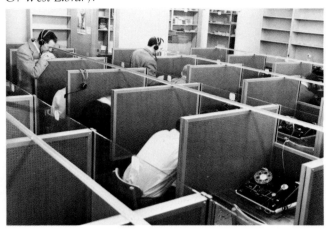

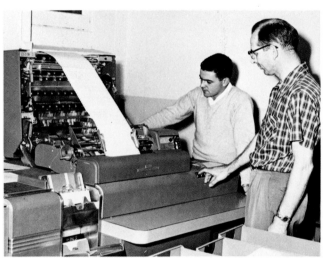

Educational foundations contributed significantly to university programs in this period. Grants from the Danforth Foundation and the Lilly Endowment made possible a pilot study for the expansion of the honors program and curricular studies in various departments which led to the introduction of such courses as Basic Beliefs of Modern Man and History of World Civilizations. The Cold War in the 1950s also inspired the addition to the curriculum of courses in Russian and Asian history and government. In 1958 the university began offering courses in the Russian language for the first time, leading eventually to the evolution of the department of German language and literature into the German and Russian department, with majors available in both languages.

Technical advances in this period included the introduction of International Business Machines computing equipment for the use of the registrar and other administrative offices in 1956. As a student publication complained, the IBM computer was becoming the "god of registration." A gift from alumna Anne Hogate Hamlet made possible the installation of tape recorders in semi-soundproof booths for use in a language laboratory in 1957. This

Hubert Smaltz (1951-66) was the Assistant Director of the Computer Center and the first to introduce the university to the computer in the basement of the Administration Building. Here he is shown with a student and an early machine. Robert Thomas of the mathematics department was the director and first gave courses in the subject.

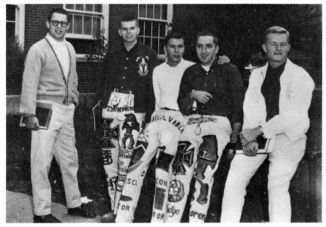

Some senior men wore yellow corduroy trousers with elaborate designs painted by underclassmen. These ATOs sport their "cords" in front of Asbury Hall.

Lilian Pierce (Taylor) and Evalena Williams were fraternity house cooks. In the middle is Adam (John Quincy) Wagner, who owned a shoe shine parlor in Greencastle for nearly 50 years. He was also a favorite doorman and fraternity houseman until his death in 1965 at 87.

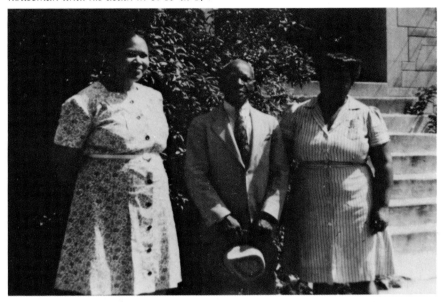

Professor Frederick Bergmann and DePauw students on the European Studies Program at the Berlin Wall.

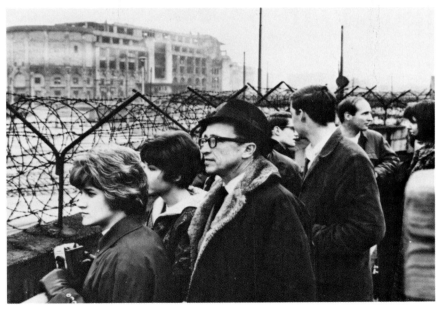

and secondary school teachers. In 1956 the Coe Foundation sponsored the first of a series of American Studies Institutes for high school teachers. Similarly the National Science Foundation funded a Science and Mathematics Institute for teachers of science in the fifth, sixth, seventh, and eighth grades for several summers. Other summer programs brought high school juniors and seniors to campus for college preparatory work and career planning.

DePauw joined with other colleges and universities in the state to advance their mutual interests. In 1953 the university became a member of the Indiana Collegiate Conference, which included Butler, Evansville, Valparaiso, St. Joseph's, Indiana State, and Ball State. DePauw continued to compete with these institutions in athletic contests for a number of years. It also had an active role in the Associated Colleges of Indiana, which was primarily a fund-raising group, as well as the lobbying association, the Independent Colleges and Universities of Indiana.

In 1959 the university joined with 11 other liberal arts colleges in Indiana, Ohio, and Michigan to form a broader type of organization which became the Great Lakes Colleges Association. The GLCA, comprised of Earlham, Wabash, Antioch, Denison, Kenyon, Oberlin, Ohio Wesleyan, Wooster, Albion, Hope, Kalamazoo, and DePauw, adopted a constitution in 1961 setting forth its objectives, which included holding conferences on educational matters and undertaking cooperative programs in teaching, research, college administration, and student activities.

Modest improvements were made in faculty compensation during this administration. The average salary for full professors rose from $5,279 in 1951-52 to $9,700 in 1961-62.

laboratory, located at various times in either the Roy O. West Library or East College, helped to improve oral teaching methods and revitalize the study of foreign languages at the university.

DePauw's foreign study program expanded to include sending groups of students under the supervision of a faculty member to various European cities as part of a Junior Semester Abroad plan. Professor Bergmann of the English department led the first group to Zell am See near Salzburg, Austria, in 1959. This program was later shifted to Vienna. In 1960 Professor Fuller of the zoology department initiated a similar program in Freiburg, Germany. Later Athens, Greece became the center for another program.

Regular summer sessions were discontinued in 1951. Instead DePauw began offering special summer programs for high school students and for both elementary

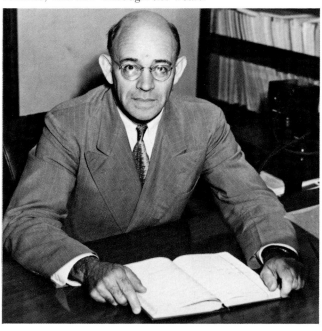

Fringe benefits were increased to include major medical insurance and minor changes in the faculty pension system administered by the Teachers Insurance and Annuity Association. A generally inflationary period also brought higher charges to students. By 1961-62 tuition had reached $1,150, approximately double the amount charged 10 years before.

A large number of new instructors joined the faculty as student enrollments grew during the period. Among them were Raymond E. Mizer, Edward K. Williams, Conrad A. Hilberry, Marian Shalkhauser (Brock), Norman Carlson, Clem C. Williams, Roger L. Cox and Fred N. Nelson in English; Robert O. Weiss, James F. Elrod, John R. Foxen, and Darrell H. Gooch in speech; Marjorie Lane (Baerg), Carl E. Steinhauser, and Glenn E. Welliver in German; Morris Wachs, C. Hal Albro, and William J. Driscoll in Romance languages; and Edwin L. Minar and Brandt N. Steele in classical languages.

Others were John J. Baughman, Clifton J. Phillips, Dwight L. Ling, John B. Wilson, James F. Findlay, and Norman K. Risjord in history;

Stephen T. Early, William L. Morrow, and Robert S. Sullivant in political science; W. Russell McIntyre and John T. Reiling in sociology; Russell J. Compton, Robert S. Eccles, H. John Eigenbrodt, Robert D. Newton, Leon Pacala, Roger Gustavsson, William E. Farley, and Elmer D. Klemke in philosophy and religion; Joseph P. Allen and Fred S. Silander in economics; and Charles K. Moore, Muriel Holland, Donald E. Orlosky, and Florence Guild in education.

Also joining the faculty were Frank S. McKenna, Barron B. Scarborough, Charles E. Platt, Curtis E. Thomsen, Felix E. Goodson, John E. Exner, Jr., Rex Rector, and Philip C. Diem in psychology; Clinton B. Gass, Charles H. Johnson, Robert J. Thomas, and John C. Anderson in mathematics and astronomy; Malcolm Correll, Hugh F. Henry, and Paul B. Kissinger in physics; John A. Ricketts and John W. McFarland in chemistry; Robert I. Fletcher and W. Preston Adams in botany and bacteriology; James A. Madison in geology; James R. Gammon in zoology; Robert R. Harvey, James C. Loveless, Elmer McCall, Theodore

Katula, and Thomas Mont in physical education; Garret J. Boone and Richard Peeler in art; Betty J. Staggs in home economics; and Anna J. Evans and Marion B. Crandall in secretarial science.

The School of Music added Daniel H. Hanna, Floyd H. Peterson, and Milton S. Trusler. Among the first instructors in the School of Nursing were Jessalyn M. Allen, Wanda Plunkett (Craddock), Carmen Sharp, Virginia Kremer, and Patricia A. Ritter. In 1954 John C. Wright began his long service as assistant director of the Bureau of Testing and Research, which was headed during this period first by Professor Scarborough and then by Professor Exner of the psychology department. New members of the library staff included Elizabeth Bowden (Baughman), J. Marian Mullendore, Suzanne Johnson (Early), Eleanor Cammack, Russell S. Dozer, and Eleanor J. Carmichael.

In January 1962 Founders' and Benefactors' Day was celebrated with special ceremonies marking the

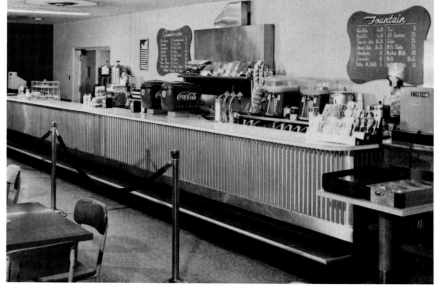

View of the food counter of the Hub in the basement of the Memorial Student Union in 1958.

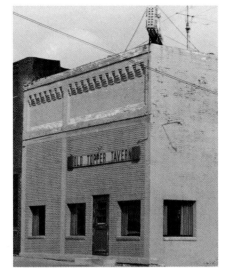

In the last 20 years the Old Topper Tavern became the favorite hangout.

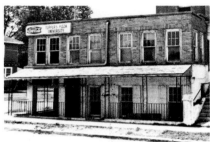

The Subway under many managers provided "short orders" for about 40 years.

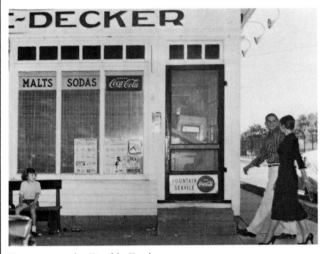

Entrance to the Double Decker.

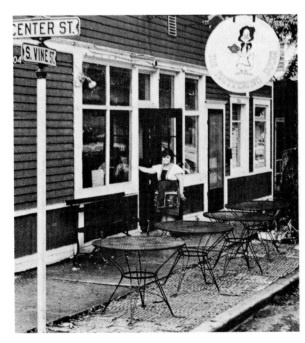

STUDENT HANGOUTS

Before the completion of the Memorial Student Union and its cafeteria, the Hub, in 1951, DePauw students found a variety of other places for eating and hanging out. Some persisted to a later period and several new establishments have opened in the meantime. Located on Anderson Street was the Rendezvous, servicing the fraternities and sororities on the east side of campus and operated first by Bruce and Sylvia Shannon and later by Glenn and Leone Deem.

Across from the Alpha Chi Omega House on Locust Street was the Double Decker, begun by a man named Decker and carried on by George Williams, Chuck Phillips, Glenn Deem, and finally by Bob, Bill, and Richard Jackson. Students from sorority row, the Music School, and faculty members patronized the Double, which outlasted the Rendezvous and survives today in an eastside Greencastle location.

On the northwest corner of Seminary Street and College Avenue was a rather unprepossessing structure standing in front of the Baynes House, one of Greencastle's finest old homes used at one time as the DKE chapter house. A popular eatery located there was the Subway, which offered hamburgers, Hostess cupcakes, and breakfast for single members of the faculty. It was run by a succession of managers, including Bill Trinkle, Mable and Fred Monnett, and Evan Crawley, the last of whom also served for a time as mayor of Greencastle. Other shops in the complex were Bernie Smith's barbershop, John Tzouanakis' shoe repair shop, later run by John Due, and Drake's Jewelry Store.

Several blocks south on College Avenue at the intersection of Hanna Street stood another row of commercial buildings. Included were a small grocery called the Campus Market, owned by Lester Conrad and his son Richard and an ice cream shop once known to students as Stinky's. The latter eventually became the U Shop, a variety store presided over by the ubiquitous Glenn and Leone Deem. For a short time doughnuts were available from the Spudnut Shop next door.

After the Second World War a small student hangout called the Fluttering Duck, located behind Asbury Hall on Vine Street, enjoyed a high level of popularity before it burned to the ground in 1979. Its proprietor, Maybelle Hamm, served short orders, an occasional more substantial meal, and specialties of the house such as hot cider. Some faculty members – sociologists in particular – also held informal seminars. Students presented plays and musical performances in the Duck. A faculty instrumental group, the Ducks of Dixieland, was often featured. Today the name is perpetuated in the Fluttering Duck bar and lounge in the Walden Inn, recently erected on the same site.

For the drinking crowd, including the Black Friars and other clandestine groups, there was Dutch Hoffman's, or simply Dutch's on South Indiana Street near the town square. Located in the same 19th century building that once housed Emanuel Marquis' music store, this establishment later became Moore's Bar. In the 1950s and 1960s the most popular tavern catering to the student trade was Topper's on the Greencastle southside. DePauw men and women resorted to this watering place in throngs, especially on Thursday, Friday, and Saturday evenings. For a while it included a small restaurant, the Annex, next door. Other drinking oases in the southend were the 713 Bar, once called D. B. Cooper's, and Charlie Brown's Bar-B-Q.

Five miles south of Greencastle Marion and Virginia Wilson were genial hosts at the Old Trail Inn for two decades, offering faculty, students, and their families old-fashioned Indiana fare in the tradition of the Halfway House in Mt. Meridian. Pearl O'Hair operated a well-known gift shop in the lobby. The Monon Grill and Mama Nunz still attract student patronage, as does Marvin's, a pizza and burrito shop that evolved from an earlier place called Topper's Pizza University, successor to the Subway. Its proprietor, Marvin Long, became a favorite student confidant, whose restaurant was advertised briefly on Red Square in Moscow in 1985 by touring DePauw undergraduates.

The Fluttering Duck in the 1970s with owner-manager Maybelle Hamm at the entrance.

STUDENTS

No coed room in the '50s was minus a radio or two, but lampshades hung as crooked as in the 19th century.

A Sigma Chi project for "Hell Week" or "Help Week" could probably be considered both.

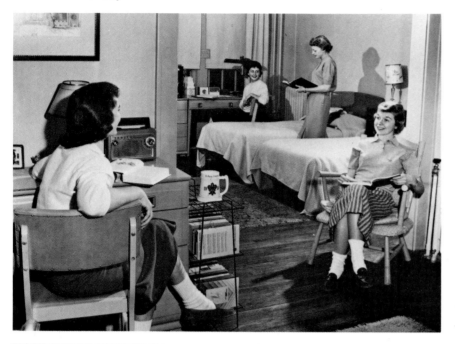

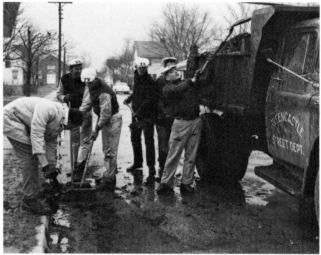

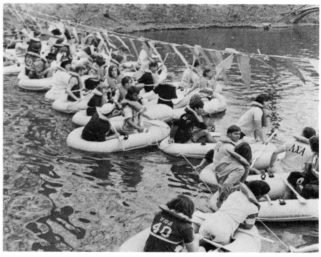

In 1976 and 1977 competitive raft races in the spring on Big Walnut River outside Greencastle became an exciting student activity.

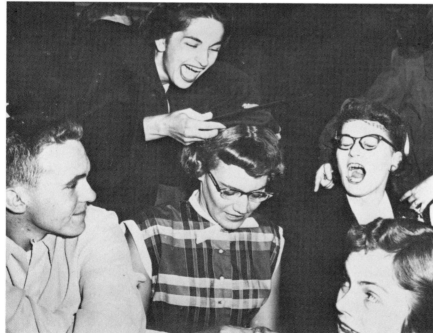

Above: Being "capped" for Mortor Board, the national scholarship-leadership society, was a "coed" highlight on May Day before the society became officially coeducational. Ann Stillwell received her honor in 1953. To the right is her mother and Methodist Student Movement Director Pat Kyle.

At right: The year 1972 was the heydey of the Boulder run, a ritual for Phi Kappa Psi members of that period to celebrate the year's first snowfall. Dean of Students William McK. Wright, after an illustrated article appeared in Playboy in September 1972, announced that "the boulder run is not a common occurrence, and is specifically a violation of a university regulation and local law."

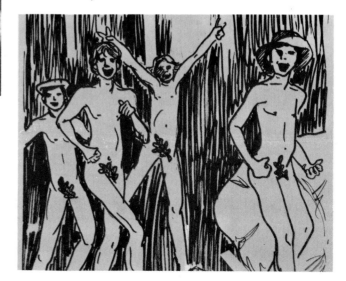

The dining room of Mason Hall in the 1940s when dining still continued to be rather dignified and refined. Student waiter Richard Smith later became chairman of the history department at Ohio Wesleyan University.

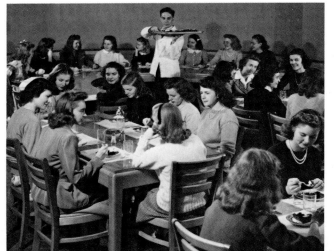

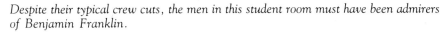
Despite their typical crew cuts, the men in this student room must have been admirers of Benjamin Franklin.

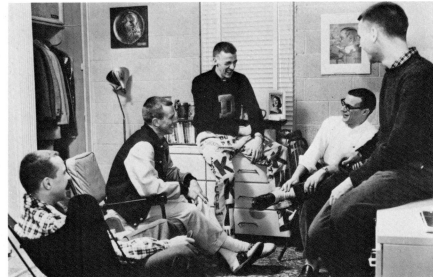

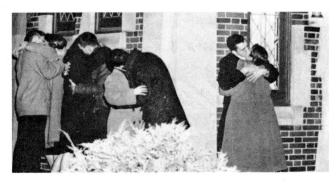

Late "hours" for coeds produced an era of prolonged goodnights. Behind the door is a housemother frantically ringing a bell.

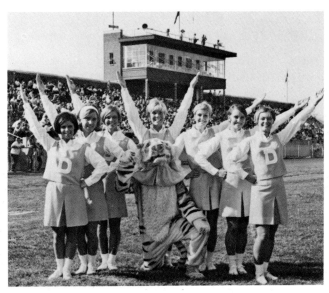

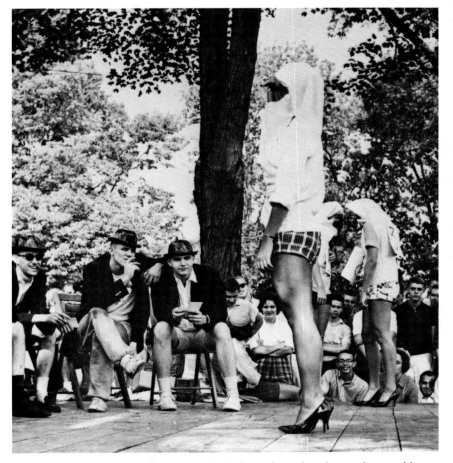

Cheerleaders and the Tiger Mascot at Blackstock Stadium for a football game.

This sexist picture from Derby Day in 1960 shows the male judges oggling coed legs in a student competition. By 1987 this type of activity would probably be illegal as an example of sexual harassment.

STUDENTS (continued)

A formal spring dance in the "Big Band" era in Bowman Gymnasium before the student world became casual.

Below: This group picture of fraternity men from the 1975 Mirage demonstrates how far some student lifestyles had evolved from 1837. Center of page: The Kappas have a song practice in 1953.

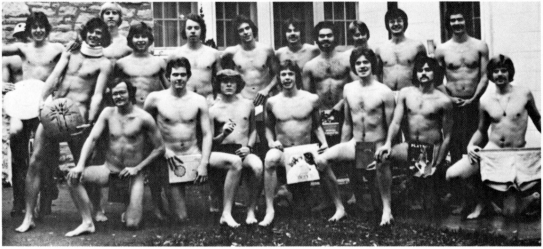

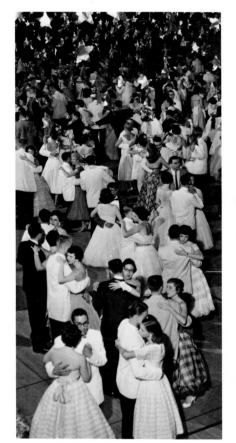

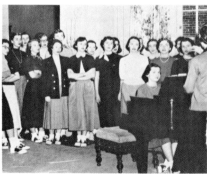

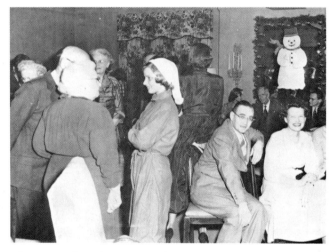

Above: Sunday afternoon faculty teas in the winter months found the students on their best behavior. Here, at a Christmas party, a student chats with Professor and Mrs. Earl Bowman. Others include Professor Welch, Mrs. Fulmer, Professor and Mrs. Clark Norton, Professor Wallace Carson, and Assistant Professor Otto Sonder.

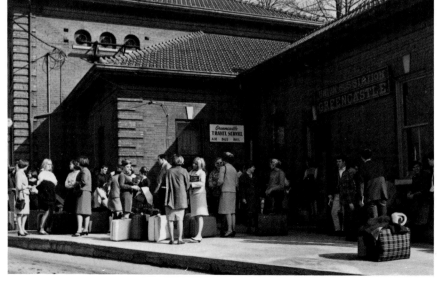

The buses still stopped in Greencastle in the '70s to take students into the "real world" for brief holidays from their strenuous scholarship.

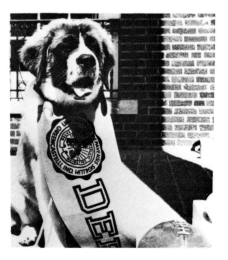

Thibideau was the name of generations of St. Bernards owned by the Sigma Nus.

Coeds descend the famous Alpha Phi staircase in baroque splendor to meet their dates, perhaps for a prom.

The naming of the Old Gold Day Queen in the early 1970s reflects the eclectic student styles of that era.

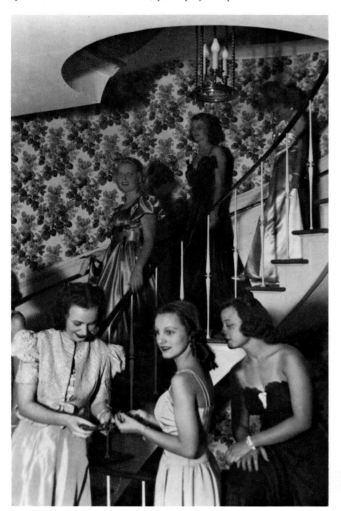

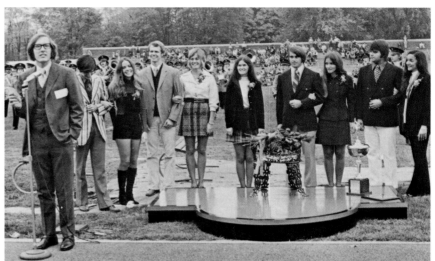

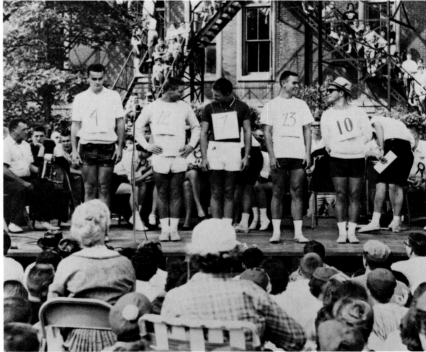

A sign of decline in women's beauty contests was this competition for the best male legs. One wonders how much the students on the East College firescapes saw, but the two seated housemothers got a good view.

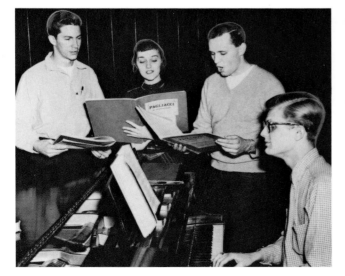

Larry Clarkson, Julie Harris, David Cryer are preparing for their roles in the opera workshop production of "Pagliacci" in 1958 accompanied by Joseph Flummerfelt.

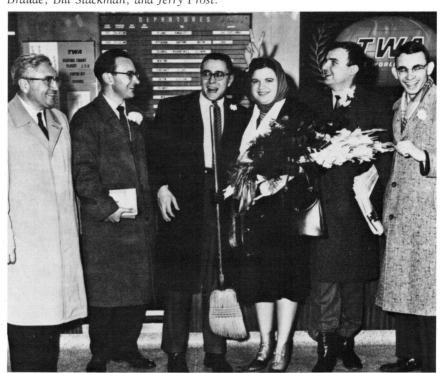

125th anniversary of the founding of DePauw University. Later that year Professor George Manhart published his monumental two-volume historical work, *DePauw Through the Years*. Adding an unexpected fillip to the celebrations was the series of five victories in a row won by DePauw students in the General Electric-sponsored College Bowl television quiz show. When the four DePauw representatives returned to campus undefeated after the final contest, hundreds of students and others came out in the rain to greet them in a gesture harking back to similar receptions given to the victors in oratorical and debating competition of an earlier era.

The sudden death of President Humbert in June 1962 cast a pall over the Commencement exercises and caused a hiatus in university leadership. His death came at the height of his career at the age of 56 and in the midst of a major fund-raising campaign. His widow, Margaret Lundy Humbert, continued to reside in Greencastle for some years and later married Professor Emeritus Jerome Hixson, with whom she now makes her home in Florida.

There followed a year's interlude during which Glenn W. Thompson, president of the board of trustees, was named chief executive of the university while Dean Farber acted as chief administrative officer. Among those appointed to the faculty during this period were Richard Kelly in psychology, who also became the director of the Bureau of Testing and Research; William J. Petrek in philosophy and religion; Ruth L. Lester in physical education; James A. Martindale and Daniel L. Smith in the library; Ned B. MacPhail in education; Zita D. Dabars in Russian; Eugene P. Schwartz in chemistry; and Edward M. Dolan, an anthropologist who began teaching that subject in the sociology department.

Minor construction projects were completed, including additions to the Bookstore and the Administration Building. A larger project was the construction of the Burkshire

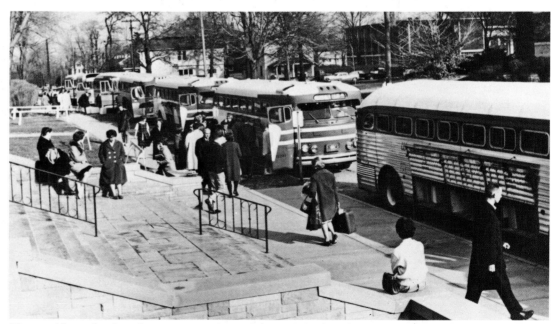

Chartered buses lined up for vacation in front of the Memorial Student Union in the 1960s.

William E. Kerstetter was president of DePauw from 1963 to 1975. Here he is shown with his wife Leona Bateman Kerstetter and daughter Laura and son William.

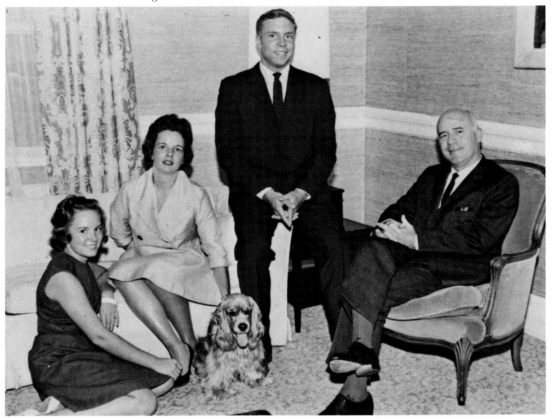

A primary objective of the Kerstetter administration was to modernize and expand the university's physical facilities. This entailed the purchase of scores of residential properties covering several city blocks south of Hanna Street to make room for projected buildings. The cost of this far-sighted move exceeded $1 million and was written into the construction budgets of the buildings to be erected there. Besides enlarging the campus considerably, the administration also took a special interest in its beautification, carrying out an extensive landscaping effort that won the university national recognition.

The first new building erected was Hogate Hall, a women's dormitory named for two alumni, the late Kenneth C. Hogate and his widow, Anne Hogate Hamlet. The latter had contributed $1 million to the Design for a Decade and also made DePauw the beneficiary of another $1million in her will. Located on land already owned by the university near the Dells on South Locust Street, Hogate Hall was designed by the Chicago architectural firm of Holabird and Root in an unusual accordian-like configuration that set the building apart from other campus structures. Its attractive brick, stone, and glass walls enclosed a lounge, reception area, and kitchen and dining facilities on the first floor, with 24 six-person suites in place of the usual rows of double rooms in its two upper stories. The new, air-conditioned dormitory opened for occupancy in the fall of 1968, providing upperclass independent women with some of the best living arrangements on campus as well as a focus for non-sorority oriented activities.

In seeking and obtaining grants from private foundations and the federal government, the administration was faced with the task of redefining the university's relationship with the United Methodist Church. In 1968 the board of trustees agreed to a partial

Apartments on the site of the former Barnaby home and Art Center on East Washington Street. The gift of alumni John and Ardath Burkhart, these two handsome buildings provided nine air-conditioned, two-bedroom apartments for faculty newcomers, a decided improvement over the barracks and prefabricated structures previously serving that purpose.

With the advice of a joint faculty-trustee committee the board of trustees conducted a presidential search that led to the election of William E. Kerstetter in 1963. A graduate of Dickinson College, he possessed both the S.T.B. and Ph.D. from Boston University, making him the eighth DePauw president in succession to have been educated at that institution. The new president was an ordained Methodist minister but had spent almost his whole career in college teaching and administration, having been a professor of philosophy at Hamline College before becoming president of Simpson College.

Shortly after his arrival on campus President Kerstetter took up the challenge of the unfinished Greater DePauw Program by persuading the trustees to launch a much more ambitious campaign to raise $30 million in 10 years. Called Design for a Decade, this campaign was led by a steering committee of DePauw trustees and other supporters headed by John Burkhart of Indianapolis.

At the end of the first five years contributions in cash and pledges reached a total of $23 million, including a contingency grant of $2 million from the Ford Foundation. Moreover, in 1966 the board of trustees finally reversed a long-held position by voting to adopt a "policy of accepting, selectively, federal funds in support of the general program of the university." As a result the university applied for and received a $2,396,454 federal allocation covering one-third of the cost of a new science building, an action unprecedented in the history of the privately-funded institution.

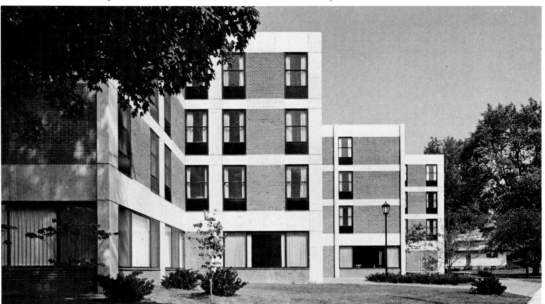

revision of the longstanding arrangements for the oversight of the university that emphasized its nonsectarian stance without disavowing the historical ties with Indiana Methodism.

The amended by-laws reduced the number of trustees from 40 to 33, with nine (counting the bishop of the Indiana area) elected by the Indiana conferences of the Methodist Church, eight by the alumni, and the remaining 16 by the board of trustees itself. The board of visitors, which was composed of nine delegates from the Indiana conferences and had already lost most of its importance, was eliminated, further reducing the official Methodist representation in the university's governing body.

The $1,736,000 cost of Hogate Hall was amortized over 20 years in order to conserve funds for other purposes, including paying off the remaining construction debts for the Memorial Student Union Building, the Roy O. West Library, the Art Center, and the Faculty Office Building. The next major project was the construction of a modern facility to replace the obsolete Minshall Laboratory. Designed by Holabird and Root as a massive concrete-and-brick block with a cantilevered upper story and a broad, open-air deck, the new science and mathematics center was completed in 1972 at a cost of $7,299,000. The main floor contained a theatre-style auditorium, classrooms, the Edgar A. Prevo Science Library, and a large Computer Center, with faculty offices, seminar rooms, and laboratories on the two upper floors.

In addition to housing the departments of mathematics and astronomy, chemistry, physics, and geology and geography, it provided office space for the School of Nursing and the Bureau of Testing and Research. In 1982 the building was rededicated as the Julian Science and Mathematics Center in honor of the distinguished DePauw alumnus and industrial chemist, Percy L. Julian.

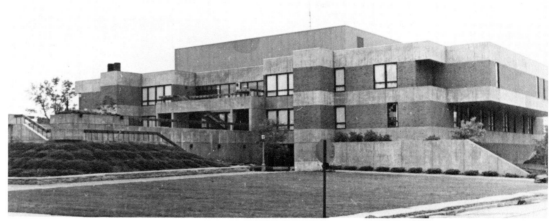

In 1973 it was decided to terminate the Design for a Decade campaign with about $3 million remaining to be raised. In its place was launched a Second Design for a Decade drive with a goal of $69 million. Alumnus and trustee Fred C. Tucker, Jr. was named to head the new campaign, which in the next five years made considerable progress toward its objective.

Among physical plant improvements carried out at this time was the complete refurbishing of the interior of McKim Observatory and the installation of a motor-driven aluminum dome to replace the original hand-operated iron one. The 90 year-old building was eventually placed on the National Register of Historic Places.

The question of what to do about an even older structure, East College, posed a serious problem for the university. It was long debated whether to raze or restore the physically weakened building, which was in imminent need of expensive repairs. A strong wave of alumni

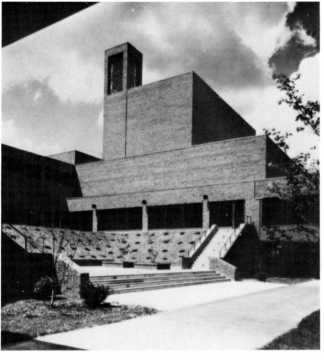

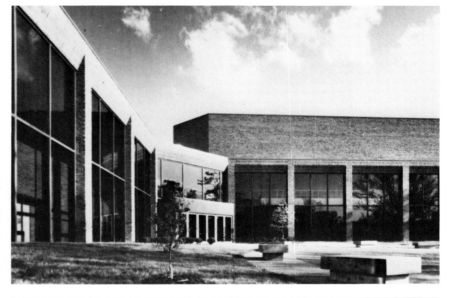

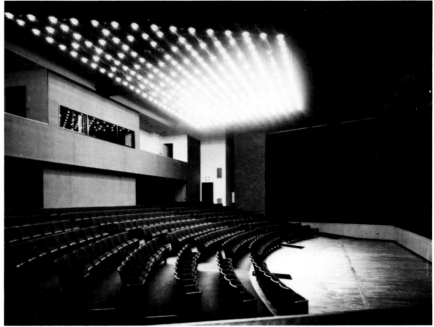

support for retaining the memory-laden campus monument along with its inclusion on the National Register of Historic Places in 1975 turned the tide in favor of restoration, which was finally accomplished at the beginning of the next decade.

The last building project completed in the Kerstetter administration was the $8.5 million Performing Arts Center which opened in 1976. The elegant multi-story complex was designed by Holabird and Root architects in a modernistic style with lavish use of glass and plain red-brick facing on both exterior and interior walls. The three-story academic building housing the offices and classrooms of the department of communication arts and sciences as well as the teaching studios of the School of Music, 53 music practice rooms, and a music library. The academic wing was named Burkhart Hall in honor of Ardath Y. and John Burkhart.

Elevated passageways connect it with the performing component, which contains the 1500-seat Kresge Auditorium named for donors Dorothy M. and Stanley Kresge, the

The Performing Arts Center was completed in 1976. The front entrance view (upper right) shows the auditorium on the right and the theatre on the left. The Moore Theatre (above) has seating for 400. The landscaped amphitheatre (upper left) is overlooked by a 37 bell carrilon. DePauw's Performing Arts Series began when the center opened, and has continued ever since, largely under the direction of Professor Robert Grocock of the School of Music.

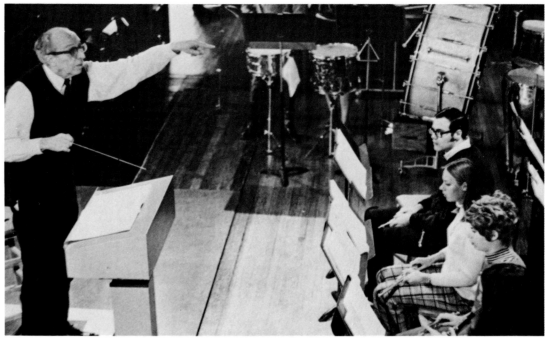

Composer-conductor Aaron Copland rehearses the DePauw Symphony during a three-day guest appearance at DePauw's first Winter Term in 1971.

400-seat Moore Theatre named for Frank M. Moore, and the 200-seat Thompson Recital Hall named for Van Denman Thompson, longtime director of the School of Music. The center also includes a landscaped amphitheatre and courtyard provided by Kappa Alpha Theta, along with a graceful tower holding a 37-bell carillon donated by Alpha Chi Omega. Both national sororities were founded at DePauw seven decades earlier. The largest single gift making the building possible was $2 million from the Krannert Charitable Trust, the creation of Herman C. and Ellvora Decker Krannert of Indianapolis.

The spirit of educational experimentation and reform was strongly evident at DePauw during the first half of the Kerstetter administration. In 1964, after extensive study and discussion, the faculty approved a major overhaul of the class schedule. No longer was credit to be awarded in "hours," based on the number of hours spent in class each week; instead a new system was adopted in which credit for one "course" was given for a class which met for a maximum of four hours per week during a single semester.

This was intended to provide students with greater opportunity for independent study and instructors with more flexibility in organizing their class work. A few half- and quarter-courses were included, chiefly in the School of Music and the art and physical education departments. The normal student load was set at four courses and the faculty teaching load at three courses a semester, with adjustments for laboratory periods in the natural sciences.

Another major change in the organization of the academic program took place in 1970. After some discussion of an alternative three-term system, the faculty voted to adopt a 4-1-4 academic calendar, made up of two slightly shortened semesters and a four-week Winter Term in January. The first semester was scheduled to begin in late

August and end just before Christmas eliminating the two-week hiatus formerly interrupting the first semester. In addition to the 31 courses needed for graduation, students were required to take four Winter Term offerings, which consisted of specially designed faculty-directed projects either on or off campus.

The first Winter Term in January 1971 featured such special events as lectures by architect R. Buckminster Fuller and the conducting of composer Aaron Copland at a Contemporary Music Festival sponsored by the School of Music. Winter Term eventually proved to be a convenient opportunity for professional internships, volunteer work projects, and study abroad. The program was later amended to include two-week as well as four-week projects, and the graduation requirement was reduced to seven two-week projects or three and one-half Winter Terms.

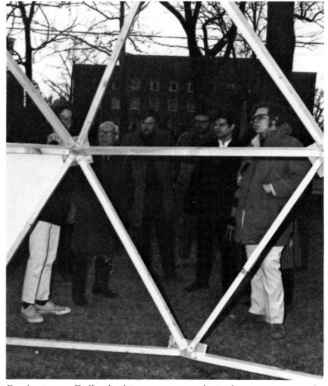

Buckminster Fuller looking over a geodesic dome constructed for his visit to the campus during the first Winter Term in 1971.

In 1971 a DePauw father, Associate Justice of the United States Supreme Court Harry A. Blackmun, received an honorary Doctor of Laws degree from DePauw. He is shown here with University Chaplain Marvin Swanson, President William E. Kerstetter, and Professor of Botany Howard R. Youse, university marshal.

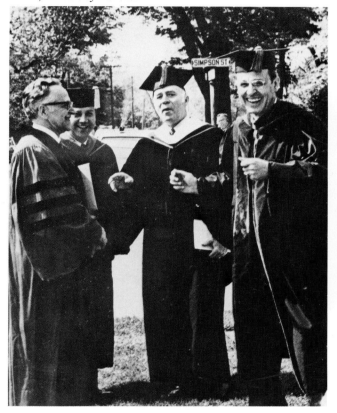

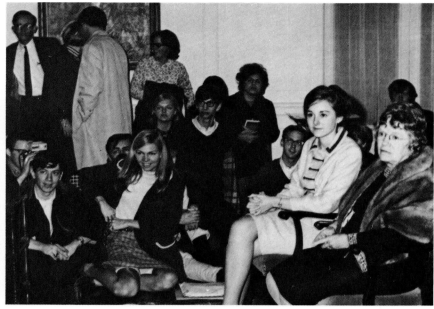

Anthropologist Margaret Mead is shown with a group of students in a visit to the campus in 1973. She attended DePauw for a year in 1919 and, after finding campus social life distasteful, transferred. In later years she returned to the campus to stimulate intellectual life.

A number of interdisciplinary courses were introduced either through the cooperative efforts of two or more departments or under the auspices of the ongoing General Studies program. The establishment of the Experimental Curriculum in 1966 also encouraged the faculty to try out new ideas for course offerings.

In 1970 the faculty approved another experimental project called the Liberal Studies program, under which up to 50 selected freshmen were permitted to choose, with the advice of a faculty counselor, an individualized course of study without following the normal graduation requirements. This program was carried out from 1971 to 1974.

In 1967 the university initiated an African Studies program at the urging of President Kerstetter, who had recently visited several countries in that continent and advocated DePauw's assuming a special academic interest in that part of the

world. The first director of the program, anthropologist Svend E. Holsoe, established an African anthropological museum in the basement of Asbury Hall and published the *Liberian Studies Journal* from his DePauw office. His successors, historians Walter T. Brown and John E. Lamphear, expanded the program to include on-campus institutes and study tours in Africa.

To encourage the study of Africa, Asia, Eastern Europe, and Latin America the faculty also adopted a non-western graduation requirement and began to add more courses in the history, language and literature, and general culture of those areas. Chinese, Japanese, and Swahili were taught for several years, and growing numbers of foreign students and visiting professors were brought to the campus.

To help achieve the administration's goal to offer every student an opportunity to become acquainted with another part of the world, a greater variety of foreign study programs was made available. In addition to DePauw's own two

Contemporary Europe Semester programs, one based in Freiburg and the other in Vienna, and the Mediterranean Studies program based in Athens, there were several GLCA-sponsored programs located in Africa, Colombia, Hong Kong, India, Japan, Scotland, and Taiwan.

DePauw students also had the option to enroll in a foreign university on an individual basis or participate in an overseas program administered by another institution. Though not everyone took advantage of these opportunities, a large majority of the student body participated in some kind of off-campus educational experience, either abroad or in one of the various domestic programs located in New York, Philadelphia, Washington D.C., Oak Ridge (Tennessee), and other cities.

An interdisciplinary program in Black Studies was inaugurated in 1972, with an area major available in that field by the following year. With the aid of a grant from the Lilly Endowment a special program

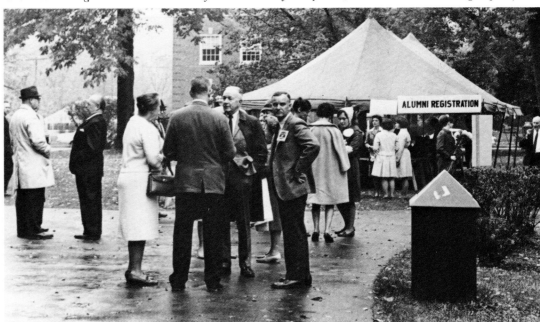

entitled Careers in Business and Public Service came into existence in 1973 under the direction of the economics and business department. It consisted of a set of core interdisciplinary courses plus specific offerings related to five career options: business, public administration, institutional management, mental retardation and mental health training, and musical arts management. Each student enrolled in this program also participated in a supervised field internship.

The university sponsored several academic symposia in various fields during these years, including one held on Old Gold Day weekend in October 1972 to celebrate the 100th anniversary of the birth of the distinguished historian Charles A.

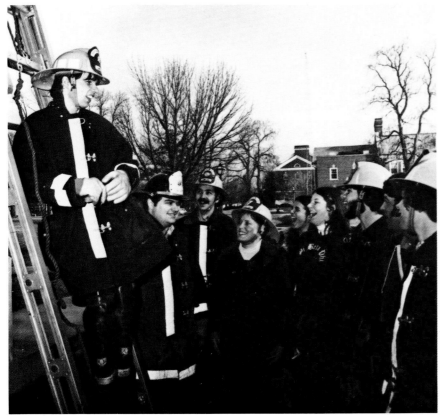

In 1971 student firefighters created the DePauw Fire Company which for over a decade ably assisted the Greencastle Fire Department and for a time had its own auxiliary truck and training program.

Beard. Both he and his wife and co-worker, Mary Ritter Beard, were native Hoosiers and Phi Beta Kappa graduates of DePauw University.

Some changes were effected in departmental organization including the elimination of the home economics and secretarial science departments. Anthropology was added to the title of the sociology department and economics became economics and business. Similarly earth sciences replaced the former departmental title geology and geography, while classical languages was renamed classical studies.

In 1974, after having begun to offer courses in digital computers shortly after the establishment of the university's Computer Center a decade earlier, the mathematics and astronomy department incorporated computer science in its title. The next year the speech department became the department of communication arts and sciences.

The aerospace department was discontinued in 1973, when the federal government withdrew the Air Force R.O.T.C. program because of lagging enrollments and budgetary restraints. Three years

The Percy L. Julian Science and Mathematics Center became the headquarters for a growing computer program for both academic study as well as in-house university needs. This shows the PDP 11/45 in use in the 1970s.

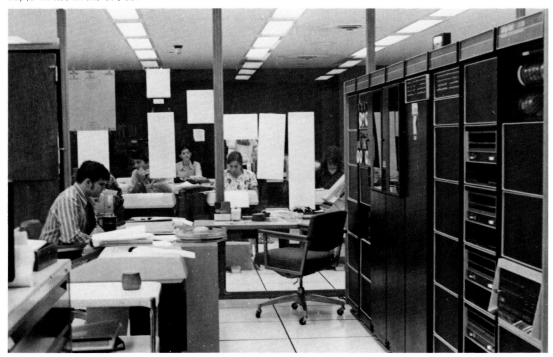

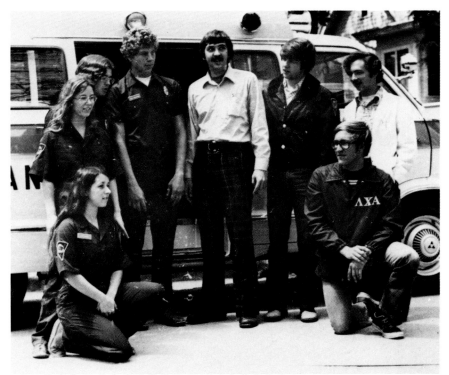

In the mid-70s student volunteers with para-medical training initiated an ambulance service for the community. The operation grew until in the the 1980s it became Operation Life, an independent ambulance service for Putnam County with local government support. It still relies heavily on trained DePauw volunteers.

later, however, the university was able to make arrangements with the Air Force department at Indiana University for DePauw students to enroll in aerospace courses on the Bloomington campus. A similar arrangement was made a year later with the Army R.O.T.C. unit at Rose-Hulman Institute in Terre Haute. The Army eventually sent an R.O.T.C. detachment to Greencastle to offer basic military courses on the DePauw campus.

The administrative offices also underwent a series of title and personnel changes, partly directed toward strengthening public relations and fund raising. In 1966 Norman Knights was named assistant to the president for planning and development, and Robert Crouch became vice president for development. After Crouch, an indefatigable fund raiser for his alma mater, retired in 1970, the former Air Force R.O.T.C. commander, Frederick Sanders, became director of development.

From 1969 to 1973 Knights served as executive vice president with broad responsibilities for the non-academic aspects of the university. James Cook was made associate director, then director, of alumni services; Patrick Aikman, director of publicity and the news bureau; Glenn T. Job, director of publications; and Marian Hoffman Maloney, assistant editor (later editor) of university publications.

In 1967 William Wright succeeded Riggs as dean of students. Oliver C. Rice came in 1969 as an assistant to the dean of students with additional responsibilities in the admissions office related to the recruitment of minority students. A new associate dean of students in 1971 was Brian R. Enos. The retirement of Value Williams in 1972 brought in Eleanor Sisson Ypma as registrar, the first in that post to possess a doctorate. Dr. Roger E. Roof succeeded Dr. Arthur W. Smith as university physician and director of health services in 1966.

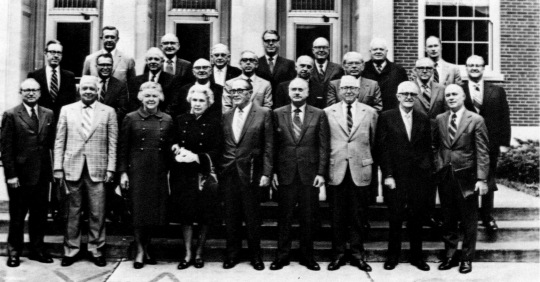

In the financial affairs office Lawrence C. Elam became the new comptroller in 1974, with William P. Marley as director of personnel and purchasing and Edward N. Pearson as chief accountant. Virginia S. Byrkit was named director of residence halls and university food service in 1976. Robert Farber, who remained as academic dean throughout the Kerstetter presidency was aided by a series of assistant and associate deans. The first assistant dean was Clark F. Norton, who also acted as director of graduate studies while continuing to teach part-time in the political science department. When he resigned to join Senator Birch Bayh's staff in Washington in 1965, Dwight L. Ling of the history department assumed the office of the assistant dean while Professor Emeritus Herold Ross took temporary charge of graduate studies.

In 1966 John A. Ricketts of the chemistry department was named director of graduate studies. Ling, whose responsibilities grew to include such matters as faculty development and the oversight of the Experimental Division, was promoted to associate dean in 1972. Other faculty members continued to hold the post of assistant dean with varied functions: Thomas A. Davis and John R. Anderson, of the mathematics department, were successively directors of graduate studies. William J. Petrek and Marvin Swanson served successively as directors of international study and off-campus programs. And for a briefer period with more generalized duties, Stanley Caine and John McFarland of the history and chemistry departments, also served as assistant deans.

Faculty ranks continued to grow in this period, along with student enrollment. Annual tuition increases as well as a rise in annual giving made possible somewhat higher levels of faculty salaries at all ranks. Newcomers to the teaching faculty in

this period tended to represent a more diverse pattern of geographical, religious, cultural, and educational backgrounds, as departments conducted national searches for the most highly qualified candidates.

Although the university endeavored to follow federal guidelines concerning affirmative action and equal opportunity, there was only slow progress in the employment of women and minorities. Increasing specialization in the training and interests of many younger intructors made for a less unified outlook and intellectual focus in the teaching faculty. By the mid-1970s it was becoming clear that DePauw was moving away from the ideal of a tightly knit, relatively homogeneous academic community toward a wider vision of a more diversified, profession-oriented, and world-minded university.

New additions to the faculty in this period were Larry G. Sutton in speech; William D. Meehan and David W. Herrold in art; William C. Cavanaugh, Elizabeth A. Christman, Cynthia E. Cornell, Thomas A. Emery, F. Walker Gilmer, Keith M. Opdahl, and Robert P. Sedlack in English; Marcia A. McKelligan in philosophy and religion; James L. Cooper, Norman Levine, Roderick A. Clifford, and

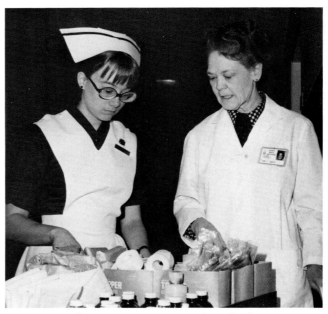

A nursing student receives instruction from Professor Wanda Craddock (1955-78).

Stanley P. Caine in history; and Ralph Gray, Alan E. Pankratz, and Gary D. Lemon in the economics department, to which former staff member Gerald E. Warren returned as head in 1966.

Also added were James E. George in chemistry; Daniel A. Sullivan and Katherine Price in earth sciences; John E. Morrill,

THE HISTORY QUARTET

Four men dominated the DePauw history department from the post World War I years through the first decades after World War II. Two Europeanists and two Americanists, diverse in temperament and interests and rivals in popularity, they worked together harmoniously enough to create a strong history program.

The first to join the DePauw faculty was William Wallace Carson, a North Carolinian with a B.A. from Wofford and M.A. from Trinity in his home state and a Ph.D. from the University of Wisconsin. He was appointed instructor in history and political science in 1916. The longtime head of both departments, Carson combined his teaching with various administrative responsibilities, including membership in the university senate in the Oxnam years and the post of university marshal, stage-managing commencements and other public occasions.

In his popular course on the American west he elaborated on the frontier thesis of Frederick J. Turner; his lectures on steamboating on the western waters were long remembered by students. The tall, courtly southern gentleman and his wife, Louella, were frequent chaperones at fraternity and sorority dances. His deafness made him appear prematurely old, but he remained a vigorous teacher until his retirement in 1953. He was a familiar figure on his walks about Greencastle until his death in 1967.

George Born Manhart came to DePauw in 1919 straight from civilian war service in army camps in Texas and Arkansas. A graduate of Susquehanna College with an M.A. and Ph.D. from the University of Pennsylvania, Manhart was a Wilsonian idealist with fervent faith in the League of Nations. He taught modern European history in the conviction that rational men might find a way to prevent world conflict by studying the causes of the two great wars of the 20th century. The most scholarly and demanding of the quartet, he encouraged many students to take up graduate studies and enter the teaching profession. He was active in the honors program and the major proponent of general education in the university, introducing and leading the teaching of the popular History of Civilization course.

A socialist and pacifist in the 1930s, he enlisted in the Air Force in 1943 at the age of 53, leaving the service as a captain in 1945. After official retirement in 1956, he kept busy with part-time teaching and the research and writing of the two-volume *DePauw Through the Years* to mark the university's 125th anniversary. He died in Greencastle in 1970, not long after the death of his wife, Florence Heritage Manhart, who had been an instructor in physical education at DePauw.

Andrew Wallace Crandall was a "son of the middle border," who came to DePauw in 1921 with a B.A. from Central College and M.A. from the University of Chicago. An officer in Europe during World War I, he remained in the Army Reserve for the rest of his life and served overseas as a member of the office of military history in World War II, retiring with the rank of major. He earned a Ph.D. at Pennsylvania with a dissertation published under the title *Early History of the Republican Party*, reprinted in 1960.

A folksy lecturer – "Don't monkey with the tariff or you'll cause hard times" – A.W., as he was generally known, captivated his students with his stories and anecdotes. His annual lecture on the battle of Gettysburg became a DePauw legend. He retired in 1960 but continued to teach as the Pulliam Professor of American History until his death three years later. He is survived by his wife, Marion Bradford Crandall, who had been DePauw's first full-time registrar and later an instructor in secretarial science.

Coen Gallatin Pierson, one of the first Rector scholars at DePauw, returned to his alma mater as an instructor in history in 1926. Holder of the M.A. from the University of Illinois and the Ph.D. from the University of Wisconsin, he specialized in British history; pre-law students flocked to his course in English Constitutional History. An ardent Anglophile, Pierson was an exchange professor at Exeter University in 1954 and frequently visited Britain with his wife, Viva Bolin Pierson, who earned two degrees from DePauw. A British publisher issued his *Canada and the Privy Council* in 1960. Pierson was active in promoting honors work and the general studies program and helped to institute the program in African Studies. After retirement in 1966 he taught briefly at Illinois State University and died in 1972. His tombstone in Greencastle is in the appropriate form of a Celtic Cross.

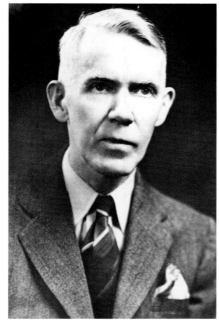

Professor William Wallace Carson was a favorite professor of history.

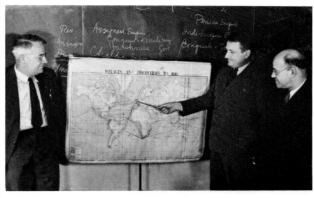

Left to right: Professors A. Wallace Crandall, Coen Pierson, and George Manhart of the history department posing before a map of the world.

Underwood Dudley, Joseph W. Corbett, Louis F. Smogor, and Carl P. Singer in mathematics, astronomy, and computer science (the last also succeeding Robert J. Thomas as director of the Computer Center); B. L. Garrett, Michael P. Silver, Edward G. Ypma, Margaret Berrio, and Steven R. Raines in psychology; Charles E. Mays and Michael D. Johnson in zoology; Ernest R. Henninger in physics; and Saad E. M. Ibrahim, John E. Kaemmer, and James M. Mannon in sociology and anthropology.

Other new faculty members were Vincent A. Serpa, Agnes Porter(Beaudry), James R. Curry, Kent B. Mecum, James S. Rambo, and Gordon B. Walters in Romance languages; Cornelius Van Zwoll, Darryl E. Gibson and Edward E. Mayer in German and Russian; Roy L. Swihart, Mildred L. Wills, Stanley Warren, and Judith A. Raybern in education; Robert E. Calvert, Amir Rafat, O. Ralph Raymond, and Byron W. Daynes in political science; and Judith Jenkins (George), Leroy Schoenfeld, Edward H. Meyer, Barbara Rae Federman, S. Page Cotton, and Mary Murphy (Bretscher) in physical education.

The School of Music added Thomas D. Fitzpatrick, Eunice A. Wilcox, John R. Sox, Mary A. C. Heller, Lorna B. Griffitt, Orcenith G. Smith, Claude Cymerman and Stanley R. Irwin. The School of Nursing hired Catherine L. Powell, Eleanor J. Miller, and Doris J. Froebe, the last of whom succeeded Catherine Friddle as director in 1974. New members of the library staff included Mary Jane Carr and Catherine A. Bean. David E. Horn followed David J. Olson as archivist in 1974.

The 1960s and early 1970s constituted one of the most turbulent periods in the history of the university. It began with the strong impact on campus of the national civil rights movement led by Martin Luther King Jr. and others. Concerned students and faculty members began to question, more urgently than ever before, the racial discrimination

After the early 1960s, DePauw blacks became organized into the Association of Afro-American Students, which supported academic and social programs, promoted black concerns, and provided camaraderie.In this picture for the Mirage of 1972, the students are shown with Assistant Professor of Art Willis "Bing" Davis standing on the far left and Oliver C. Rice, admissions counselor and assistant to the dean of students, on the far right.

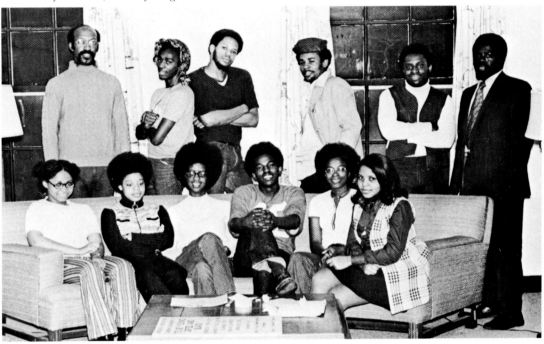

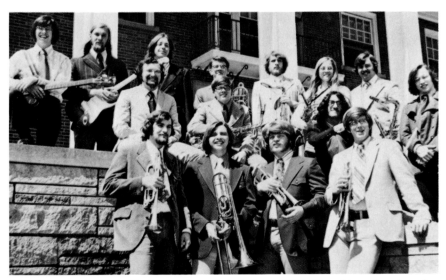

John Sox was Assistant Professor of woodwinds from 1967-80 and introduced work in the modern music media. Here he is shown on the steps of the Union (far left of the second row) with his jazz combo.

practiced by the social fraternities and certain commercial enterprises in the city, especially the barber shops patronized by DePauw students. In 1963 the Greencastle chapter of the National Association for the Advancement of Colored People was organized with considerable representation from the DePauw community. Both

students and professors took part in its activities, which included demonstrations and protest marches on campus and downtown.

The student senate responded to the rising social consciousness on campus by forming an interracial study committee, and the administration added to the statement of purposes and aims in

A TRIUMVIRATE OF SPEECH PROFESSORS

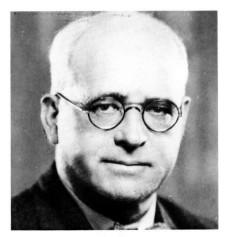

Harry B. Gough, 1907-36

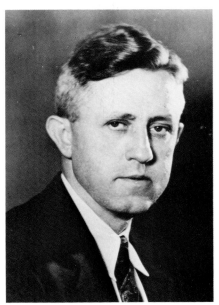

Robert E. Williams, 1921-57

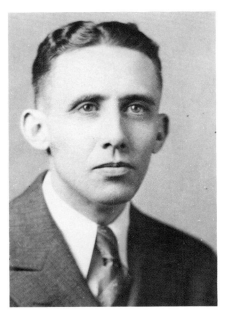

Herold T. Ross, 1927-61

Three men molded the speech department in the modern period, Harry B. Gough and his two protégés, Robert E. Williams and Herold T. Ross. The Kentucky-born Gough, who earned both an A.B. and A.M. from Northwestern University before serving as a Methodist pastor in Illinois and as president of Hedding College, was named DePauw's first professor of public speaking and debate in 1907. He soon became a popular figure on campus, known among other things for his booming voice and his unusual locutions. "By the great horned spoon" was one of his favorite expressions.

In addition to training outstanding orators and debaters, Gough had a large part in introducing theatre to DePauw in an era when its Methodist constituency still tended to frown on stage performances. In 1914 he founded the dramatic society Duzer Du, which survives to the present. The author of two books on public speaking, Gough was elected president of the National Association of Speech Teachers in 1923. After 29 years as head of the speech department at DePauw he retired in 1935 but lived on in Greencastle until his death 10 years later.

In 1921 Gough brought one of his students, Robert E. Williams, back to DePauw as the second member of the speech department. Williams, who graduated in the class of 1916, enlisted in the American Ambulance Service and saw action on the North Italian front in World War I. After teaching briefly at Knox College and the University of California, he earned an A.M. at the University of Wisconsin in 1921. His forte was oral interpretation and dramatics, and he became director of the Little Theatre. He organized a chapter of the National Collegiate Players at DePauw and was elected its first national treasurer. Like his mentor, Gough, he was a popular chapel speaker, known especially for his entertaining dialect stories. Retiring in 1957, he taught part-time for another decade. He died in Greencastle in 1982 at the age of 91.

The third man to join the department was another of Gough's students, Herold T. Ross, who came to DePauw as a freshman in 1914 from his hometown of Rochester, Ind. He later recalled how he was met at the railroad station by a group of Sigma Nus, who transported him by horse and buggy to their house and immediately pledged him to the fraternity. Near the end of his senior year he joined the Army and saw active service in France in the Argonne. After the war, he taught briefly in high schools and at Iowa State University, was English master at Cutler Preparatory in New York for a year, and earned an M.A. at Columbia University.

Ross began teaching at DePauw in 1927 and five years later completed his Ph.D. from the State University of Iowa with a dissertation on DePauw graduate Senator Albert J. Beveridge. He was active in the university's program in oratory, debate and drama and became head of the speech department on Gough's retirement in 1935. He was chiefly responsible for inaugurating DePauw's radio station WGRE-FM and also introduced work in television programming. He served a term as national president of the speech honorary society Delta Sigma Rho. After his retirement in 1961 he served one year as assistant dean of the university and taught at Butler, Hanover, Wabash, and Central Missouri. In 1986 the *Indianapolis Star* granted him the Jefferson Award for community service, especially in his leadership role in the American Association of Retired People. At present he is a vigorous 91 and rarely misses a university function.

the college catalogue the sentence: "DePauw University, in the Judeo-Christian tradition, believes that discrimination on the basis of race, creed, or nationality is incompatible with its principles." Not long after the organization of a local chapter of the Association of Afro-American Students, the university converted Locust Manor into the Afro-American House, which served variously as a residence for black students and a center for Afro-American social and cultural affairs. In the meantime a few fraternity and sorority chapters opened their membership to blacks.

The second phase of the student rebellion arose in reaction to the United States military intervention in Vietnam in 1965. Passionate debate of the issues took place, both in and out of class. Anti-war protestors participated in the Washington Peace March in October 1966, organized teach-ins on campus, and observed National Moratorium Day in 1969. President Richard Nixon's decision to send troops into Cambodia in April 1970 brought matters to a boiling point.

On May 1 the DePauw community was alarmed and shaken upon learning of an arson fire at the Air Force R.O.T.C. building. Two students were later tried and convicted on charges connected with this incident. A contrast to that isolated case of violence was the large peaceful demonstration on May 6 in the academic quadrangle. It was organized to protest the Cambodian invasion and the Ohio National Guard's firing upon student demontrators that left four persons dead on the Kent State University campus two days before.

A third aspect of the student movement has been called a cultural revolution, affecting such matters as living arrangements, dating and sexual behavior, clothing styles and the like. Proms and other formal events lost favor with undergraduates, who chose to pursue personal fulfillment and sought relevance rather than tradition. A principal demand of many students

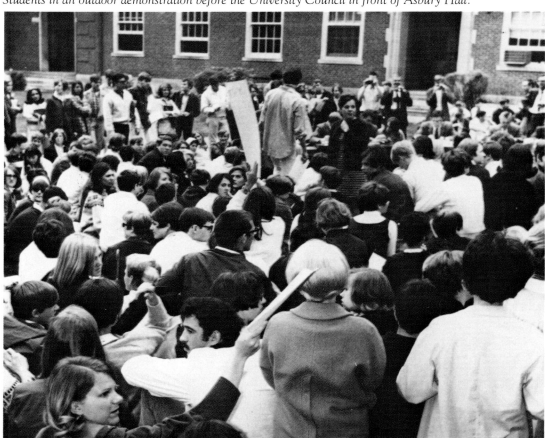

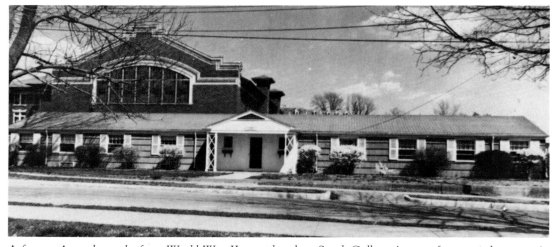

A former Army barracks from World War II was placed on South College Avenue for married veterans' apartments. In 1950 it was converted into the food laboratories for the home economics department and classes of Professor Audrey Beatty. Later it served as headquarters for the Air Force ROTC and Foreign Student Program. After the American invasion of Cambodia in May 1970 it was the scene of student arson.

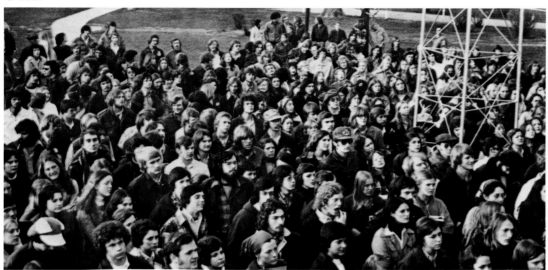

Another student demonstration in the 1970s on the East College lawn back of the Memorial Student Union.

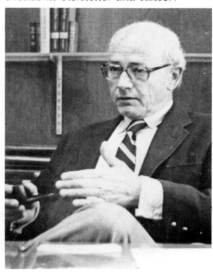

Thomas Wyatt Binford, an Indianapolis entrepreneur and civic leader, served as acting president of DePauw in 1975-76, between the administrations of Presidents Kerstetter and Rosser.

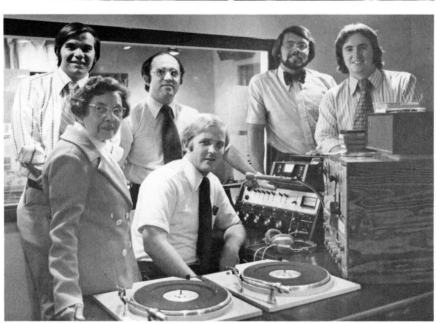

Elizabeth Turnell is shown with former students in the radio station of the campus – WGRE. Left to right are Rick Gudal, Bayard Walters, John Midbo, Larry Trimmer, Rick Warner. Professor Turnell taught speech communication and especially radio and supervised the station for 25 years, from 1946-71.

was for relaxation of the university's social and parietal regulations, especially in regard to closing hours for women's residences and coed visitation privileges. After a series of confrontations with student groups during the 1968-69 academic year, the administration made significant concessions on these questions that virtually ended the university's longstanding *in loco parentis* role.

The board of trustees authorized the creation of a Community Concerns Committee composed of students, faculty, administration and trustees which was to approve "all basic policies and minimum standards, enforcement procedures, and responsibilities relating to the social activities and other nonacademic interests and pursuits of the DePauw students." The committee delegated to the Association of Women Students the authority to recommend closing, or lock-up, hours for women's residences and made each living unit responsible for implementation and enforcement of the new privileges.

Compared with many other college and university campuses at this time, DePauw experienced a rather calm, nonviolent student rebellion. There were no riots, building-seizures, or similar incidents. Yet the student movement left a permanent mark on the institution, which ended the era more committed to antidiscriminatory practices, freedom of student expression, and social autonomy. One major long-term result was the election of student representatives to the board of trustees.

In October 1975 Kerstetter resigned from the presidency and was appointed to the long-dormant position of chancellor, with responsibilities chiefly for development and fund raising. The board of trustees named Indianapolis businessman Thomas W. Binford acting president while the search for a new chief executive was conducted. Princeton graduate Binford, who was a successful financier but lacked experience in managing academic affairs,

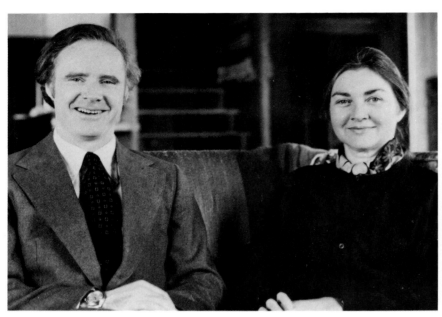

Richard Franklin Rosser was president from 1977-86 and chancellor in 1986. Here he is shown with his wife, Donna Eyssen Rosser.

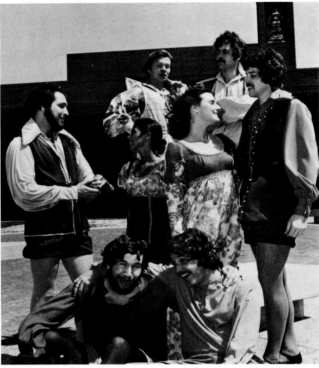

In 1976 the first production in the Performing Arts Center's Moore Theatre was the "Two Gentlemen of Verona," directed by Associate Professor Larry Sutton and including in the cast John Bower, Paul Case, Eli Gould, Dick Johnson, Liz Ogilvie, Betsy Rubino, David Schutz, and Tim Siner.

maintained an office on the DePauw campus several days a week during the next few months before resigning in August 1976 to return to his Indianapolis business enterprises.

At that point Dean Farber, who was given the additional title of vice president, assumed academic leadership of the university on an interim basis for the second time. At the end of the 1977-78 academic year Chancellor Kerstetter retired to his home on Cape Cod in Massachusetts. With his wife Leona Bateman Kerstetter, he presently resides in Sandwich, MA, where he is engaged in preparing a memoir of his DePauw years.

After an extensive search conducted by a joint faculty-trustee-alumni-student committee, the board of trustees named to the vacant presidency Richard F. Rosser, dean of faculty and professor of political science at Albion College, a member with DePauw of the Great Lakes Colleges Association. Rosser, a graduate of Ohio Wesleyan with both a master's degree in public administration and a Ph.D. from Syracuse University, had retired

from the Air Force after serving as professor and head of the department of political science at the Air Force Academy. Though a Methodist layman, he was the first non-ordained president of DePauw. He brought to his new post in February 1977 a brisk, energetic, and forceful administrative style.

One of President Rosser's first tasks was to reorganize the administrative departments of the university. Dean Farber remained in office until his retirement in 1979, but Donald Dodge Johnson was brought from Lawrence University in the summer of 1978 to take over responsibility for academic affairs with the new title of provost. In January 1979 Fred Silander of the economics department was named dean of the university. After Silander was transferred to the post of vice president for finance in 1981, his place as academic dean was taken first by Mildred Wills of the education department and then by James Cooper of the history department, who had been serving as faculty development coordinator since 1978. Upon the resignation of Provost Johnson in 1983, Cooper was advanced to the chief academic

leadership position with the title of vice president for academic affairs. Named to assist him were John Morrill of the mathematics department as director of academic planning and James Rambo of the Romance languages department as coordinator for special academic programs.

Other faculty members named to part-time administrative posts were the following: Robert H. King of the philosophy and religion department as assistant to the president; John White of the philosophy and religion department as faculty development coordinator; Amir Rafat of the political science department as director of foreign study and off-campus programs, succeeded later by Darrell La Lone of the sociology and anthropology department; Margaret E. Catanese of the economics and business department as coordinator for individual Winter Term off-campus projects; and Myra J. Rosenhaus of the philosophy and religion department as director of convocations.

RELIGIOUS LIFE AND THE UNIVERSITY CHAPLAINCY

Of the major religious organizations on campus in the early 20th century the YMCA and the Student Volunteer Movement had disappeared before the Second World War, while the YWCA lingered on another decade or two before fading from view. In their place were the denominational clubs and programs sponsored by various local churches, especially Gobin Memorial Methodist Church, in a time when Methodism still remained the largest single religious preference among DePauw students.

The Rev. John Tennant, pastor of Gobin in the 1940s, was especially active in organizing and supporting the work of the Methodist Student Movement and assigned an assistant, Barbara Daniels, as official adviser of the group. Among her successors as advisers or directors of the MSM, known later as the Methodist Student Federation and finally as the Christian Action Movement, were Patricia B. Kyle (1950-1954), Kermit B. Morrison (1954-1958), John Dorr (1958-59), Jack T. Hanford (1959-60), Samuel Kirk (1961-66), and Donald E. Bossart (1967-70). In 1967 the Indiana Methodist conferences financed the construction of a modernistic aluminum-and-glass building in the rear of Gobin Church to serve as the University Christian Center. Later reverting to the use of the church and its congregation, it has been renamed Wesley Hall.

In the meantime Orville L. Davis, a former Methodist missionary in India who had been a member of DePauw's department of religious education since 1946, was named director of church relations in 1952 with the additional responsibility of coordinating religious activities on campus through the interdenominational Council on Religious Life. Finally, in 1962, after a brief hiatus following the death of Davis, President Russell Humbert appointed Elmer E. Carricker to the newly created post of university chaplain. Carricker, a DePauw alumnus who had served as a military chaplain during the war, carried on the somewhat vaguely defined duties of that office until 1967, when he resigned to accept the vice presidency of Baker University.

The next year President William Kerstetter named to the vacated chaplaincy Marvin E. Swanson, who had graduated from Simpson College during Kerstetter's presidency there and earned an S.T.B. and Ph.D. from Boston University. One of Swanson's tasks was to define the chaplain's role on campus, especially in relationship to the director of the Methodist Christian Action Movement. A continuing responsibility was the organization of the university's weekly chapel services and such programs as the annual Mendenhall Lectureship.

In 1971, however, Swanson accepted the additional post of director of international studies. By 1973 it was clear that one person could not perform the duties of both offices simultaneously, and the state conferences of the United Methodist Church were approached with a request for assistance in funding a full-time chaplain at the university. The result was the appointment of William Fred Lamar as university chaplain in 1974. Under Lamar, a graduate of the University of Alabama with a B.D. from Eden Theological Seminary and Ph.D. from St. Louis University, the chaplaincy took on both an interdenominational and a Methodist character. Headquarters was established at first in the Methodist conference-financed University Christian Center. Later its activities were transferred to Locust Manor and then to the present location in O'Hair House.

Through the Chaplain's Living Unit Council, the social service program was particularly expanded, with student work projects initiated in the community, nation, and many parts of the Third World. Under Chaplain Lamar's direction the popular Winter Term in Mission program has taken approximately 1450 students on 61 different projects, providing health services and constructing church buildings and other facilities in various sites in Central America and the Caribbean, Africa, and the Philippines during the past decade. Since 1977 a series of assistant chaplains has been appointed to help carry on the increased functions of the office, including Mary Stubbs, James B. Lemler, Bruce R. Coriell, Terence Jones, and Kevin B. Armstrong. Currently the chaplain's staff also includes a chaplain intern and two retired professors from the philosophy and religion department on a part-time basis. Providing continuity to the office since 1958 has been its efficient secretary, Frances O'Neal.

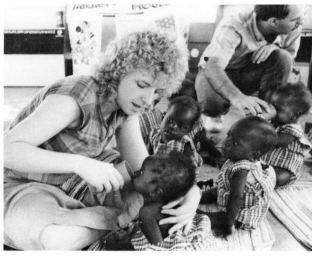

Chaplain Fred Lamar is shown making a contribution to a service project sponsored by the Chaplains' office.

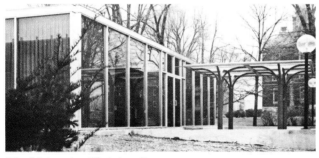

Students Christy Schleuter and Ernie Limbo working in a nursery for malnourished children in Haiti during the Winter Term Project in 1987.

The University Christian Center was constructed behind Gobin Memorial United Methodist Church for the offices and reception rooms for the University Chaplain. It later became known as Wesley Hall and furnished offices for the church while the chaplains moved to O'Hair House.

When White was named special assistant to the vice president for academic affairs in 1985, Anthony Catanese of the economics and business department became faculty development coordinator. Marion K. McInnes succeeded Rosenhaus as director of convocations in 1985 and the next year was given the additional task of coordinating the celebration of the university's sesquicentennial. Ray H. French, as university curator, made a detailed inventory of the institution's extensive art collection before his retirement in 1984. His successor was Mary La Lone of the sociology and anthropology department.

In 1978 Robert G. Bottoms was appointed to the position of vice president for university relations, a title changed to vice president for external relations in 1980 and executive vice president in 1983. His chief responsibilities lay in the planning and implementation of the university's development and fund-raising programs. In a reorganization of this department Frederick

Sanders was named director of planned giving, James N. Kleinschmidt director of development and alumni relations. Theodore Katula became associate director of alumni relations in addition to his post as director of student activities, formerly known as director of the Memorial Student Union Building.

Other appointments in development and alumni affairs over the next few years included John McConnell, John D. Fetters, Debra L. Haerr, Bruce E. Ploshay, Linda M. Katula, Marsha J. Brown, and Ann Daly. In the expanded office of public relations under the direction of Patrick Aikman were Gregory Rice, director of publications and later university editor; Dian D. Phillips, who succeeded Rice as director of publications in 1985; Judith C. Magyar, director of summer conferences; and John McGauley, director of news services.

David C. Murray became director of admissions in 1978, later adding the title of assistant provost and

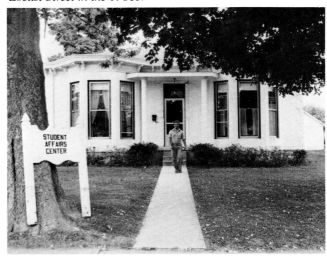

A crowded Administration Building forced the Student Affairs Office to relocate in this former residence on South Locust Street in the 1980s.

finally assistant vice president. Assisting him in that important office have been William D. Berg, longtime staffer Richard E. Lyons as associate director of admissions, Elizabeth A. Napoli, Polly A. Coddington, Veda R. Robinson, and a series of young admissions counselors, mostly recent DePauw graduates. Kenneth R. Ashworth succeeded Charles W. Bruce as director of financial aid in 1982. Registrar Eleanor Ypma added the title of assistant provost and director of graduate studies.

In its new location in a remodeled residence on South Locust Street, the student affairs office underwent considerable reorganization. In 1979 Joan M. Claar became the new dean of students after Associate Dean Patricia E. Domeier had served as acting dean the previous year. John R. Mohr continued as an associate dean of students and director of placement from 1977 to 1982. His successor, Robert G. O'Neal, was replaced the next year by Thomas R. Cath, who took the title of director of career planning and placement. This office also relocated to more spacious quarters in the Student Union Building, where it is much

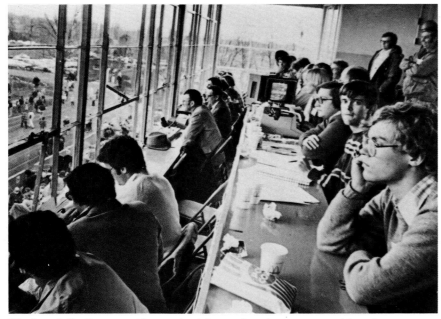

Blackstock Stadium provides a splendid press box for viewing and broadcasting football games.

Students use computers in the Rainbow Room in the basement of the Roy O. West Library.

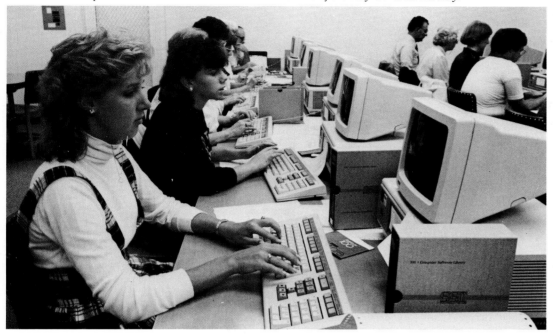

frequented by job-conscious students. Rebecca S. Lamb was named assistant director of career planning and placement in 1985.

Other members of the student affairs staff in this period have been husband-and-wife team Carol A. Arner and Thomas D. Arner, presently associate dean and assistant dean of students, respectively, Vic Boschini, Janice Simmons, and James W. Schlegel. Supervising the work of the student dormitory counselors are three residence life directors, formerly called head resident advisers.

In 1978 the office of comptroller was changed to vice president for finance, a position filled first by Lawrence Elam and after 1981 by Fred S. Silander. Richard Conrad was manager of the DePauw Book Store from 1978 to 1986, when he took over the same position in the Book Store Annex. Successive directors of the physical plant during this period have been Robert D. Gaston, Bruce V. Collins, and James Daugherty. In 1984 John Henry was named to the new post of director of personnel, later adding the title of assistant vice president for support services.

President Rosser initiated a major change in departmental governance, replacing a time-honored system of near-permanent, seniority-determined department heads with chairmen appointed for a three-year term. In its place he established a system where reappointment was subject to departmental evaluation and recommendation by the committee on faculty. This system, which had been foreshadowed by rotating headships in the history and chemistry departments earlier, brought about many shifts in departmental leadership and widened participation in faculty decision-making. The administration also placed strong emphasis on periodic evaluation of faculty members, both by peers and by students. It also attempted to establish a program of merit raises in recognition of superior teaching and professional attainments that was never fully implemented.

Some departments acquired new titles to reflect more closely the nature of their course offerings. Physical education was broadened to health, physical education, and recreation. Economics and business became economics and management. Earth sciences reverted to its former

title of geology and geography, and astronomy was shifted from mathematics to the physics department by mutual agreement. In a return to an older terminology at DePauw, zoology merged with botany and bacteriology to form the department of biological sciences. Two casualties of changing student interests and budgetary restraints were the programs in African Studies and Black Studies, both of which were phased out early in the Rosser administration.

The Rosser presidency was a time of rethinking the university's goals and restructuring the curriculum to re-affirm the liberal arts ideal. In 1979 the faculty adopted a new statement of purpose and aims, the first such in nearly six decades. While continuing to stress intellectual inquiry, clear thinking, and effective expression, the statement also made reference to students' lifestyles, emotional needs, and career choices. Its philosophy was summed up in the reaffirmation of a commitment to "academic excellence, growth in personal and social awareness, and preparation for leadership."

After prolonged committee consideration and faculty debate, a new set of graduation requirements was put into effect for the College of Liberal Arts. It involved a division of the distribution requirements into six newly defined groups: 1) natural sciences and mathematics; 2) social and behavioral sciences; 3) literature and the arts; 4) historical and philosophical understanding; 5) foreign languages; and 6) self-expression. Students were to choose two courses from each of the first five groups and one and a half courses from the sixth, which included physical education, applied music, studio art, and certain extracurricular activities. In a compromise, the original proposal was amended to permit students to omit any two courses from the six groups. The School of Nursing adopted a slightly modified version of these graduation requirements.

FRATERNITIES/SORORITIES

Greek houses and the years in which
they were chartered at DePauw.

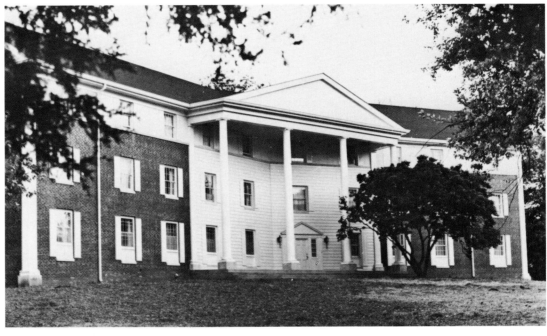

Alpha Omicron Pi – 1907

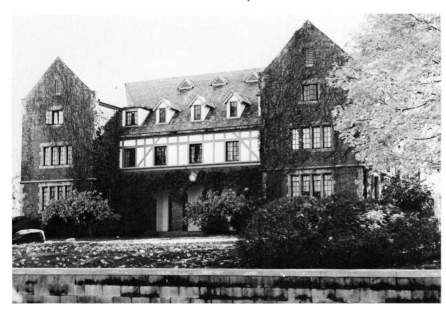

Phi Delta Theta – 1868

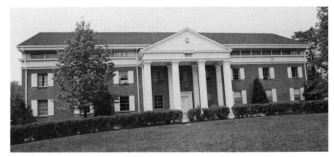

Beta Theta Pi – 1845

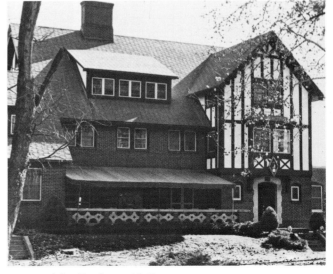

Sigma Alpha Epsilon – 1949

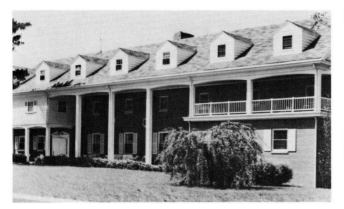

Alpha Chi Omega – 1885

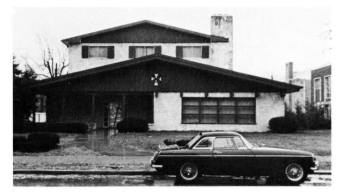

Sigma Chi – 1859

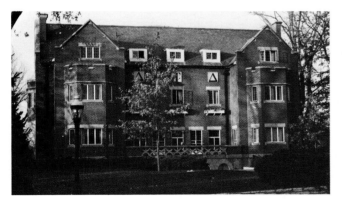

Delta Tau Delta – 1871

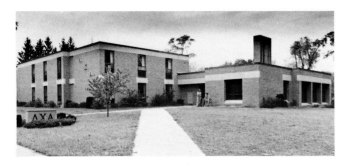

Lambda Chi Alpha – 1915

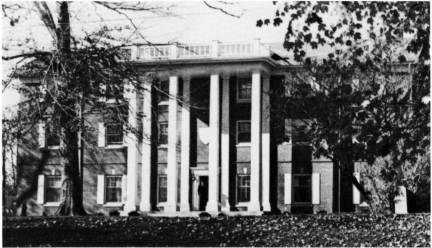

Phi Gamma Delta – 1856

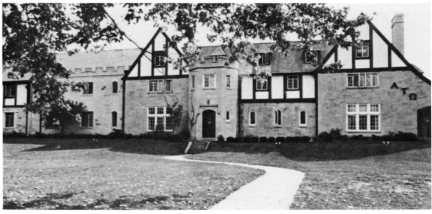

Alpha Tau Omega – 1924

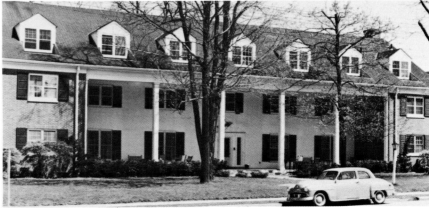

Pi Beta Phi – 1942

FRATERNITIES/SORORITIES
(continued)

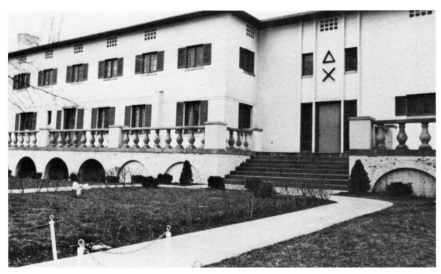

Delta Chi – 1928

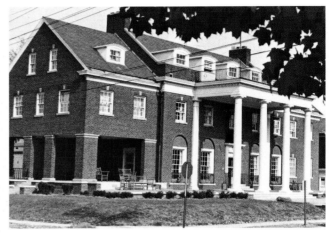

Sigma Nu – 1890

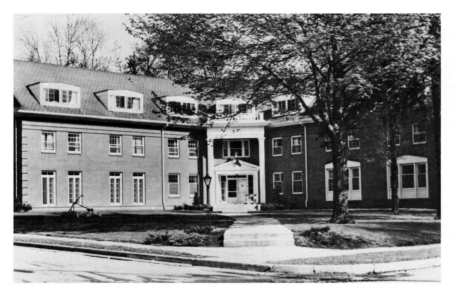

Delta Gamma – 1949

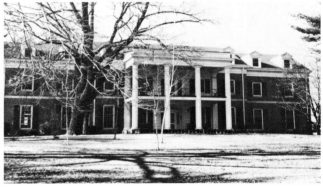

Kappa Alpha Theta – 1870

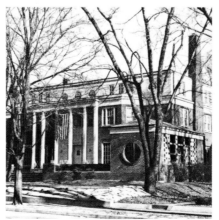

Kappa Kappa Gamma – 1875

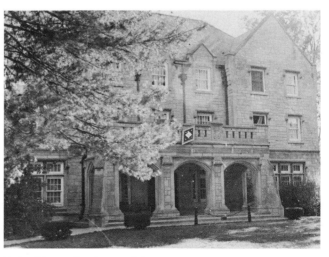

Delta Kappa Epsilon – 1866

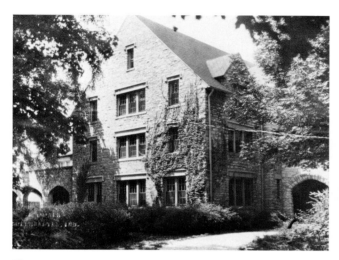

Phi Kappa Psi – 1865

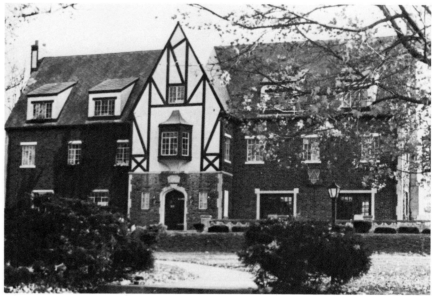

Delta Upsilon – 1887

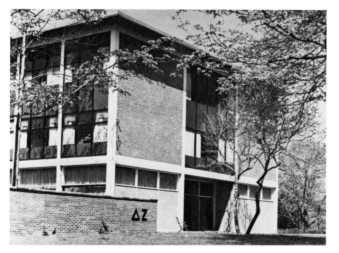

Delta Zeta – 1909

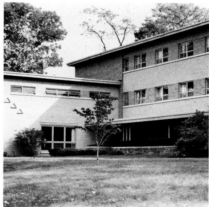

Delta Delta Delta – 1908

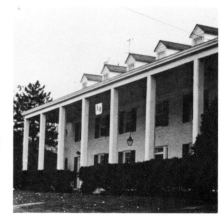

Alpha Phi – 1888

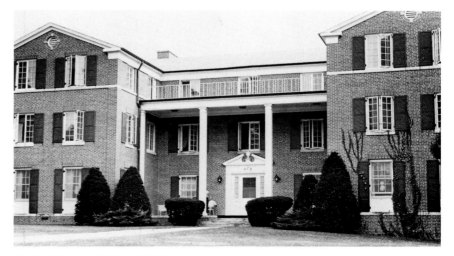

Alpha Gamma Delta – 1908

A more radical innovation was the addition of competence requirements for graduation from both the College of Liberal Arts and the School of Nursing. Three areas of competence were identified: writing, quantitative reasoning, and oral communication. Students were required to demonstrate competence in each of these in various ways, including passing courses in regular departmental subject areas. These courses were designated for that purpose by the letters W (writing), Q (quantitative reasoning), and S (speaking) to indicate the appropriate competence.

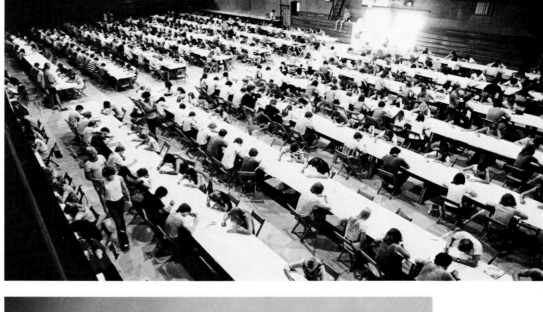

In 1979 the DePauw Honor Scholar program was introduced, offering special opportunities for intensive intellectual experience to 20 carefully selected freshmen each year. Members of each honors class enroll in a cross-disciplinary seminar during the first four semesters and in the last two years pursue independent study culminating in an honors thesis prepared under the direction of one or more members of the faculty. The organizer and first director of the program was Robert E. Calvert of the political science department. Other faculty members assisted in the program from the beginning, and in 1985 Eugene Schwartz of the chemistry department succeeded Calvert as director.

The Center for Management and Entrepreneurship came into existence in 1980 to "prepare liberal arts students for leadership roles in private and public sector management and to encourage the spirit of entrepreneurship." Among the center's activities have been an executive-in-residence program that brings business leaders to campus for presentations and round-table discussions, a series of symposia, and an annual Small Business Conference. The center also supervises the DePauw Management Fellows program for exceptional students planning careers in management, either in large corporations, small business firms, or non-profit organizations. Its

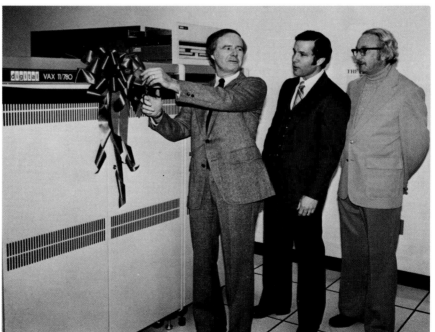

President Richard Rosser, along with Carl Singer, director of academic computing, and Robert Thomas, professor of mathematics and computer science, celebrate more computer equipment, a VAX 11/780.

Professor John B. Wilson of the history department teaching in the restored main floor classroom of East College.

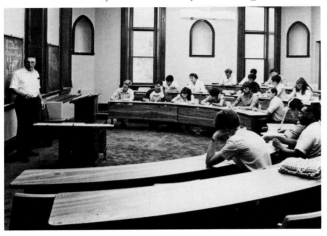

directors have been John S. McConnell, Charles R. Tilden, and B. Thomas Boese. Vincent Serpa of the Romance language department was acting director in 1985-86 and assistant director for the following year.

Two unfinished construction projects reached completion in the early part of the Rosser presidency. A campaign headed by Trustee Ardath Burkhart to raise funds for the restoration of East College culminated in the bequest of an estate valued at $2.7 million from alumnus Philip St. John Charles in memory of his parents and his sister, Emilie Charles, also a DePauw graduate. The bulk of it was designated for the restoration of East College. A gift from alumna Caroline Hughes Crummey in honor of her father, Edwin Hughes, former DePauw president and Methodist bishop, went toward the restoration of Meharry Hall.

Under the direction of Indianapolis architects H. Roll McLaughlin and Forrest Camplin the majestic old building was meticulously refurbished and

restored to approximately its original appearance, but with the addition of such modern appurtenances as wall-to-wall carpeting, air conditioning, and an elevator. In Meharry Hall, the structure's centerpiece, the organ was removed from the stage, which was itself restored to the smaller size and curved front seen in early illustrations, and a replica of the small balcony that originally extended over the stage was built. The elimination of the iron fire escapes from the outside wall at the rear of the hall, however, led to a fire marshal-imposed ban on occupation of the distinctive sloping balconies favored by freshmen in the old daily chapel days.

The new East College also contained remodeled classrooms, faculty studies, the offices of the Center for Management and

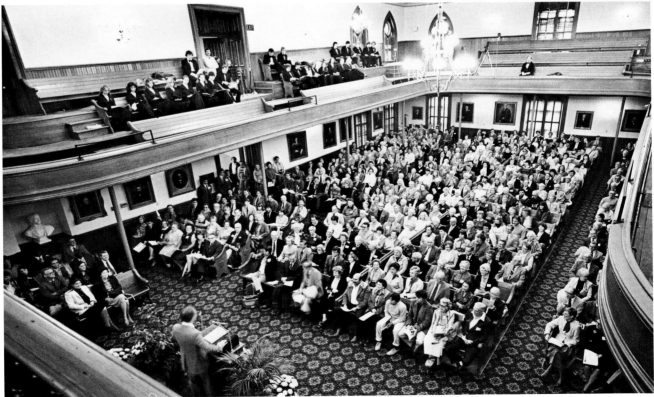

A capacity audience was present for the rededication of Meharry Hall in the restored East College on Old Gold Day, 1981. The fire marshal prevents use of the balcony except for the choir. Descendants of the original Meharry family occupy the front right pews

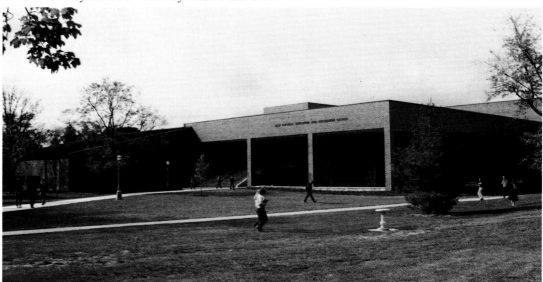

Entrepreneurship, a Hall of Donors, a faculty lounge, and the depository of the Indiana Journalism Hall of Fame, established earlier by Sigma Delta Chi. The dedication of the restored East College on Old Gold Day 1981 was a celebration of the spirit of Old Asbury in the midst of an extensive modernization of the DePauw University campus.

The next year the Lilly Physical Education and Recreation Center was completed at a cost of $7.2 million. Located just south of the Julian Science and Mathematics Center it was designed by Herbert R. Thompson of the Indianapolis architectural firm of James and Associates and named collectively for Josiah K. Lilly Jr., Josiah K. Lilly Sr., and Colonel Eli Lilly– the father, grandfather, and great grandfather, respectively, of Ruth Lilly Van Riper, the chief donor. The imposing structure contained a spacious fieldhouse, natatorium, auxiliary gymnasium, and numerous smaller facilities, as well as classrooms and offices for the coaching and physical education staff. The fieldhouse itself was named in honor of Raymond "Gaumey" Neal, who coached the famous championship football team of 1933. Surviving members of the team contributed $2.3 million to its construction, Chester Elson and Norman Frees of the class of 1936 each pledging $1 million.

The razing of Music Hall and Bowman Gymnasium presented a unique opportunity for the creation of a beautifully landscaped plaza in the three-acre empty space between Hanna Street and the new Performing Arts Center. Bowman Park, complete with a natural amphitheatre, reflecting pool and fountains, curving walks, and a patio furnished with tables and chairs for outdoor refreshment, came into being in 1983. It provided an open-air recreational area located conveniently near the center of the campus.

Other additions to the physical plant included the purchase of Charter House from Gobin United

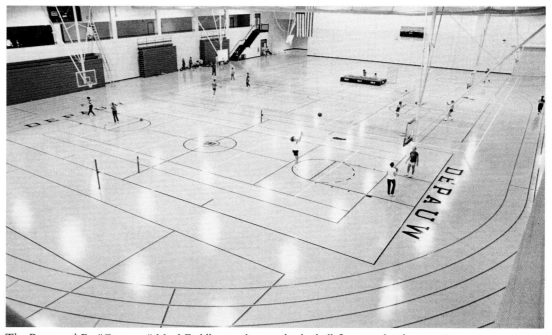

The Raymond R. "Gaumey" Neal Fieldhouse showing basketball floors and indoor track.

A view across the pond with fountains in Bowman Park at the Performing Arts Center.

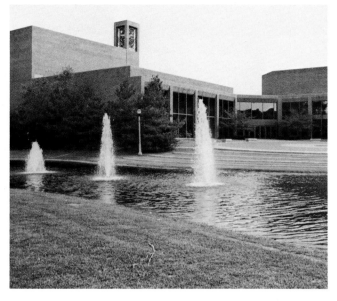

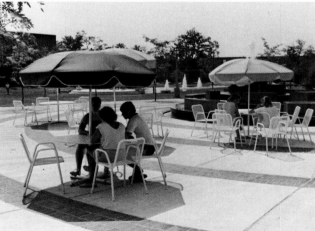

Bowman Park on the site of Bowman Gymnasium has become a favorite hangout for students, who gather around the fountain in warm weather.

HIRAM L. JOME: TEACHER OF ECONOMICS

Born in Sturgeon Bay, Wis. of Norwegian immigrant parents, Hiram L. Jome spoke fluent Norwegian, which he taught along with the English language at parochial schools during summer vacations as a college student. During World War I he served in the U.S. Navy as a ship's radio operator and graduated from St. Olaf College in 1918. He later earned M.A. and Ph.D. degrees from the University of Wisconsin and taught there and at Denison University before coming to DePauw in 1931 to head the department of economics.

He soon became one of the most popular teachers at the university, known especially for his ability to use concrete illustrations to make abstract theory come alive. He explained profit margin by describing trying to sleep on an army cot under a blanket lacking two inches from reaching the edge of the bed. Often covered with chalk dust from his lavish markings on the blackboard, Jome illustrated the primitive "barndoor" sort of bookkeeping by writing on the classroom door. "His graphs explode beyond the confines of the blackboard," one former student wrote.

A kind and considerate teacher, much sought after by students for advice and guidance on career planning, he was also an inspirational chapel speaker and a productive scholar. He wrote over 30 magazine articles and several books on subjects ranging from the radio broadcasting industry to the Securities and Exchange Commission.

An avid home gardener, music lover, and baseball fan, Jome was a sometime catcher on the Greencastle Kiwanis nine and occasionally played the violin, or fiddle, as he called it. In April 1958 he suffered a stroke in his classroom in Asbury Hall and died the next day. He was survived by his wife Martha Fjelde Jome and two daughters, Helen Jome Houck '43 and Florence Jome Donner '44. His death came just as the department was sending out a letter to economics graduates seeking contributions to purchase a special collection of books to be placed in the library in Jome's name. Ironically, the letter began: "The world is full of memorials to great men. Unfortunately, in too many cases, recognition was tardy and those honored could not enjoy the goodwill expressed toward them."

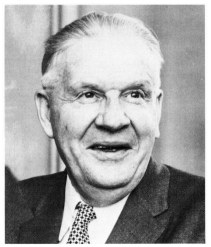

Professor Hiram Jome

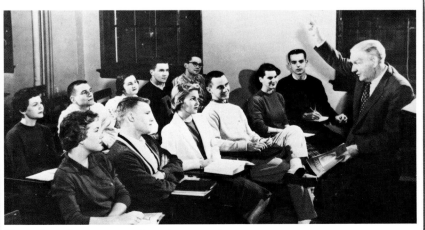

Hiram Jome lectures to students in economics.

195

ATHLETICS

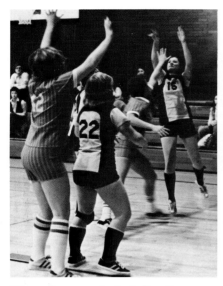

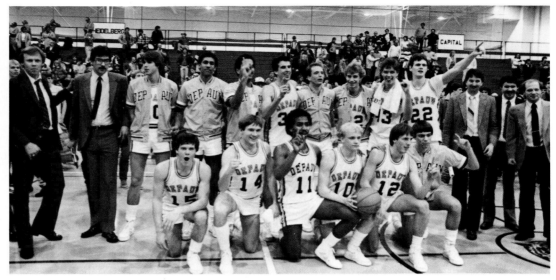

Women's varsity basketball in Bowman Gym.

The 1983-84 basketball team after winning the Great Lakes Regional Tourney in Neal Fieldhouse. DePauw went to a third place in the NCAA Division III finals.

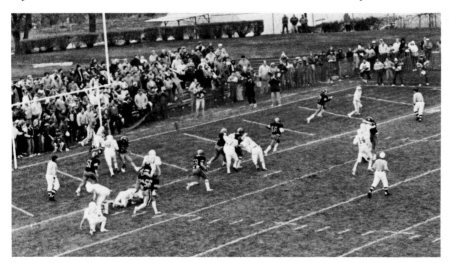

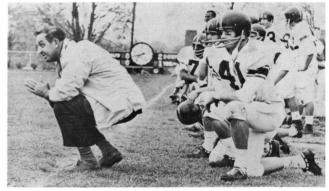

Is Coach Tom Mont praying for his team?

The game-winning play in the DePauw-Wabash contest in 1983 clinched the Tigers a 7-3 record for the season and a 24-6 record for the last three years. (Pat Aikman)

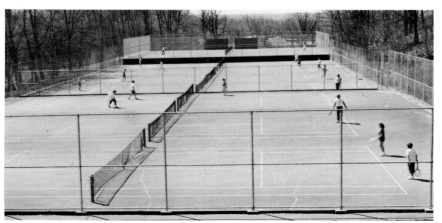

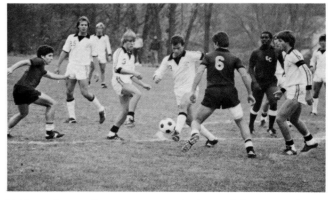

DePauw began playing soccer in 1967 as a club sport and fielded a varsity team in 1968.

The new green-topped tennis courts behind Blackstock Stadium built in 1963.

One of DePauw's best women's basketball teams, 1983.

A goal! Field hockey was DePauw's first women's intercollegiate sport.

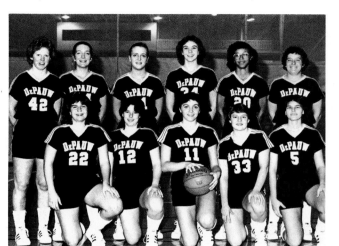

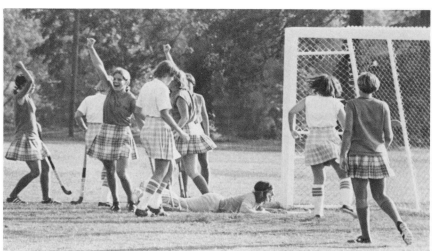

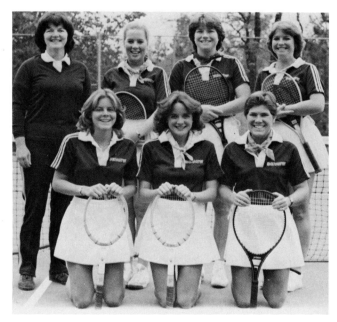

State champions 1981-82. For the third time DePauw women went to the AIAW Division III tennis tourney, returning with a fifth place finish.

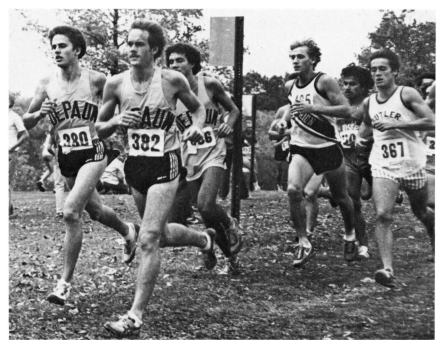

The 1979 cross-country interstate run at Windy Hill Country Club.

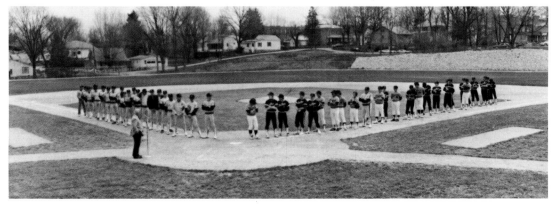

Alumni baseball game played at the dedication of Walker Field in 1984.

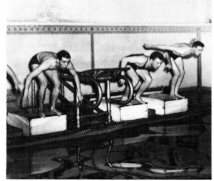

Members of the swimming team in 1944 in the Bowman Gymnasium pool.

Aerial view of the DePauw campus in 1986. Left to right in the foreground are the Walker Baseball Field, Boswell Soccer Field, Blackstock Stadium, and McKeen Field. In the center are Asbury Hall, Roy O. West Library, Harrison Hall, Percy L. Julian Science and Mathematics Center, Lilly Physical Education and Recreation Center. In the rear find East College, Mason Hall, Rector Hall, Lucy Rowland Hall, Memorial Student Union, Bowman Park, Performing Arts Center, and Bishop Roberts Hall.

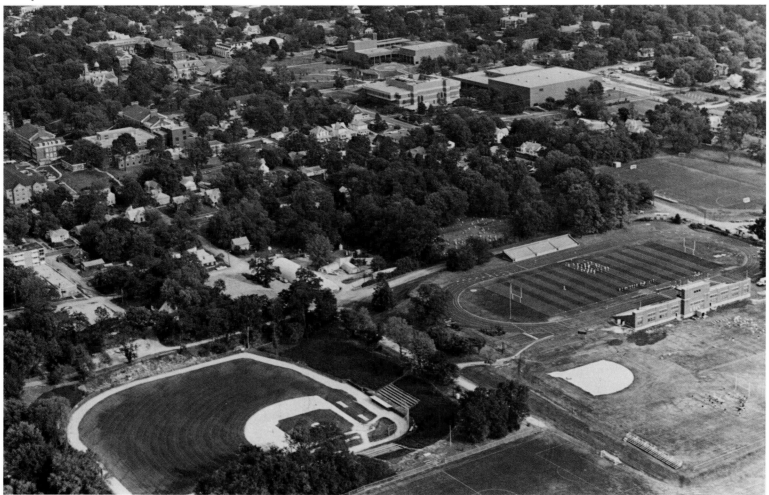

Methodist Church in 1983 and the construction of a new baseball field named for alumnus-athlete Merle "Ole" Walker in 1984. Charter House provided a centralized location for the offices of development, alumni affairs, public relations, university publications, the news bureau, and summer conferences as well as improved quarters for the university health services. The administration also planned extensive remodeling of older university facilities, especially Asbury Hall, Harrison Hall, and the Roy O. West Library. The work on Asbury Hall was completed by the fall of 1986, while the even more thorough refurbishing of the library extended through the 1986-87 academic year and into the fall of 1987.

In the meantime the development office under the leadership of President Rosser and Vice President Bottoms, had been successful in increasing the level of annual giving to the university, especially through the Annual Fund. In April 1983 Eugene L. Delves, chairman of the board of trustees, announced the launching of a $90 million campaign to be led by trustee James J. Kelly. Thirty months in the planning stage, this drive, the most ambitious ever, was to reach completion in June 1987 at the time of the celebration of the 150th anniversary of DePauw University and was accordingly known as the Sesquicentennial Campaign.

Unlike early campaigns which focused in large part on building projects, this was aimed chiefly at raising funds to endow student scholarships and academic programs. By February 1985 the campaign had made so much progress that the goal was raised to $100 million. On Old Gold Day the next fall the administration was able to announce that enough gifts and commitments had been received to ensure going over the new goal, but that the campaign would continue until its appointed end in June 1987. It was said that no other liberal arts college of DePauw's size had ever raised so large a sum in a single campaign. Gifts from alumni accounted for nearly 85% of the total.

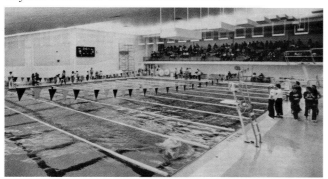

The Olympic-size pool is in the lower level of the Lilly Physical Education and Recreation Center.

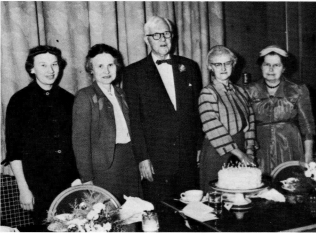

To help Dr. Worth Tippy, university archivist, celebrate his 90th birthday in 1956 were archives assistants Geneva Talbott, Catherine Tillotson McCord '18, Eleanore Cammack '28 (archivist from 1955-71), and Alma John Woodson '02, daughter of President John.

Among the immediate results of the campaign was the establishment of the Fisher Fund for faculty development and scholarly research, funded by a gift in excess of $1 million from John and Janice Fisher of Muncie, Indiana. In February 1985 the administration revealed that anonymous donors had made a multimillion dollar donation to the university for the creation of a Center for Contemporary Media. President Rosser, who described the gift as the largest in the history of the university, appointed a committee to plan for the establishment of the center, which would include resources for training undergraduates in radio, television, and print journalism within a liberal arts context. Named to head the center was Drake Mabry from the *Des Moines Register*, who set up headquarters in the former Delta

TWO DISTINGUISHED BOTANISTS

Adding luster to DePauw's reputation in the sciences were two outstanding teacher-scholars, Truman G. Yuncker and Winona H. Welch. Yuncker, a native of Carson City, Mich., who received his B.S. from Michigan State and A.M. at the University of Nebraska, taught briefly at Manual High School in Indianapolis before serving with the Army Medical Corps in World War I. After obtaining his Ph.D. from the University of Illinois he joined the DePauw faculty in 1919 and served as head of the botany and bacteriology department from its establishment in the 1920s until his retirement in 1956. During his long tenure at DePauw, Yuncker pursued his study of plant life in Europe, Central and South America, and such exotic places as the Tonga Islands in the South Pacific, often taking along student assistants from his college classes. He became the world's leading authority on the herb *Piperaceae* and published his monumental work, *The Piperaceae of Northern South America*, in 1950.

The only DePauw faculty member to this date to receive a Guggenheim fellowship, Yuncker was widely recognized for his scientific work. He served as president of both the Indiana Academy of Science and the American Society of Plant Taxonomists, and vice president and treasurer of the Botanical Society of America, which named him one of the country's outstanding botanical scientists in 1962. He died in Greencastle in 1964, survived by his wife Ethel and two daughters, Betty Jane Lee '42 and Barbara Yuncker '43.

Winona H. Welch, born on a farm in Goodland, Ind., enrolled in DePauw in 1919. A prize student of Yuncker, she graduated in 1923 and went on for advanced study in botany, receiving the M.S. from the University of Illinois and Ph.D. from Indiana University. After teaching at Indiana and the Central Normal School in Danville, Ind., she returned to her alma mater as an instructor in botany in 1930. Like Yuncker, she was an assiduous researcher and plant collector, concentrating most of her work on the water mosses *fontinalaceae*. She examined more than 15,000 collections of mosses in the United States and abroad and gathered over 39,000 specimens on her travels in Central America and the Caribbean, Alaska, Australia, and the South Pacific. Two of her major published works were *Mosses of Indiana* and *A Monograph of Fontinalaceae*.

Professor Welch followed Yuncker as head of the botany and bacteriology department in 1956, becoming the first woman to hold such a position in the sciences at DePauw. She also was the first woman to be elected president of the Indiana Academy of Science and to chair the Central States Section of the Botanical Society of America. Active in Phi Beta Kappa and such organizations as the American Association of University Women, Daughters of the American Revolution, and the national sorority PEO, she was given a special citation by the General Federation of Women's Clubs. She continued to teach part-time after retirement and served as curator of the Truman G. Yuncker Herbarium to which she and her mentor had contributed so many specimens.

Still active at the age of 91, Winona Welch was recently asked why she took up the study of mosses. "Because I felt sorry for them," she replied. "You could ask questions about trees or flowers and get answers, but not about mosses." Thanks to her work, today there are many answers to questions about the world's mosses.

Professors Yuncker and Welch trained scores of professional botanists during their teaching careers at DePauw. Two who later became their colleagues in the botany and bacteriology department were Howard R. Youse '37, who succeeded to the headship upon Welch's retirement in 1961, and Robert I. Fletcher '51, who taught bacteriology from 1957 to 1983.

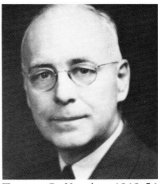
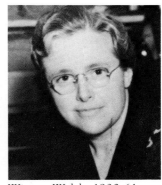

Truman G. Yuncker, 1919-56.   Winona Welch, 1930-61.

ADMINISTRATION

HUMBERT

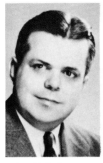

Robert H. Farber
Dean of the University

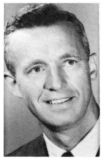

Norman J. Knights
Executive Vice President

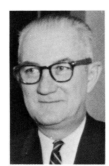

Deward W. Smythe
Comptroller

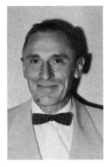

John J. Wittich
Director of Admissions

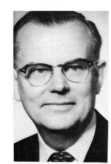

Willard E. Umbreit
Director of Admissions and
Greater DePauw Program

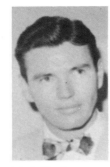

Lawrence A. Riggs
Dean of Students

KERSTETTER

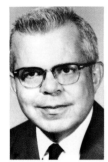

Robert H. Farber
Vice President

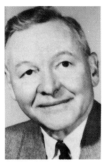

Robert E. Crouch
Sec. of Alumni Affairs
Vice President for
Development

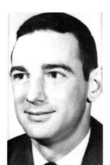

Lawrence C. Elam
Comptroller

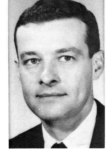

Louis J. Fontaine
Director of Admissions

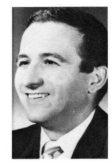

James N. Cook
Director of Alumni
Affairs

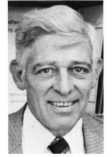

William McK. Wright
Dean of Students

ROSSER

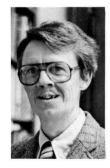

D. Dodge Johnson, Jr.
Provost

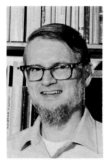

James L. Cooper
Vice President for
Academic Affairs

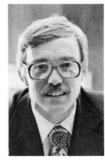

David Murray
Ass't Vice President for
Admissions

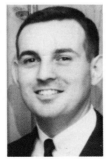

Frederick A. Sanders
Director of Planned
Giving

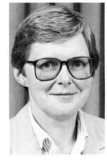

James P. Aikman
Director of Public
Relations

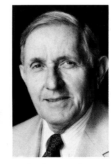

Joan M. Claar
Dean of Students

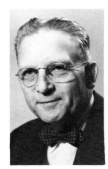

Orville Davis
Director of Church
Relations

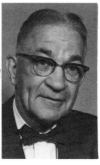

Frank DeVaney
Assistant Comptroller

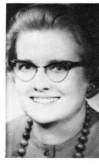

Value T. Williams
Registrar

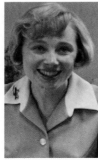

Eleanor S. Ypma
Registrar

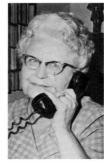

Elsie DePonte Miller
Director of Residence
Halls

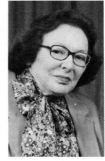

Virginia Byrkit
Director of Residence
Halls and University Food
Service

200

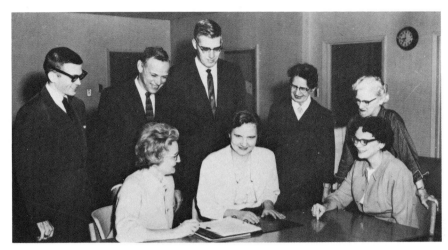

The staff of the University Library in 1962 included, (standing left to right): Larry Cunningham, James Martindale (Librarian, 1962-83), Daniel Smith, Audrey Knowlton (1943-70), Eleanore Cammack (1955-71). Seated, (left to right): Marian Mullendore, Eleanor Carmichael (1960-82), Emily Alvord.

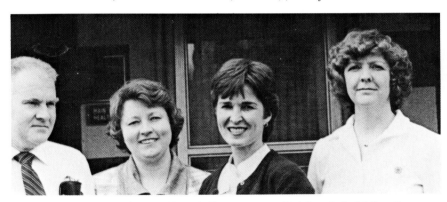

University health service staff (from left): Roger Roof M.D., Judy Miller, Jane (Sullivan) White, and Marilynn (Hunter) Sturgeon.

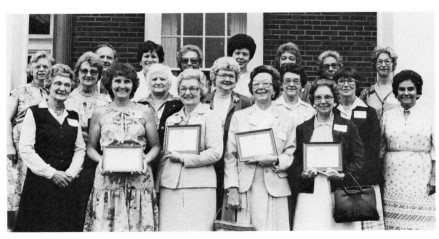

Recognized for longtime service to the university on the Support Staff in the Rosser Administration were, front row, left to right: F. Stanish, J. Stevens, V. Hanna, B. Eiteljorge, V. Callender. Row two: V. Brann, J. Applegate, E. Huber, M. Carter, G. Sublette, M. Garl, M. Harlan. Back row: R. Rosser, B. Waldron, R. Hanlon, L. Boswell, F. O'Neal, L. Hope, J. Reynolds.

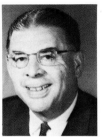

M. Arthur Perry
Superintendant of
Buildings and Grounds

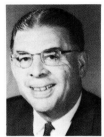

Lucille Scheuer
Associate Dean of Students

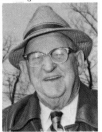

Carl "Splinter" Myers
Storeroom Manager 1950-76

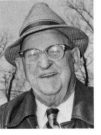

Nelle I. Barnhart
Associate Dean of Students

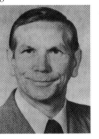

Bruce Collins
Physical Plant 1951-84

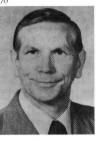

Ethel Mitchell
Associate Dean of Students

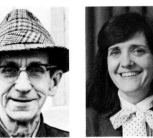

Marion "Ted" Glidewell
University Electrician
1935-82.

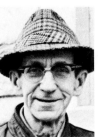

Carol Arner
Associate Dean of Students

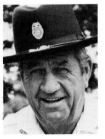

Grover A. Vaughn
Security Director 1955-86

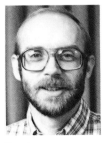

Tom Arner
Assistant Dean of Students

201

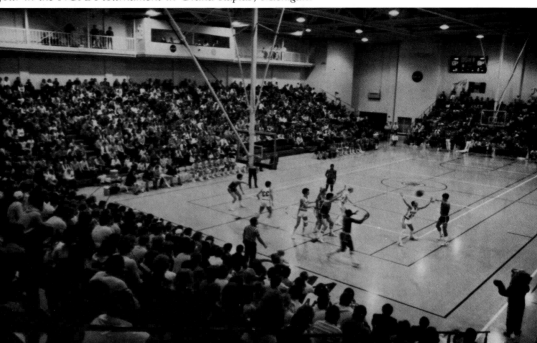

Zeta sorority house on East Anderson Street.

The Rosser administration faced continuing demands from the student body for increased autonomy in personal and social affairs. The visitation issue was finally resolved in 1978 by a plan offering all students certain visitation options for members of the opposite sex. Incoming freshman were assigned to rooms in university residences according to their stated preferences on this matter, and visitation procedures for sections of upperclass halls and Greek living units were to be determined by 3/4 vote of the residents. In the fall of 1979 an additional option was provided by making both Longden and Hogate Halls coeducational, with men and women living on alternate floors. In addition juniors and seniors could obtain permission on a lottery basis to live out in town, the number not to exceed four percent of the undergraduate student body.

For the first time all students were permitted to bring automobiles to campus, with the proviso that they register them with the Student Affairs Office and park them only in university-designated areas. The thorniest question of all was the drinking issue, long the subject of student agitation and administrative concern. By 1980, however, the administration, recognizing a significant shift in attitudes among the DePauw constituency, was ready to make an historic departure from the traditional policy of prohibition by according students over the legal age the right to consume alcoholic beverages under certain conditions. Discussions over the next four years culminated in the adoption in 1984 by the board of trustees of a new comprehensive policy "intended to promote either abstinence or responsible use of alcohol." Strict guidelines and regulations were set down concerning the serving and consumption of alcoholic beverages by students that included a complete compliance with the laws of Indiana. The administration also demonstrated its special concern in

Old Gold Day 1984 showing traditional release of the yellow balloons when DePauw first scores.

the area of alcohol abuse and reaffirmed its opposition to the possession, use, or sale of illicit drugs.

A large number of new instructors joined the ranks of the faculty. Listed below by departments, they include the following: art: Robert D. Kingsley and Catherine Fruhan; biological sciences: Robert J. Stark, Wade N. Hazel, Bruce S. Serlin, and Kathleen S. Jagger; chemistry:

A.J.C.L. Hogarth, Bryan S. Hanson, and David T. Harvey; classical studies: Carl A. Huffman; communication arts and sciences: Nancy J. Metzger, Samuel Abel, and Jeffrey N. McCall; economics and management: Anthony V. Catanese, Margaret E. Catanese, William J. Field, Shanker Shetty, Daniel R. Wachter, Wassim N. Shahin, and Lisa L. Wichser; English: Martha Rainbolt, Wayne E. Glausser, J.

THE LITTLE 500 AND NEW FESTIVE TRADITIONS

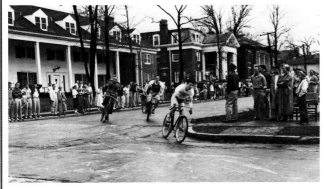

The first Little 500 turning the corner of Seminary and Locust streets in 1957.

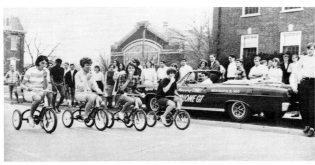

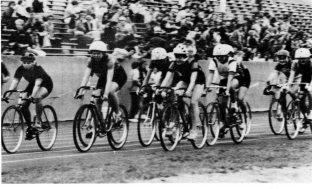

Above middle: A tricycle competition for women students was an early part of the Little 500 week.

Bottom: In recent years the women students entered the Little 500.

When it comes to student festivities, traditions rise and fall rapidly on college campuses. DePauw's oldest continuing festive tradition is probably Old Gold Weekend, which began as Old Gold Day in 1907. Even now yellow chrysanthemums are worn at the Saturday afternoon homecoming football game, balloons are released after DePauw's first score, and the Old Gold Day Queen is crowned at halftime. But gone are the class scraps, the campus bonfire, the living unit decorations, the wearing of freshman beanies and senior cords. They have all disappeared into the limbo of lost traditions, along with mock chapel, Gridiron Dinner, Monon Revue, Sigma Chi pledges ringing the East College bell after football victories, and other half-forgotten customs.

Yet students are inventive enough to create new festive traditions in every college generation. Since the close of World War II many have been instituted on the DePauw campus, including beautiful legs contests, ugly man contests, watermelon busts, rock concerts, and Octoberfests.

The most enduring festivity of all has been the Little 500, which has expanded from a single afternoon of men's bicycle racing to nearly a week of varied activities involving a large part of the student body. DePauw's Little 500 began in 1956, just five years after a similar event was held at Indiana University in Bloomington. Both were bicycle races inspired by the famous 500-mile auto race held at the Indianapolis Speedway each Memorial Day.

In the first DePauw Little 500, 14 teams from men's living units pedaled 30 miles on the streets around East College on a rainy Saturday afternoon. Lambda Chi Alpha won that race as well as the next three in succession. In the interests of safety and crowd control the race was moved in 1957 from Greencastle streets to the cinder—now Uni-Royal composition—track in Blackstock Stadium, where it has been run ever since. In the early years the late Tony Hulman, owner of the Indianapolis Speedway, drove the pace car and started the race.

In 1966 a faculty bicycle race was added to the program. Mason Hall, then a women's dormitory, entered a team in the 1973 race, and two years later the Little 500 steering committee substituted for the faculty race a women's bicycle race, which has been held every year since, just prior to the men's contest. Rector Hall was the initial victor in that event. One of the first signs of spring in and around Greencastle these days is the appearance of helmeted men and women cycling determinedly through the streets in practice for the Little 500.

Men's and women's living units have from the beginning been paired for competition in some of the ancillary events of the Little 500. Chief of these has been the Mini 500, a tricycle race taking place in the street outside the Student Union Building on Friday afternoon. Other happenings, many added in very recent years, include a tug-of-war, obstacle course run, bathtub race, pie-eating contest, a mud volleyball tournament, and an all-campus picnic.

Music has always been part of the festivities too, with either a Saturday night dance or a performance by a popular rock group. In 1987 "spirit awards" were offered for the first time for participation by the various living unit pairs, and President Robert Bottoms hosted a special awards banquet on the Sunday after the race. Thus do new traditions arise.

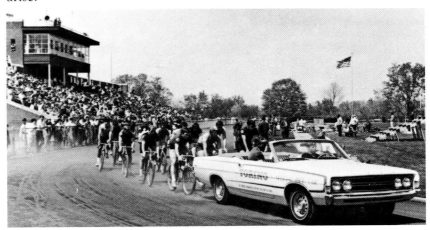

Early Little 500 bicycle race at Blackstock Stadium is led by a pace car borrowed from the Indianapolis Motor Speedway.

GREENCASTLE

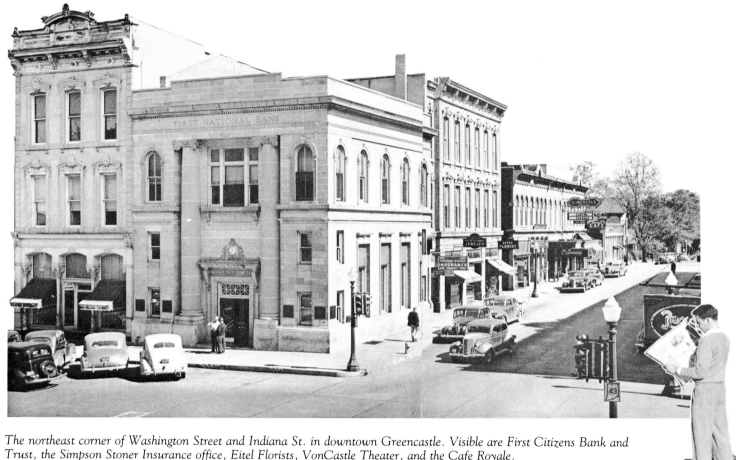

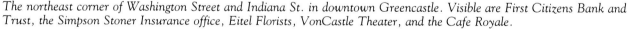

The northeast corner of Washington Street and Indiana St. in downtown Greencastle. Visible are First Citizens Bank and Trust, the Simpson Stoner Insurance office, Eitel Florists, VonCastle Theater, and the Cafe Royale.

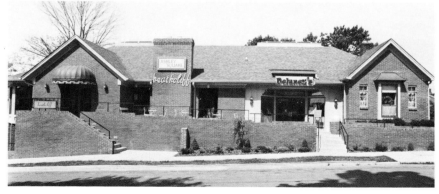

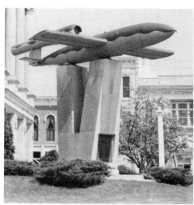

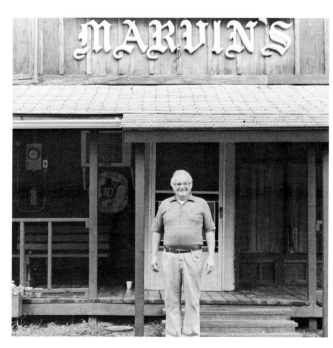

Above: Ashley Square shopping center, which opened in 1983 at Seminary and Vine streets; far right: Marvin's, a campus eatery, is famous for its garlic cheeseburgers; right: the "buzz bomb" monument on the Greencastle courthouse square.

The DePauw Chamber Symphony directed by Professor Orcenith Smith poses for a publicity photograph before its Winter Term tour in 1985-86.

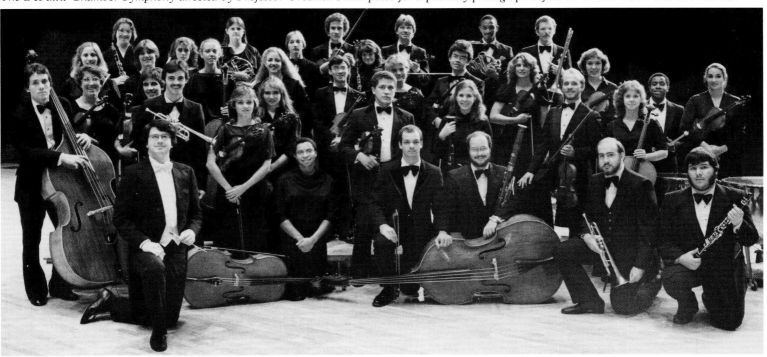

David Field, Istvan Csicery-Ronay, David Klooster, and Erin McGraw; geology and geography: Frederick M. Soster; health, physical education and recreation: Nick Mourouzis and Michael Steele; history: Barbara J. Steinson, John T. Schlotterbeck, Sharon Nolte, and John Dittmer; mathematics and computer science: Richard C. Smock, Gloria C. Townsend, Janet E. Teegarden, Susan C. Gardsbane, Mark Kannowski, Nachimuthu Manickam, Robert Hieb, and Steven Csik.

Other additions include, also by department: philosophy and religion: John B. White, Marthe A. Chandler, William P. Harmon and Naomi Steinberg; physics and astronomy: Howard L. Brooks and Victor A. DeCarlo, Jr.; political science: Sidney M. Milkis, Ngeen Sang-Mpam, James R. Simmons, and Bruce Stinebrickner; psychology: Candace J. Schulenberg, Steven R. Raines, Thomas E. Hagaman, and Donald Haruo Ryujin; Romance languages: Francoise M. Coulont-Henderson and Arthur B. Evans; sociology and anthropology: Deborah P. Bhattacharyya, Nancy J. Davis, and Darrell E. La Lone.

The School of Music: Vergene C. Miller, Randy K. Salman, Dan J. Rizner, David L. Ott, and Cleveland

T. Johnson; the School of Nursing: Sherry Smith, who became director of the school in 1979; Martha S. Avery, Carol L. Cherry, Theresa A. Kessler, Anna M. Miller, Margaret S. Hamilton, Louise Hart, and Nancy Drew. Directors of the quantitative reasoning center, the writing center, and the speaking and listening center were Susan Gardsbane, David Klooster, and Ann Weiss, respectively. Added to the library staff in this period were Loraine N. Sprague, Pei-Ling Wu, Gillian S. Gremmels, and Kathy Davis. Upon the retirement of James Martindale in 1983, Jana Bradley was named director of libraries. The next year Wesley W. Wilson became coordinator of archives and special services.

President Rosser was granted a sabbatical leave for travel and writing the first semester of the 1985-86 academic year, during which Vice President Bottoms took charge of university operations. Shortly after Rosser's return to campus in January 1986 he announced his intention to resign the presidency in July. The Board of trustees then appointed him to the post of chancellor of the university with responsibilities primarily for external relations and coordination of the upcoming

celebration of DePauw's 150th anniversary. In September, however, Chancellor Rosser resigned from the university in order to accept the presidency of the National Association of Independent Colleges and Universities. He went to Washington, D. C. to take up his new duties and soon moved with his wife Donna Eyssen Rosser to a new home in Alexandria, Virginia.

Within a few weeks of Rosser's resignation from the presidency, the board of trustees named Vice President Robert G. Bottoms as his successor, making the appointment from the current faculty and administrative ranks for the first time since the elevation of Dean Hillary Gobin to the presidency in 1896. The new president was a native of Alabama who had earned a B.A. from Birmingham-Southern College, a B.D. from Emory University, and the degree of doctor of ministry from Vanderbilt University. He served as assistant dean and assistant professor of church and ministry at Vanderbilt before coming to DePauw in 1978. A member of St. Andrews Episcopal Church in Greencastle, he became the first non-Methodist president of DePauw University.

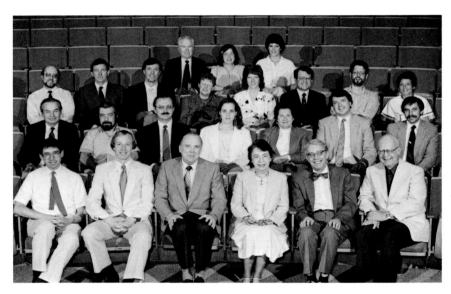

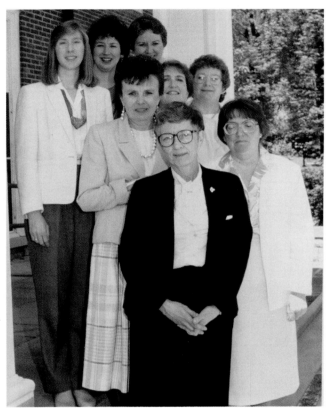

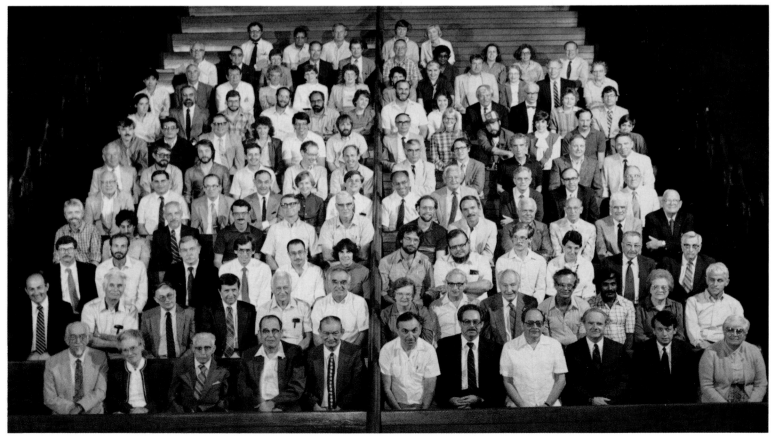

CONCLUSION

THE SESQUICENTENNIAL YEAR, 1986-1987

P resident Robert G. Bottoms entered upon his new duties at the outset of the year-long celebration of the 150th anniversary of the founding of Indiana Asbury-DePauw University. The festivities began with a formal opening convocation on September 5 addressed by President Paul Hardin of Drew University. Two weeks later the university hosted 150 descendants of the 25 original members of the board of trustees, who joined the student body, faculty and administration and hundreds of residents of Greencastle and Putnam County in celebrating Community Day with a chapel program in Meharry Hall and a picnic in Bowman Park.

The following Friday the history department presented a special convocation on DePauw's historical heritage, and a panel of local alumni reminisced about student life in earlier decades in an "Evening of Nostalgia." On Saturday morning, Barbara Blakemore '46, Vernon Jordan '57, and Joseph Allen '59 spoke eloquently about the value of a liberal arts education before a Parents' Weekend audience in Kresge Auditorium.

Chancellor Emeritus Alexander Heard of Vanderbilt University gave the principal address at the formal inauguration of President Bottoms in a Friday morning convocation at the beginning of Old Gold Weekend in October. Other participants in the ceremony were Chancellor Richard Rosser, Professor Arthur Carkeek of the Music School representing the DePauw faculty, United Methodist Bishop Leroy C. Hodapp, and the outgoing chairman of the board of trustees, Eugene L. Delves. The newly installed chairman of the board, Robert R. Frederick, presented the presidential medallion to Bottoms, who made a brief inaugural address. That evening the university instituted the DePauw Athletic Hall of Fame, naming 25 former students and coaches as its first members.

On Saturday morning Chancellor Rosser presided over the dedication of the William Weston Clarke Emison Art Center, renamed to honor the contributions of the Emison family to the university over four generations. Professor Emeritus Jerome Hixson, former Dean Robert Farber, and Athletic Director Tom Mont shared the podium at the traditional Old Gold chapel in Meharry Hall. A gala musical performance by the DePauw Symphony Orchestra and the DePauw Concert Choir and Festival Choir concluded the festive weekend, featuring the world premiere of a specially commissioned sesquicentennial composition by Paul Whear '48 entitled "Old Gold —a Celebration" and appearances by opera singer Pam Coburn '74 and guest conductor Joseph Flummerfelt '58.

A series of special events extended throughout the academic year, including lectures and symposia on scientific and public policy issues. Honorary degrees were awarded to five women religious leaders representing a broad spectrum of faith and action, Roman Catholic, Protestant, and Jewish. In addition programs were devoted to remembering the social idealism of the 1960s, Black Cultural Week, Women's Week, and a Week of the Arts. Three prominent ministers delivered sermons for "A Great Day of Preaching." DePauw also formally inaugurated the Center for Contemporary Media with addresses and panel discussions by noted journalists. The sesquicentennial celebration was brought to a grand conclusion, along with the sesquicentennial financial campaign, on Alumni Weekend in June 1987, with a succession of events culminating in an impressive display of fireworks in Bowman Park.

In his inaugural address President Bottoms set forth three important initiatives for his administration: (1) to bring about greater diversity in the student body, faculty and administrative staff, and the curriculum; (2) to give renewed emphasis to science education; and (3) to provide moral leadership in an increasingly secularized environment. With wide support from the DePauw constituency, he began implementation of these goals, both by organizing task forces to plan appropriate action and by concrete steps such as the establishment of a new minority scholarship program and a policy of increased representation of women and minorities on the university staff.

Photos on opposite page:

Top left: Faculty, School of Music, Sesquicentennial Year 1986-87. Left to right: **Row 1:** *C. Johnson, D. Rizner, R. Grocock, M. Carkeek, C. Grubb, D. Hanna.* **Row 2:** *A. Carkeek, C. Cymerman, C. Rader, S. Lange, B. Grubb, O. Smith, D. Ott.* **Row 3:** *S. Hanna, L. Philpott, S. Irwin, E. Wilcox, D. Martin, M. Borschel, J. Beckel, A. Reynolds.* **Row 4:** *T. Fitzpatrick, L. Griffitt, L. Cerone.*

Top right: Faculty, School of Nursing, Sesquicentennial year 1986-87. **Row 1** *(from left): Ritter, Powell;* **Row 2:** *S. Smith, Cherry, Hamilton;* **Row 3:** *Kessler, Drew, Hart.*

Bottom: Most of the Liberal Arts Faculty and Emeriti in the Sesquicentennial Year, 1987. Left to right: **Row 1:** *Warren, Beatty, Ross, Youse, Cook, Mayer, Gibson, Mecum, Rosser, Bottoms, Falco.* **Row 2:** *James George, Sprague, Raymond, McFarland, Fuller, Kissinger, Teeguarden, Thomas, Gass, Dudley, Manickam, V. Williams, Morrill.* **Row 3:** *W. Wilson, Yochum, Elrod, J. McCall, Abel, Metzger, Hazel, Smogor, Kannowski, Gardsbane, Garriott, Gooch.* **Row 4:** *White, Serlin, Calvert, Mays, Gammon, D. Smith, Schlotterbeck, Dittmer, Farber, R. Harvey, E. McCall, Lovelace.* **Row 5:** *Phillips, Stark, Eccles, Emery, M. Catanese, Brooks, Mourouzis, Erdmann, Wright, Henninger, Turk.* **Row 6:** *Burkett, Hagaman, Moore, Garrett, Glausser, Soster, Newton, Schwartz, Kelly, Edward Ypma, J. Wilson.* **Row 7:** *Simmons, Shahin, Carlson, Wichser, Lemon, W. Field, Sutton, Price, M. Johnson, C. Cornell, L. Cornell, Steinberg.* **Row 8:** *Jagger, Evans, Hanson, Raines, A. Catanese, Coulont-Henderson, J. Rambo, A. Rambo, Eigenbrodt, Gustavsson, Davis, Huffman.* **Row 9:** *Ryujin, Opdahl, Goodson, Biggs, Weaver, Leverenz, Erndl, E. Welliver, G. Welliver, S. J. Williams, C. Williams, Barnhart.* **Row 10:** *B. Steele, Mizer, Raybern, McPhail, Anderson, W. Gilmer, Brown, Steinson, Chandler, Baughman.* **Row 11:** *Mannon, Shetty, Curry, D. Field, Eleanor Ypma.*

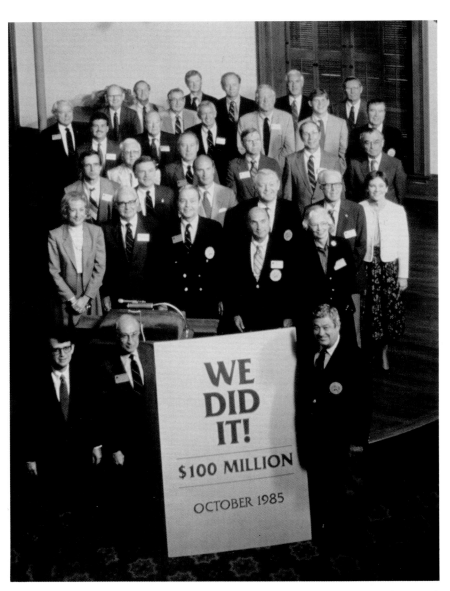

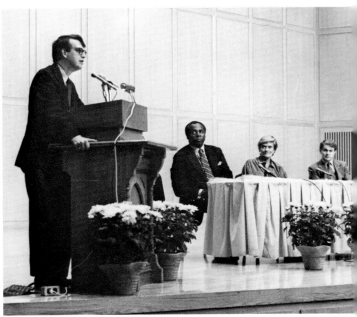

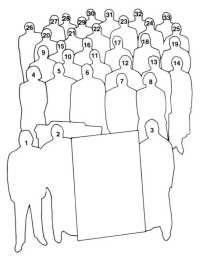

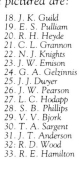

Above: On Old Gold Weekend in 1985 the DePauw trustees announced that more than $100 million had been committed to the Sesquicentennial Campaign. Those pictured are:

1. R. G. Bottoms
2. E. L. Delves
3. J. J. Kelly
4. S. B. Jones
5. W. F. Welch
6. N. B. Stephens
7. R. R. Frederick
8. J. Brady
9. D. R. Daseke
10. A. J. Paine
11. T. H. Sams
12. A. E. Klauser
13. C. N. Frees
14. G. R. Ensing
15. E. C. Boswell
16. E. E. Schulze
17. I. M. Rolland
18. J. K. Guild
19. E. S. Pulliam
20. R. H. Heyde
21. C. L. Grannon
22. N. J. Knights
23. J. W. Emison
24. G. A. Gelzinnis
25. J. J. Dwyer
26. J. W. Pearson
27. L. C. Hodapp
28. S. B. Phillips
29. V. V. Bjork
30. T. A. Sargent
31. J. T. Anderson
32. R. D. Wood
33. R. E. Hamilton

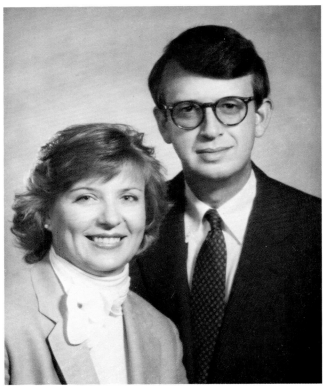

Top photo: Sesquicentennial Parents Day ceremony in Kresge Hall in 1986 with President Bottoms, Vernon Jordan '57, Barbara Blakemore '46, Joseph P. Allen IV '59.

Bottom photo: Robert G. and Gwen Vickers Bottoms

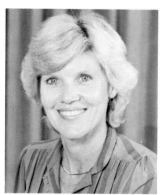
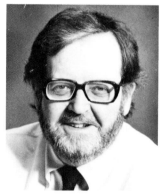
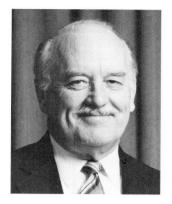
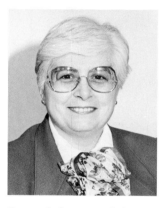

Pictured above, top left: Fred S. Silander, vice president for finance; Barbara E. Smith, vice president for external affairs; bottom left: Maria J. Falco, academic vice president; bottom right: Drake Mabry, director of the Center for Contemporary Media

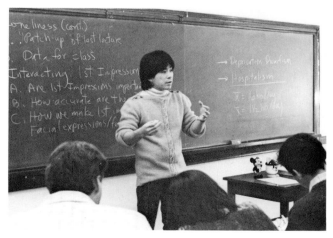

Donald Ryujin lectures a psychology class.

A major move was the appointment of three-time Olympic gold medalist Wilma Rudolph as director of women's track and consultant to the president on minority affairs. Bottoms also named Dorothy Brown, a Greencastle native who had been the first black teacher and administrator in the local public schools before becoming principal of an Indianapolis elementary school and eventually an instructor in DePauw's education department, to the post of assistant dean of students for minority affairs. Blacks were also appointed to positions in admissions, the library, the office of personnel, and campus security.

Two top administrative posts went to women for the first time. In July 1986 Maria Falco, formerly academic dean and professor of political science at Loyola University in New Orleans, came to DePauw as vice president for academic affairs. In April of the next year DePauw alumna Barbara E. Smith left an executive career in advertising to accept the post of vice president for external affairs, with responsibilities for development, alumni affairs, and public relations. The history department's Barbara Steinson was also appointed assistant to the president on a part-time basis.

When Falco was granted a special leave of absence to complete a research and writing project, Vice President for Finance Fred Silander assumed the added duties of acting academic vice president for 1987-88. John White of the philosophy and religion department, who had been assistant vice president for academic affairs, was promoted to the position of associate dean of the university.

The sesquicentennial year was not only a time for reflection upon the long historical record and proud tradition of Indiana Asbury-DePauw University, but also a time for thinking seriously about the institution's present and future direction. Over the past century and a half the university has undergone many significant changes, though perhaps none so dramatic as the transformation of Indiana Asbury into the new DePauw University in 1884. In recent decades, however the pace of change has accelerated, as the university trustees, administration, and faculty have endeavored to respond to changing conditions and meet new challenges creatively and wisely.

Like many other contemporary institutions, DePauw University has become a more complex organization than the 19th and early 20th century university, with some of the same characteristics as the modern corporation. During this time the administration and support staff, for example, have experienced unprecedented growth, while the teaching faculty, freed from much routine housekeeping detail, has become even more independent and professionally oriented. The student body itself has gained appreciable social and personal autonomy as well as a larger share in the whole educational process. At the same time DePauw's alumni have come to play a more extensive part in university affairs, through representation on the board of trustees and the newly instituted advisory board of visitors and by virtue of their loyal support, both moral and financial. Finally, the board of trustees has gained in stature as the guardian and sustainer of an educational enterprise which has grown, with the assistance of generous benefactors, to encompass a total endowment of more than $90 million and an annual budget in excess of $26 million.

Moreover, DePauw University has been able to conserve its essential spirit throughout all the changes of the past century and a half. Remaining true to its original charter, which stated that the university was to be "forever conducted on the most liberal principles, accessible to all religious denominations, and designed for the benefit of our citizens in general," DePauw has grown in service to the nation and the world while striving to maintain a renewed sense of academic community. The university, having met and overcome various crises and found successful solutions to most of the problems facing institutions of higher education in the past, may look forward confidently to a future of continuing conservation and transformation.

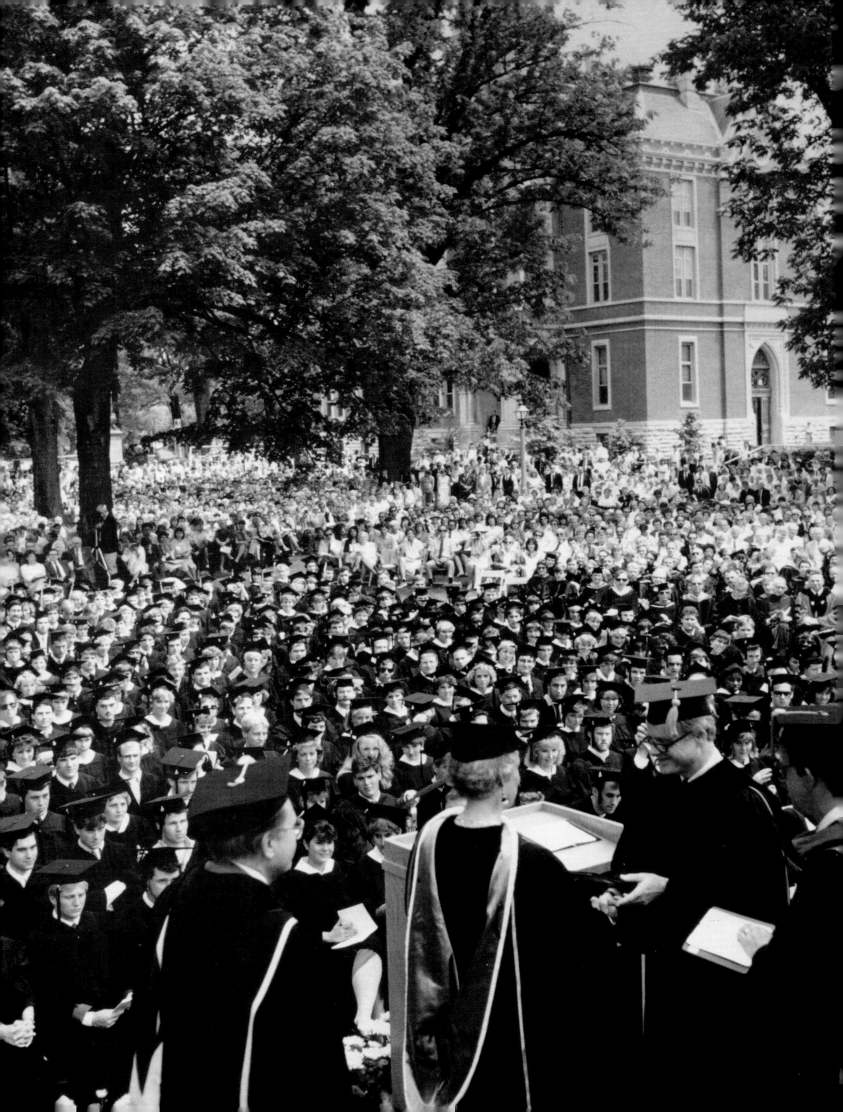

Appendix A:
A PROFILE OF DEPAUW STUDENTS

Despite the remarkable transformation of DePauw University, especially during the last one hundred years, DePauw students have remained largely white, middle-class, and midwestern. Recent decades have seen important changes in students' religious background, geographic residence, and career patterns, but the social composition of the student body and the patterns of student life have become perhaps even more homogeneous and predictable since World War II.

During the first half of DePauw's history, the institution was relatively small and recruited students chiefly from Indiana farms and small towns. Total student enrollment grew steadily from just over 200 in the 1840s to about 400 in the 1870s. After the creation of the new professional schools in the early DePauw years, student population jumped to between 700 and 800 during the 1880s and 1890s. Only about one-third to one-half of these students were engaged in college-level work. The collegiate enrollment grew gradually from 50 students in the 1840s, to just under 200 by the 1870s, to 300 students in the 1890s, and around 460 during the next decade. Graduating classes were even smaller with only seven students receiving degrees each year in the 1840s, 16 in the 1860s, 45 in the 1880s, and 69 between 1900 and 1910. Small class size and the prescribed curriculum, which insured that members of each class enrolled in the same courses, maintained an intimate and personal social environment.

DePauw students in the 19th century had very similar backgrounds. Probably three-fourths came from Methodist homes, and between 85 and 90 percent were Hoosiers, mostly from central Indiana. Antebellum transportation was too expensive or, in many cases, unavailable, preventing students from traveling long distances to obtain an education. Students' families were part of Indiana's large rural and small-town middle class that included successful farmers, shopkeepers, ministers, lawyers, and doctors. Few were wealthy, even by 19th century standards, but, as property owners, they enjoyed financial security and social respectability and held positions of leadership in their communities.

Early DePauw graduates overwhelmingly entered the professions, just as the northern middle class was shifting from property ownership to education and professional training as the main basis of its membership. Despite the university's close Methodist ties, only one-fourth of its early graduates became ordained ministers. Of all graduates between 1840 and 1905, in fact, just 16 percent were ministers or missionaries while 22 percent were educators and 18 percent lawyers. Such a relatively low proportion of alumni in the ministry may seem surprising for a 19th century church-related university, but it clearly reflects the secular career orientation of its students as well as the fact that most Methodist churches still did not demand a highly educated leadership. Only 11 percent of the pre-1905 graduates went into business, a career that eventually became much more attractive; around one-fourth of the members of each class after 1910 found employment in business and finance. Female graduates who sought careers generally became teachers.

DePauw not only promoted its graduates' social mobility but also trained leaders for the midwest's rapidly developing commercial and urban society. A DePauw degree also enhanced geographic mobility. Almost 65 percent of the 1900 and 1901 graduates were from Indiana, but by 1920, only 42 percent still resided in the state and 23 percent were living outside the midwest. By the 1950s, about half of the alumni were no longer midwesterners.

Nineteenth-century DePauw students probably came from a broader social base than is true today. Early DePauw was a remarkably open institution. There was no tuition, and incidental fees were only $24 per year in 1900. A room could be rented for $20 to $30 per year and board was $2.50 per week. The college catalogues claimed that $200 was sufficient to obtain a year's education at DePauw. Many students, in fact, were self-supporting and financed their education by taking odd jobs in Greencastle during the school year and through summer employment.

Admissions standards were also flexible. In 1840, prospective students were expected to possess "good moral character" and entrance was gained by examination. Deficiencies in specific subjects could be made up by enrolling in the preparatory department. Students thus entered Indiana-Asbury when they were prepared or had saved enough money. As a result, there was a broad range in the ages of DePauw students, with boys of 13 in the preparatory department and men in their mid-30s enrolled in the collegiate courses. The median age of graduates rose from 21.5 in the 1840s to 23.7 in the 1890s. The admission of women in 1867 and creation of music, art, and other professional schools in the mid-1880s further added to the diversity of the student population. Women were about four years younger than the men, while ministerial students were three to four years older than others. Although women were required to lived on campus after construction of Ladies Hall in 1884, most men continued to live out in town in private boarding houses or with their families or relatives. There was also a high turnover of students from one academic year to the next. Many students attended DePauw for only one or two years, and only one-fourth to one-third of entering freshmen graduated four years later. As late as the 1930s, less than 30 percent of all students who had attended DePauw since 1837 had actually graduated.

The most significant demographic change in the last seventy-five years has been the increase in the number of students. Most of this growth occurred in a brief twenty year period after 1905 when enrollment in the College of Liberal Arts soared from an average of 460 between 1900 and 1910 to almost 800 in the 1910s, and over 1400 during the 1920s. After declining by 300 during the Great Depression, enrollment again expanded to an average of 1700 students during the post war years and peaked at 2200 when the baby-boom generation entered college in the 1960s. Liberal arts students have declined slightly in the last two decades, but expansion in the School of Music and the addition of the School of Nursing in 1955 has kept total undergraduate enrollment between 2300 and 2400 over the last four decades.

The number of earned degrees has grown even more rapidly. Less than 700 degrees were awarded during the first decade of the twentieth century. In the 1920s, DePauw granted over 2200 degrees and over 5300 during the 1970s. Over half of the 30,300 degrees granted by DePauw during its 150-year history have been given since 1958, and 73 percent of the degrees have been awarded in the last 50 years (1938-87) compared to less than four percent during the first 50 years (1837-87). Only five percent of DePauw degrees have been masters degrees. Most alumni are still alive, and their vast increase in numbers after World War II has made them an influential group in shaping the life of the university.

Women achieved numerical parity with men in the early twentieth century. In the first two decades of coeducation, women comprised about one-fourth of the liberal arts students but earned only 16 percent of the degrees. By 1891, 43 percent of the students were women and they have made up 45 to 50 percent of the student population ever since. Equally significant, by 1900 women were earning degrees in proportion to their numbers, and in most decades of the 20th century, the proportion of women graduates is greater than their representation in the student population. This collective record of women's scholarship is very impressive, especially since until recently, women did not have equal access to scholarship funds.

212

The creation of the Rector Scholarship Foundation in 1919 had a revolutionary impact on the student population. Edward Rector's beneficence remade DePauw during the 1920s and 1930s. By providing 400 full scholarships to the brightest male high school graduates, Rector sustained DePauw's continued growth while raising academic standards.

About one half of the male students during these decades were Rector Scholars. The program also broadened the social composition of male students while enlarging class divisions between male and female students. Women, who were denied Rector Scholarships in these years, increasingly came from wealthier families than the men. Rector based this discrimination on the fear that DePauw was becoming "feminized." In the 1910s slightly over half of the students were women, and it was believed that if this trend continued men might avoid coming to a school with a female majority. The Rector Scholarships boosted enrollment and increased social diversity at the same time. As late as the mid-1930s, almost 44 percent of all DePauw students were still first-generation college students. Only one-third had at least one parent with a college degree, while only 12 percent had a parent who had attended DePauw. More youths were coming from midwestern cities like Chicago, Indianapolis, and St. Louis, but even in 1931, one fifth of the students still came from farm families.

The Rector money also broadened the geographic and religious origins of DePauw students. In 1911, 88 percent of the students were Hoosiers; this fell to 38 percent by World War II. The share of Illinois students jumped from 5 to 36 percent and students from other midwestern states grew from two to 17 percent, while students from outside the midwest doubled to eight percent. DePauw in the 1920s and 1930s was moving beyond its traditional Indiana origins and was on the threshold of becoming a truly national institution in terms of student enrollment. There was an even more dramatic shift away from DePauw's traditional Methodist base. In 1916, about three-fourths of DePauw students were Methodists; this had plummeted to 40 percent by 1941. Presbyterians, Congregationalists, Episcopalians, and Lutherans achieved significant representation in the student population, growing from a combined total of 13 to 36 percent. There was even a small Roman Catholic population (about 4 percent) for the first time, but no significant increase in the number of Jews or blacks.

Student career patterns have changed over the last 75 years. In the 1930s students continued to move from families engaged in business and trade to professional careers. Teaching was the most popular choice (40 percent) for graduating seniors, while only 20 percent indicated a preference for business and 6 percent for the ministry. Business and banking, however, became more attractive to male graduates beginning around 1910, a trend that accelerated after World War II. In 1962, about one-third of the alumni who were gainfully employed reported careers in business and industry.

After World War II the GI Bill temporarily maintained opportunities for young men of varied social backgrounds to obtain an education at DePauw. The Great Depression had reduced the impact of the Rector Scholarships, however, and there were few changes in the residence or religious preferences of DePauw students during the 1940s and 1950s.

Other long-term developments were helping to stabilize the social composition of students and the campus culture at DePauw. More and more students came from similar social backgrounds and had increasingly predictable academic patterns. The age range of the student body had narrowed considerably by the early 20th century. The Academy, successor to the preparatory department, closed, and a minimum age of 16 was established for admission as college freshmen.

After 1915 all students admitted were high school graduates who came to DePauw with similar educational experiences. The closing of the professional schools also eliminated most older students from the campus. Accordingly, the student body became increasingly concentrated in the 18 to 22 year range.

Family backgrounds of the students became more homogeneous. By the 1930s, over 70 percent of DePauw students' fathers were professionals or businessmen. Recent students were also more likely to have college-educated parents, many of whom had attended DePauw. Today about one-fourth of the entering freshmen have some family ties to the university.

The steady rise in tuition, which has increased more than 20-fold from $350 in 1945 to $8200 in 1986, along with a quintupling of living expenses in the same period–not quite matched by gains in scholarship and loan funds–has meant that many students today come from more affluent families and are financially dependent upon their parents. For these young men and women the "DePauw experience" has become a continuation of, rather than a departure from, family tradition.

Contributing to the growing homogenity of the student body was the fact that a larger proportion of the student body remained on campus for four years. In the 1920s only about 40 percent of the entering freshmen stayed until graduation; this became 55 percent by the end of World War II and reached 70 percent in the 1980s. By the early 20th century DePauw had become a predominantly residential campus, with virtually all freshman women and unaffiliated students in university dormitories and fraternity and sorority members living in nearby chapter houses. Approximately three-fourths of the student body were affiliated with national fraternities and sororities, a proportion that has remained remarkably steady down to the present. Peer culture and the campus social environment, including Greek living units, athletics, and students activities of all kinds, increasingly shape the undergraduate experience as much as does the classroom.

The most important changes in the last two decades have been in students' geographic origins and religious preferences. Although the proportion of Hoosiers has risen from 35 percent in 1961 to 42 percent in 1986, partly because of the availability of Indiana state scholarships, DePauw students in general come today from a broader geographic base than ever. For example, 24 percent are from midwestern states outside of Indiana and Illinois and 16 percent from states outside the midwest. Foreign students comprise only 1.4 percent of the population, but this is a higher proportion than any other period. Even more dramatic is the decline in students claiming a Methodist religious preference, from 36 percent in 1961 to under 20 percent in 1986. There has also been a significant drop in the proportion of Presbyterians and Congregationalists. On the other hand Roman Catholics students have increased from only seven percent in 1961 to slightly more than 22 percent today, making them the largest single religious group in the student body. Since most of them share similar backgrounds with their Protestant counterparts, it seems likely that this newest wave of students will enhance rather than transform the dominant contours of campus life and social organization at DePauw.

Appendix B:
FROM PIETY TO PROFESSIONALISM: A PROFILE OF DEPAUW FACULTY

Over the past 150 years there has been an enormous increase in the number of DePauw faculty members and radical changes in their professional training. Before 1880 the Liberal Arts faculty never numbered more than 10. In the last two decades of the 19th century, despite a 50 percent growth in student enrollment, faculty size averaged about 17. The ranks of the teaching faculty grew rapidly during the next quarter of a century, tripling to 50 by 1921 and to 88 five years later. Financial stringency during the Great Depression reduced the number of faculty by 15, but DePauw entered another period of expansion of instructional staff in the late 1930s. Soon after World War II the number of faculty members reached 100 and by the late 1950s grew to 150. In the last decades faculty ranks have continued to expand to approximately 170, but mostly by means of increased employment of part-time instructors.

DePauw has long celebrated its small classes and close student-faculty relations. This feature was more characteristic of the Indiana Asbury and early DePauw period than of the present century. In 1881 there were just 11 liberal arts students for each member of the faculty. Since faculty growth did not keep pace with rapid increases in the student population, there were 26 students per faculty member by 1911. The student-faculty ratio gradually fell over the ensuing decades, reaching 15 to 1 in the early 1950s and has remained more or less stable down to the present.

The backgrounds of DePauw faculty members have also changed dramatically. Indiana Asbury University sought to instill Christian piety in its students while transmitting a common classical culture through memorization and recitation from textbooks. Christian character, not professional training, was demanded of professors, who in the 19th century were chiefly Methodist ministers or devout laymen engaged in teaching a wide variety of subjects. Sometimes they were assisted by recent graduates of the institution. A striking example of such virtuosity was Professor James Riley Weaver, who came to the university in 1885 with an A.B. and S.T.B. to teach German and French. During his 30-year tenure he also offered courses in history, political science, economics, and sociology. But the next year, representing the wave of the future, Oliver P. Jenkins arrived with a Ph.D. to teach biology. President John P.D. John's "new education" required a faculty with professional training in a specific academic subject. Almost all new instructors appointed after 1890 had at least a master's degree in their specialty and many had earned doctorates. At the same time the teaching faculty was divided into definite ranks; associate professors appeared in the 1890s and assistant professors in the 1910s.

The "Ph.D. revolution" spread from the top down. The Ph.D. degree gradually became a prerequisite for appointment to a full professorship in the College of Liberal Arts (except in fields such as studio art, where the terminal degree was at the master's level). In 1881 less than one-fifth of all full professors possessed Ph.D.s; this proportion grew to one-third by 1891 and one-half by 1911. It continued to climb at an even faster rate in later decades, reaching over 80 percent by the 1940s and 96 percent in 1986. Eventually the same Ph.D. standard was applied to the entire liberal arts faculty. In 1986, 82 percent of all full-time members of the teaching faculty in the College of Liberal Arts held doctorates.

The arrival of coeducation in 1867 did not bring equitable female representation on the faculty. While frequently engaged as instructors in the Schools of Music and Art, women were notably absent in the College of Liberal Arts. In 1881, when women comprised one-fourth of the liberal arts enrollment, there was only one woman, Alice Downey, an instructor in the preparatory department, among the 17 faculty members listed in the college catalogue. Only three women appointed to the faculty before 1900 ever attained full professor rank: Alma Holman (1882-1885) in modern languages; Belle A. Mansfield (1886-1911) in history and aesthetics; and Minna Kern (1895-1932) in German and French. By the 1910s there was a female student majority in the College of Liberal Arts but less than one-fifth of the faculty were women. The proportion of female instructional staff gradually increased to about one-fourth of the liberal arts faculty in the 1920s and nearly 30 percent after World War II, when the absence of men provided temporary opportunities for women to enter the college teaching field. Representation of women on the faculty, however, declined to about 16 percent by the late 1960s and has only reached 28 percent in 1986 after a gradual increase in the last decade. Women members of the faculty have also been clustered disproportionately in the junior ranks of instructor and assistant professor. Although one-fourth to one-half of all instructors have been women, they have rarely comprised as much as 15 percent of full professors. In the 1970s and 1980s, in fact, less than four percent of all full professors in the College of Liberal Arts have been women, their lowest representation since the 1920s.

These patterns reflect national trends. Although education has long been a field open to women, they were often discouraged from obtaining the graduate training that was increasingly necessary for a career in college teaching. Female instructors were more likely than men to lack the advanced degrees required for promotion to higher academic ranks. Unlike their male colleagues women faculty members often had to choose between marriage and a family and the pursuit of a teaching career. These social constraints discouraged many women from entering the academy in the immediate post-World War II period.

INDEX

222

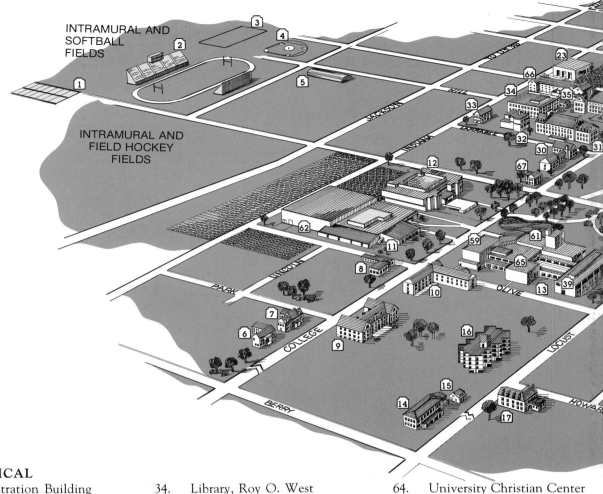

INTRAMURAL AND SOFTBALL FIELDS

INTRAMURAL AND FIELD HOCKEY FIELDS

ALPHABETICAL